UNDERSTANDING LABORATORY INVESTIGATIONS FOR NURSES AND HEALTH PROFESSIONALS

D0878842

UNDERSTANDING LABORATORY INVESTIGATIONS FOR NURSES AND HEALTH PROFESSIONALS

Second edition

Chris Higgins MSc FIBMS DMLM

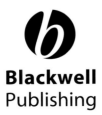

Blackwell
Publishing

First edition published 2000
This edition first published 2007
© 2007, 2000 Blackwell Publishing Ltd

Blackwell Publishing was acquired by John Wiley & Sons in February 2007.
Blackwell's publishing programme has been merged with Wiley's global Scientific,
Technical, and Medical business to form Wiley-Blackwell.

Registered office
John Wiley & Sons Ltd, The Atrium, Southern Gate, Chichester, West Sussex, PO19 8SQ,
United Kingdom

Editorial office
9600 Garsington Road, Oxford, OX4 2DQ, United Kingdom

For details of our global editorial offices, for customer services and for information about
how to apply for permission to reuse the copyright material in this book please see our
website at www.wiley.com/wiley-blackwell.

Library of Congress Cataloging-in-Publication Data
Higgins, Chris, FIBMS.
   Understanding laboratory investigations : a text for nurses and healthcare professionals / Chris
Higgins. – 2nd ed.
     p. ; cm.
   Includes bibliographical references and index.
   ISBN-13: 978-1-4051-3127-8 (pbk. : alk. paper)
   ISBN-10: 1-4051-3127-6 (pbk. : alk. paper)   1. Diagnosis, Laboratory.   2. Nurses.   3. Allied
health personnel.   I. Title.
   [DNLM: 1. Laboratory Techniques and Procedures–Nurses' Instruction.
QY 25 H6356u 2006]
   RB37.H544 2006
   616.07′56–dc22

                                                                              2006014423

A catalogue record for this book is available from the British Library.

Set in 10/12pt Sabon by Graphicraft Limited, Hong Kong
Printed in Singapore by Fabulous Printers Pte Ltd

2   2008

CONTENTS

PREFACE TO THE FIRST EDITION

The purpose of this book is to help nurses to understand better how the work of clinical laboratories contributes to patient care. It answers the following questions:

- Why is this test being ordered on my patient?
- What sort of sample is required?
- How is that sample obtained? And most importantly:
- What is the significance of the test result for my patient?

Answers to these questions must be based on an understanding of basic science. Care has been taken to introduce this science, which includes some basic biochemistry, physiology and anatomy, in a way which is accessible to all those with an interest in how the body works. Much will be familiar to nurses.

The format of the book is simple. After two introductory chapters (one of which emphasises the role of nursing staff in the process of laboratory testing), each chapter is devoted to consideration of a single test or group of related tests. Each of these chapters begins with some relevant biochemistry, physiology or anatomy to put the substance being measured (i.e. the test) in some physiological context. A consideration of the sample requirements follows, and finally interpretation of the test results. Wherever possible patient pathology, symptoms and test results are related. A mock case history is included at the end of each chapter to illustrate the practical clinical use of the test being discussed and give a human face to the science.

It is not possible in a book of this size to discuss all the tests performed in clinical laboratories in this degree of detail, so it has been necessary to be selective. The tests discussed are the most commonly requested, and those that nurses are most likely to encounter. Taken together the tests discussed in this book account for around 70–80% of the total workload of clinical laboratories in the average district general hospital.

Although the primary audience for this book is nursing staff, it should be of interest to other healthcare workers and also students of biomedical sciences interested in pursuing a career in laboratory medicine.

PREFACE TO SECOND EDITION

The aim of this second edition remains the same as for the first: to provide nurses with as much relevant information as is possible, within the constraints of book size, about the most commonly requested tests performed on patient samples in clinical laboratories.

The general format remains the same as that of the first edition but significant changes have been made. Two additional chapters have been included: the first on measurement of calcium and phosphate in blood and the second on dipstick testing of urine. The whole text has been reviewed and updated in the light of changing practice and new knowledge. Extensive revision of some chapters has been necessary; for example, the chapter dealing with laboratory diagnosis of myocardial infarction has been rewritten.

Artwork has been improved, and more extensive up-to-date suggestions for further reading have been added at the end of each chapter. These, combined with miscellaneous additions (glossary, list of reference ranges) at the back of the book are intended to make the book more attractive and user-friendly.

ACKNOWLEDGEMENTS

Very special thanks to my son Jon Higgins who has transformed the artwork so wonderfully for this second edition, and always gets my computer to work!

Thanks also to everyone at Blackwell involved in the production of the book, especially Beth and Katharine for commissioning it and waiting so patiently, as each deadline passed.

For Mary, Tom & Jon again

PART 1

Introduction

Chapter 1

INTRODUCTION TO CLINICAL LABORATORIES

Patients may be subjected to many investigative procedures. These range in complexity from ward or clinic-based measurements familiar to all nurses, such as determining body temperature, pulse and blood pressure, through monitoring of heart function by electrocardiographic (ECG) machines to complex body imaging techniques, such as X-ray, computed tomography (CT) and magnetic resonance imaging (MRI) scan. All of these require the presence of the patient; they are performed on the patient, if not by nurses, at least often in their presence. In contrast, all the investigations described in this book are performed on samples removed from the patient. The remoteness of patients from the site of laboratory testing helps to engender the understandable though misguided perception that laboratory testing has little to do with nursing care and therefore need not concern nurses. In fact, an understanding by nursing staff of the work of clinical laboratories is important for several reasons.

Nurses are in a unique position to satisfy the need that many patients express for information about the tests to which they are subjected. This may be to allay fears and anxieties among those who have never undergone such a test before, or it may simply reflect a right to know. Most laboratory tests are only minimally invasive but can only be done with a patient's informed consent. Of course many patients will express no interest but some have questions that must be addressed.

Nurses often have responsibility for the collection and timely, safe transport of specimens. It is vital that anyone collecting samples is aware of the importance of good practice during this pre-testing phase.

Some blood and urine tests (e.g. blood glucose testing and urine dipstick testing) are performed by nurses at the point of care. It is important that the pitfalls, limitations and clinical significance of such testing are appreciated by those performing these investigations. Development of technology has allowed the introduction of chemical analysers into intensive care and emergency room settings, and an already established trend of increasing point of care testing is set to continue, with more nurses becoming involved in the analytical process.

Nurses are frequently involved in the reception of laboratory results. It is important that they are familiar with the terminology and format of laboratory reports

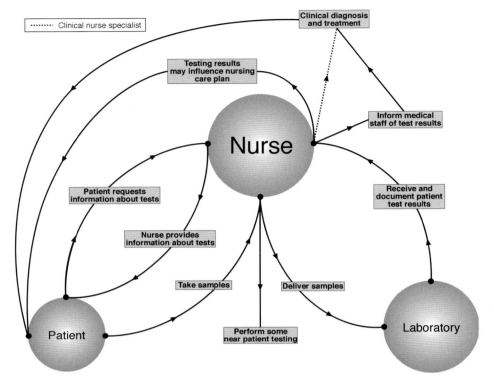

Figure 1.1 Nursing staff involvement in testing of patient samples.

and are able to identify abnormal results, particularly those that warrant immedi-ate clinical intervention. Traditionally, doctors have had sole responsibility for both requesting and interpreting laboratory test results, but the developing role of the clinical nurse specialist and nurse consultant has required that nurses become involved in both of these processes. In any case, all qualified nursing staff have to make judgments about how the results of laboratory tests might impact on the formula-tion of nursing care plans for their patients.

Finally, there are those nurses whose professional role requires especially detailed knowledge of the work of the laboratory as well as close co-operation with labor-atory staff. These include haematology nurse specialists, blood transfusion nurse specialists, infection control nurses and diabetic nurse specialists.

All the tests described in this book are performed – although not exclusively so – in clinical pathology laboratories. The final part of this introductory chapter serves to describe in outline the work of the five subdisciplines of clinical pathology, the range of patient types and samples tested (Table 1.1).

Table 1.1 Range of samples useful for laboratory investigation.

	Sample type
Chemical analysis	Usually blood or urine Less commonly: ● Faeces ● Cerebrospinal fluid (CSF): the fluid which surrounds the brain and spinal cord ● Pleural fluid: the abnormal accumulation of fluid in the pleural cavity of the lungs ● Ascitic fluid: abnormal fluid which accumulates in the peritoneal cavity
Haematological analysis	Usually blood only Occasionally bone marrow biopsy also useful
Microbiological analysis	Urine ● Blood ● Faeces ● Sputum Swabs from almost any accessible site including nose, throat, eye, ear wounds, vagina etc. Less commonly: ● Cerebrospinal fluid ● Pleural fluid ● Skin scrapings ● Nails ● Vomit
Histopathological examination	Tissue specimens only
Cytopathological	Cells recovered by scraping the surface of tissues (e.g. cervix) or aspirating abnormal fluids (e.g. cysts) Also urine and sputum are useful
Immunological analysis	Usually blood only

The clinical chemistry laboratory

(also known as chemical pathology, clinical biochemistry)
Clinical chemistry is concerned with the diagnosis and monitoring of disease by measuring the concentration of chemicals, principally in blood and urine. Occasionally, chemical analysis of faeces and other body fluids, for example cerebrospinal and pleural fluid, is useful.

Blood is a chemically complex fluid containing many inorganic ions, proteins, carbohydrates, lipids, hormones and enzymes, along with two dissolved gases, oxygen and carbon dioxide. In health, the blood concentration of each substance is maintained within limits that reflect normal whole body and cellular metabolism. Disease is often associated with one or more disturbances in this delicate balance of blood chemistry; it is this general principle that underlies the importance of chemical testing of blood in the diagnostic process. The range of pathologies in which chemical testing of blood and urine has proven diagnostically useful is diverse and includes disease of the kidney, liver, heart, lungs and endocrine system. Some cancer cells release specific chemicals into blood. Measurement of these so-called tumour markers allows a limited role for the clinical chemistry laboratory in the diagnosis and monitoring of malignant disease. Nutritional deficiencies can be identified by chemical analysis of blood.

In addition to its diagnostic role, clinical chemistry is also involved in the monitoring of treatment. This role is most evident among patients receiving intravenous fluid replacement therapy or parenteral nutrition, who require regular monitoring of some aspects of blood chemistry. The blood concentration of some drugs must be monitored to ensure maximum therapeutic effect and minimum toxicity.

Most chemical testing of blood and urine is performed on highly sophisticated, automated machinery. A typical modern clinical chemistry analyser can process around 200–400 samples an hour with the option to perform up to 20 or more tests simultaneously on each sample. Results of the most commonly requested tests are usually available within 24 hours of receipt of the specimen. Some more specialised tests are performed only once a week. All laboratories offer an urgent 24-hour service for a limited range of tests; results of such urgently requested tests are usually available within an hour.

Intensive care patients often require frequent and urgent monitoring of some aspects of blood chemistry. In these circumstances, limited blood testing is performed by nursing staff using dedicated analysers sited within intensive care units; this represents one aspect of so-called point of care testing.

The haematology laboratory

Haematology is concerned principally with the diagnosis and monitoring of diseases that affect the number, size and appearance of the cellular or formed elements of blood. These are: the red blood cells (erythrocytes), the white blood cells (leucocytes) and platelets (thrombocytes). The full blood count (FBC) is the most frequently requested laboratory test, reflecting the range of common and less common disorders which affect both the numbers and appearance of these cells. It is in fact not one but a battery of tests.

The modern haematology analyser is able to process FBC tests at the rate of 100 samples per hour. The detailed information about the blood cells which these analysers provide has dramatically reduced the number of specimens which need to be examined under the microscope, but the microscope remains an essential tool to the haematologist for examination of bone marrow biopsy specimens and, in some circumstances, blood.

Apart from the cells in blood, haematology is also concerned with measurement of the concentration of some of the proteins present in blood which are involved in the process of blood coagulation.

Disorders of the blood in which haematology testing is important include: haematological malignancy (e.g. the leukaemias, Hodgkin's disease, myeloma), anaemia and diseases such as haemophilia in which disturbances of blood coagulation result in an increased tendency to bleed. Some haematology tests, including the FBC, are useful in the diagnosis or clinical management of some common, non-haematological diseases. For example, infectious disease is usually associated with an increase in the number of white blood cells. Anaemia is often a feature of many chronic inflammatory disorders such as rheumatoid arthritis, or may result from diseases of nutritional deficiency.

Many patients at risk of heart and blood vessel disease are given tablets, which tend to prevent the blood from clotting. This anticoagulation therapy must be monitored by regular blood testing to prevent excessive bleeding, a potentially dangerous side effect of such therapy.

Most haematology test results are routinely available within 12–24 hours. However, if the need is clinically justified, results of some haematology tests, including FBC, can be made available within an hour or so, at any time of the day or night.

The clinical microbiology laboratory

Clinical microbiology is concerned with the diagnosis of disease caused by infective agents, mostly bacteria but also viruses, fungi and parasitic worms. Much of the work involves isolation and identification of bacteria from many sorts of sample, including urine, sputum, faeces, blood, cerebrospinal fluid and swabs taken from a variety of infected sites. Bacteria can sometimes be seen by examining these specimens under the microscope, but more precise identification can only be made after culture, or growth of bacteria on nutrient-enriched media. One of the problems encountered by the microbiologist when dealing with clinical specimens is that many bacterial species are normally present in many sites around the body; indeed in some cases are essential for normal health. The microbiologist must isolate those that are pathogenic (i.e. cause disease) from those that are normally present, and from any environmental bacterial contaminant introduced during sample collection. Some body fluids are normally sterile; these include blood, cerebrospinal fluid, and fluid aspirated from joints and the pleural cavity. Bacteria isolated from these sites are always pathogenic.

Having isolated and identified a species of pathogenic bacteria, the next step is to test the sensitivity of the organism to a range of antibiotics. This information helps in deciding which antibiotic therapy is likely to be most effective in eradicating the infection.

Blood testing plays a limited but important and evolving role in detecting infections that are caused by organisms difficult to isolate by culture. During any infection the immune system produces specific antibodies directed at specific antigens present on the surface of the invading organism. A rising amount of the antibody in blood provides evidence of current infection.

Specific antigens present on the surface of organisms also provide a means of identifying infective agents. Testing blood for the presence of viral antigens is an important means of diagnosing viral infections such as those that cause hepatitis and acquired immune deficiency syndrome (AIDS).

Microbiological investigation may take from several days to several weeks to complete; this delay is governed largely by the speed of bacterial growth in culture. Initial microscopical examination can be performed immediately on receipt of the specimen if clinically necessary, and results can usually be made available on the day the sample is received in an interim report.

Clinical microbiology laboratories operate a 24-hour service for the rare cases when urgent culture and microscopical examination of samples is necessary. These include suspected cases of immediate life-threatening infections of blood (septicaemia) and central nervous system (meningitis).

Quite apart from their diagnostic role, hospital microbiology laboratories play an important role with infection control nurses in the monitoring and prevention of nosocomial infectious disease, that is infectious disease acquired by patients while in hospital, an ever present problem, which impacts on the working life of all nursing staff.

The blood transfusion laboratory

Blood transfusion is concerned with the provision of a safe supply of blood and blood products. In contrast to other pathology departments, blood transfusion has limited diagnostic function. In some senses its function more resembles a pharmacy in that its main purpose is to supply therapeutic products. With the possible exception of very severe blood loss involving more than half the total blood volume, the transfusion of whole blood is rarely necessary. The most frequently needed blood product is red cells, to correct anaemia and to replace blood lost during surgery or as a result of trauma. Much less commonly, the white cells of blood, platelets and the proteins present in blood plasma are therapeutically useful.

The National Blood Service (NBS) is responsible for the collection and supply of safe (disease free) donated blood to hospital blood transfusion laboratories. Here, each donated unit of red cells must be tested for compatibility with the patient's blood before it can be transfused. The transfusion of incompatible blood products can have very serious health consequences and is potentially fatal. Advances in compatibility testing have ensured that compatible red cells can be made available for transfusion usually well within an hour of a patient's blood sample arriving in the laboratory; this service is available 24 hours a day.

The blood transfusion department also has an important specific diagnostic role for some forms of haemolytic anaemia, in which the body produces antibodies against its own red cells. One important aspect of this work is haemolytic disease of the newborn, a potentially fatal condition in which the red cells of the developing fetus are destroyed by antibodies present in the mother's blood. All pregnant women are routinely tested for the presence of such antibodies.

The histopathology laboratory

(also known as morbid anatomy, cellular pathology)
Histopathology, the oldest of all pathology disciplines, is concerned with the diagnosis of disease by microscopical examination of tissue samples (biopsies). The rationale for this approach is that disease processes, e.g. malignancy, inflammation, infection, etc. are characterised by specific changes at the tissue and cellular level which are evident when tissue is viewed under the microscope. There are many ways of recovering tissue samples from the body. Tissue from the gastrointestinal tract, lungs and urinary tract are commonly sampled at the time of endoscopic examination. An endoscope is an instrument used to visually examine internal organs directly by fibre optics. The instrument includes small forceps, which can be used to remove small pieces of tissue during the examination. Tissue may be taken during surgery by incision or excision biopsy. Incision biopsy is the removal of a sample cut from an area of diseased tissue, whereas excision biopsy involves removal of the whole area of diseased tissue.

Before transport to the laboratory, biopsy samples must be 'fixed' in a chemical fixative, usually formalin, to preserve structure. This process can take from a few hours to a whole day depending on the size of the specimen. In the laboratory, 'fixed' specimens are impregnated with paraffin wax, allowed to harden and then cut into very thin sections just 3–5 µm thick. These wafer thin sections are then mounted on glass microscope slides and stained with chemicals, before examination under the microscope. The whole process from reception of specimen to issue of a histopathological report can take from one to three or four days depending on the size of the biopsy sample. Sometimes it is important to make a diagnosis very quickly, and in these circumstances a frozen section is performed. Tissue is 'fixed' immediately by freezing. This process allows sections to be cut almost immediately the sample is removed from the patient. The sections are stained and examined under the microscope. This rapid technique allows a diagnosis of, for example breast cancer, to be made in a half an hour or so while the patient remains anaesthetised on the operating table. Armed with a laboratory report that confirms malignant disease, the surgeon can proceed immediately to surgical treatment.

Microscopical examination of tissue removed from the patient is probably most widely used in the diagnosis and staging of malignant disease in organs throughout the body. It is also used in the differential diagnosis of non-malignant disease of the liver, kidney, lungs and gastrointestinal tract. It has a role in the diagnosis of connective tissue and skin disorders. More recently it has been used in the early diagnosis of tissue rejection among patients who have received transplanted organs.

All histopathological tests are invasive, often requiring surgical intervention to recover samples. Both financial and patient safety considerations ensure that, unlike other laboratory investigations, histopathological investigations are reserved for those patients in whom there is a strong suspicion of serious disease. In many cases, this suspicion will have been raised by the abnormal results of blood and urine tests performed in other pathology laboratories, so histopathology can represent the final stage in laboratory diagnosis.

Finally, post mortem examinations, to determine cause of patient death, are conducted in the hospital mortuary, which is administratively part of the histopathology department.

Cytopathology is a sub discipline of histopathology. Whereas histopathology is concerned with microscopical examination of tissue samples, the focus of the cytopathologist is the cells that are normally exfoliated from the epithelial surface of organs. Sample recovery is less invasive than that required for histopathological investigation. Typically cells are scraped from the surface of organs such as the cervix of the uterus, the mucosal surface of the duodenum and stomach and lungs. Cells can also be recovered by aspiration using a fine needle and syringe, from the pleural and peritoneal cavities, or from solid tumours, for example in the breast. The cells are spread onto a glass microscope slide, fixed and stained and then examined under the microscope. Cytopathology is almost exclusively concerned with diagnosis of pre-malignant and malignant disease. The cervical smear test, used to screen women for cervical cancer, accounts for a large proportion of the workload of the cytopathology laboratory.

The immunology laboratory

Clinical immunology laboratories are concerned principally with blood testing for the diagnosis of autoimmune diseases, in which the body's normally protective immune system produces antibodies against its own tissue antigens. These self-reacting, destructive antibodies are called autoantibodies. The detection in blood of organ specific autoantibodies is helpful in the diagnosis of many diseases with an autoimmune component including some thyroid disorders, pernicious anaemia, and some forms of kidney and liver disease. More rarely, tissues may be microscopically examined for the presence of the complex formed when an autoantibody reacts with its complementary antigen. For example, the autoimmune disease systemic lupus erythematosus (SLE), which affects many organ systems, can be diagnosed by microscopical examination of a skin biopsy for the presence of such complexes.

Laboratory staffing

Clinical laboratories are staffed by graduate trained biomedical scientists (BMS) who are responsible for the analysis of samples. They are helped in this task by medical laboratory assistants (MLAs). Cytoscreeners are a specially trained group whose work is confined largely to the examination of cervical smears. Each pathology department is headed by a medically qualified doctor of consultant status who has specialised in one area of laboratory medicine (in some cases a non-clinical scientist fulfils this role). They provide a consultancy for clinicians on all aspects of laboratory medicine, so they might advise both on the most appropriate laboratory investigation in particular cases, and the clinical significance of test results. Haematology consultants also have clinical responsibility for the care of patients suffering haematological disease (e.g. leukaemia). Medical consultants attached to clinical chemistry departments are often responsible for the clinical care of patients suffering diabetes and other metabolic and endocrine disorders, while a microbiology consultant is responsible with the control of infection nurse for the formulation and implementation of the hospital control of infection policy.

Histopathological diagnoses are made by a consultant histopathologist who also performs all post mortem examinations with the assistance of a mortuary technician

The future

Around 70% of patient diagnoses depend on the results of pathology laboratory tests. Recognition of the central role that pathology provides in the delivery of medical care to patients has led to a government-initiated programme of modernisation of pathology services.[1] One of the principal aims is to identify novel ways of delivering pathology services that are more responsive to patient needs. This may well include an expansion of point of care testing, that is the delivery of pathology services by non-laboratory staff at sites outside the laboratory (e.g. pharmacies, GP surgeries, outpatient departments) with nurses and other non-laboratory healthcare professionals becoming more involved in patient testing.

A report by the Audit Commission in 1993 revealed that around 85 million pathology test requests were being processed annually by around 400 NHS clinical pathology departments in England and Wales.[2] In doing this work, pathology laboratories consumed an estimated 3.3% of total NHS expenditure.[2] Over the intervening years workload has continued to rise, currently at the rate of 10% per annum.[3]

As in all other areas of patient care, successful laboratory investigation depends on teamwork; nurses are important members of that team. Good communication between nursing and laboratory staff can help to ensure that resources consumed in delivery of pathology services are used to best effect for the patient.

References

1. Department of Health (2005) *Modernising Pathology: Building a Service Responsive to Patients*. London, The Stationery Office.
2. Audit Commission (1993) *Critical Path: An Analysis of Pathology Services*. London, HMSO.
3. Beastall G (2004) The impact of the General Medical Services Contract: national evidence. *Bull R Coll Pathol* 128: 24–27.

Useful websites

www.ibms.org Institute of Biomedical Sciences – the professional organisation that represents biomedical scientists – the largest group of pathology laboratory staff.

www.rcpath.org Royal College of Pathologists – the professional organisation that represents pathologists – medically qualified laboratory staff.

www.acb.org.uk Association of Clinical Biochemistry – the professional organisation that represents non-clinical scientists working in clinical chemistry laboratories.

www.labtestsonline.org.uk website for patients about laboratory tests – includes a wealth of information about the work of pathology laboratories.

Chapter 2
SOME PRINCIPLES OF LABORATORY TESTING

Laboratory investigation of patients can be divided into three distinct phases:

- pre-testing, which includes collection and transport of specimens to the laboratory
- analysis in the laboratory
- post-testing, which includes reporting and interpretation of results.

In this second introductory chapter, some general principles relating to pre-testing procedures are discussed. Then four general topics relating to the post-testing phase are considered. They are: units of measurement; the concept of normal or reference range; the concept of sensitivity and specificity of test results, and finally critical values.

Pre-testing procedures

It is difficult to overemphasise the importance of good practice during the pre-testing phase of laboratory investigation. The production of high quality, accurate results which are clinically useful depends as much on practice before the sample reaches the laboratory as it does on the analytical process within the laboratory. Aspects of the pre-testing phase that need to be considered are:

- the pathology request form
- the timing of sample collection
- sampling technique
- collecting the right amount of sample
- sample containers and labelling
- safety during collection and transport of samples.

This chapter is concerned with principles only. The detail of pre-testing will be considered again under each test heading. However, it must be remembered that practice, although based on the principles in this book, does vary between laboratories. There is no real substitute for consultation with your local laboratory.

Pathology request form

Each patient sample must be accompanied by the appropriate fully completed pathology request form, signed by the doctor – or in some instances where that responsibility has been delegated – the specialist nurse practitioner making the request. Poor documentation can result at the very least in delay of pathology reports and may result in reports never being filed in patient records. Attention to detail is particularly vital for blood transfusion requests. Most cases of incompatible blood transfusion are the result of documentation errors. All pathology request forms should include the following information:

- patient details, including full name, date of birth and hospital number
- hospital ward, clinic or GP surgery
- nature of specimen (e.g. venous blood, urine, biopsy, etc.)
- date and time of sample collection
- name of test requested (e.g. blood glucose, full blood count, etc.)
- clinical details (these should very briefly explain why the test is being requested and may include a suspected or provisional diagnosis or symptoms)
- details of any drug therapy that might affect test or interpretation
- an indication, where relevant, of the urgency of the request
- some health authorities request details about budget cost centres.

Timing of sample collection

Whenever possible, samples should be taken to coincide with routine transport to the laboratory, so that they can be processed by the laboratory without undue delay. It is not good practice to leave samples for more than a few hours or overnight before sending them to the laboratory; in many cases the samples will be unsuitable for analysis. For a few biochemical tests, e.g. blood hormone levels, it is vital that blood is sampled at a particular time of the day. For others (e.g. blood glucose) it is simply important to know what time the sample is collected. Some tests (e.g. blood gases) require that samples be processed immediately they are taken. Collection of these must be timed by prior agreement with the laboratory. Samples for microbiological investigation are best taken before antibiotic therapy is started, since antibiotics will inhibit the growth of bacteria in culture.

Sample collection technique

Venous blood collection

Most blood tests are performed on venous blood collected by a technique known as venepuncture, using either a needle and syringe or more commonly, an evacuated tube system (Figure 2.1).

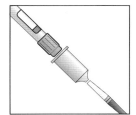

Vacutainer® System comprises:
- Sterile, double ended needle
- Needle holder
- Blood collection tube containing a pre-set vacuum

Additional equipment required:
- Disposable gloves
- Tourniquet
- Sterile alcohol-soaked swab
- Cotton wool

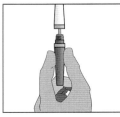

- Hold the coloured section of the needle and break the white paper seal.
- Remove and discard the white plastic needle shield. DO NOT USE if paper seal already broken.

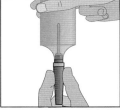

- Screw needle into needle holder and leave coloured shield on needle.

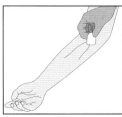

- Apply tourniquet about 10 cm above elbow to make veins visible and locate a suitable site for venepuncture.
- Clean site with alcohol-soaked swab. Allow to dry.

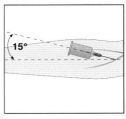

- Remove needle shield.
- Ensure patient's arm is supported and straight at the elbow.
- Insert needle bevelled side uppermost into the vein.

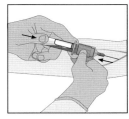

- Insert blood collection tube into the needle-holder.
- Ensuring needle does not move within the vein, push tube to the end of the needle holder, gently but firmly.
- Release tourniquet as blood flows into tube to fill vacuum.

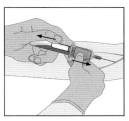

- Withdraw blood collection tube when blood flow ceases.
- Continue to hold needle and needle holder in position. (For further samples, insert next blood collection tube as before)

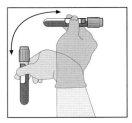

- Withdraw tube from holder.
- Invert tube 8–10 times to ensure mixing of blood with any additives in tube.

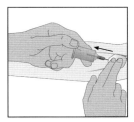

- Withdraw needle holder with needle attached.
- Cover injection site with cotton wool and apply gentle pressure for a minute or two.

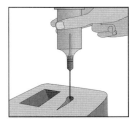

- Dispose of needle and needleholder (if disposable) in accordance with manufacturer's instruction/local safety policy.
- Label all tubes fully in accordance with local laboratory policy.

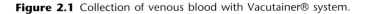

Figure 2.1 Collection of venous blood with Vacutainer® system.

- Patients may be anxious at the prospect of a venepuncture. A calm, confident manner is important. Explain in simple terms what is involved and that mild discomfort or pain is usually felt as the needle is inserted.
- If there is a history of fainting during blood collection, take the sample with the patient lying down.
- When performing venepuncture on a patient receiving intravenous (IV) fluids, do not take blood from the arm used for IV administration. This avoids the risk of IV fluid contamination of the sample.
- Haemolysis, the rupture of red cells during blood collection, may render the sample unsuitable for analysis. This may occur if blood is forced at speed through narrow gauge needles or if the sample is shaken vigorously. When using syringe and needle technique, remove the needle before expelling the blood into the sample container.
- Prolonged use of a tourniquet can affect laboratory results. Avoid the use of a tourniquet if possible and do not collect blood if tourniquet has been in place for more than one minute. Release and try the opposite arm.
- Although the cephalic or basilic vein are the preferred site, the back of the hand or the foot provide alternative sites for those with 'difficult' veins.

Capillary blood collection

Capillary blood can be recovered by a simple skin puncture with a lancet, usually on the fingertip or, in the case of babies, the heel of the foot. It is useful if only very small sample volumes (less than 1 ml) are required. The technique can be performed by patients themselves and is routinely used, after training, by diabetics to obtain samples for monitoring their blood glucose concentration.

- The fingertip, or heel in the case of neonates and babies, is wiped with alcohol. A sterile lancet or autolet device is used to puncture the cleansed skin on the side of the finger tip or heel. Puncturing the ball of the fingertip is more painful.
- Undue pressure to squeeze blood out, can cause inaccurate results – blood must flow freely.
- Blood should be collected immediately into an appropriate container, designated for capillary samples and mixed gently by inversion.
- Pressure must be applied to the puncture site with a sterile gauze until blood flow ceases.

Arterial blood collection

The only test that requires sampling of blood from arteries is blood gases. The technique, which is more hazardous and painful than venepuncture, is described in Chapter 7.

Urine collection

Four kinds of urine collection are commonly made:

- midstream urine (MSU)
- catheter specimen urine (CSU)
- early morning urine (EMU)
- 24-hour urine, i.e. all the urine passed during a 24-hour period.

The test requested determines which of these is appropriate. For most non-quantitative purposes, such as dipstick testing and microbiological testing, an MSU is necessary. This is a small (10–15 ml) sample of urine, collected part way through micturition, which can be collected at any time of the day. A CSU is the urine sample collected from a patient who has an indwelling urinary catheter. The detail of collecting an MSU or CSU for microbiological examination is given in Chapter 21.

The first urine passed in the day, the so-called EMU, is the most concentrated and an EMU provides the best method of detecting substances in the urine which are present only in low concentration. An example of its use is pregnancy testing. The urine pregnancy test is based on detection of a hormone, human chorionic gonadotrophin (HCG), which is not normally present in urine, but is excreted in increasing concentration during the first few months of pregnancy. Early in pregnancy, the concentration is so low that unless a concentrated urine test (i.e. an EMU) is used, the result may be falsely negative.

Sometimes it is useful to know exactly how much of a particular substance (e.g. sodium, potassium) is being lost from the body in urine on a daily basis. Quantification of this urinary loss can only be made by collecting all the urine passed during a 24-hour period. The detail of collecting a 24-hour urine is provided in Chapter 5.

Sputum, swab collection

All these specimens are destined for microbiological examination and the object is to sample only from infected sites, while avoiding bacterial contamination from other sites on the body or from the environment. For example, a sputum specimen is intended to reflect the environment of the respiratory tract, not the mouth. Saliva is not sputum. Sputum is best collected first thing in the morning and must be coughed up from the lungs. Washing out the mouth before sampling reduces the risk of salivary contamination.

When collecting throat swabs, it is important to ensure that the swab does not come into contact with the tongue or sides of the mouth. This can be avoided by use of a tongue depressor. The swab should be gently rubbed only over the area at the back of the mouth (pharynx) and tonsils, especially inflamed areas.

Wound swabs are obtained by sampling the affected site only, avoiding contact with surrounding normal skin or tissue. When collecting any microbiological specimen, it is important to minimise environmental contamination by using aseptic technique and replacing swabs back in sterile containers or transport medium immediately.

Tissue (biopsy) collection

A very brief reference to tissue sampling techniques, necessary for histopathological examination has already been made (Chapter 1). Such sampling is always the responsibility of doctors and is beyond the scope of this book. Nurses are, however, involved in sampling of cervical cells for the cervical smear test (Chapter 23).

Collecting the right amount of sample

The amount of blood required for laboratory testing is governed largely by local laboratory equipment and is therefore a matter of local laboratory policy. In general, continuing technological advance significantly reduces the amount of blood required for many tests. All laboratories supply a list of tests with the minimum blood volume requirements. Anyone responsible for blood collection must become familiar with this local list. Some blood specimen bottles contain pre-weighed amounts of chemical preservatives and/or anticoagulants which determine the optimum volume of blood which the bottle should contain. This volume is stated on the side of the bottle. Erroneous results may occur if these blood volume instructions are not observed.

While the volume of urine collected for MSU and CSU is not critical, it is vital, when collecting 24-hour urines, that all the urine passed in the collection period is collected, even if a second collection bottle is required.

In general, the size or amount of sample is important for successful isolation of bacteria. For example, it is more likely that bacteria will be isolated from a large specimen of sputum than a small specimen. Aspiration of pus with a needle and syringe is more likely to result in isolation of the causative organism than a swab of the pus. Falsely negative blood culture results can occur if insufficient blood is added to culture bottles.

Sample containers

Pathology laboratories supply a bewildering array of sample bottles and containers. Each container has specific uses; it is vital for accurate results that the correct container is used for the test requested.

Some blood containers contain chemicals (Table 2.1) either in liquid or powder form. These chemicals serve two purposes: they prevent the blood from clotting and preserve either blood cell structure or the concentration of some blood constituent. It is important that these chemicals are mixed with the blood sample.

A preservative may be necessary to preserve urine during collection of 24-hour urine. The need for a preservative is determined by the substance in urine to be measured.

All sample containers for microbiological examination, e.g. urine, swabs, blood culture bottles, etc. are sterile and should not be used if seals are broken. Some bacteria will only survive outside the body if preserved in special transport media.

The structure of tissue samples is preserved by 'fixing' the tissue in formalin. Biopsy sample containers contain this preservative.

Table 2.1 Some common additives present in blood collection tubes.

Additive	Purpose
Ethylenediaminetetraacetate (EDTA)	An anticoagulant which prevents blood from clotting by binding to and effectively removing the calcium present in blood plasma (calcium is required for clotting to occur). EDTA also preserves the structure of blood cells. Present in bottles (usually purple/lavender tops) for full blood count and some other haematology tests.
Heparin (present as either the sodium or potassium salt of this acid i.e. sodium or potassium heparin)	An anticoagulant which prevents blood from clotting by inhibiting the formation of thrombin from prothrombin. Present in bottles (usually dark green or orange tops) for chemistry tests that require blood plasma. The anticoagulant properties of heparin are used therapeutically (p. 233).
Citrate (present as the sodium salt of this acid, i.e. sodium citrate)	An anticoagulant, which prevents blood from clotting by precipitating calcium (similar in action to EDTA). Present in bottles (usually light blue top) reserved for coagulation studies.
Oxalate (present as either the sodium of ammonium salt of this acid, i.e. sdium or ammonium oxalate)	An anticoagulant which prevents blood from clotting by precpitating calcium (similar in action to EDTA). Used with sodium fluoride (see below) in bottles specifically for blood glucose estimation (usually yellow or grey tops).
Sodium fluoride	This is an enzyme poison and prevents the continued metabolism of glucose in blood after collection, i.e. preserves blood glucose concentration. Use with oxalate in bottles specifically for blood glucose (usually yellow or grey tops).

All sample containers must be fully labelled, including the patient's full name, date of birth and location of patient (ward, clinic or GP). Laboratories receive many hundreds of specimens every day, which may include specimens from two or more patients with the same name. It is vital if results are to find their way back to the correct patient's records that specimen labels accurately and fully identify the patient. The laboratory may reject inadequately labelled specimens, resulting in the need for the patient to be retested – an entirely avoidable waste of time and resources to both patient and staff.

Safety during sample collection and transport

All laboratories have a locally written safety policy relating to the safe collection and transport of patient specimens, based on the premise that all patient specimens are potentially hazardous. Anyone involved in sample collection should be familiar with this policy. Among the many hazards which may be present in pathological specimens are viruses that cause AIDS and hepatitis, both of which can be transmitted by contact with infected blood. Tuberculosis can be transmitted by contact with infected sputum and gastrointestinal infections by contact with infected faeces. Good practice can have a major impact in reducing the risk to all staff and patients. The detail of good practice should be included in local safety policy. Some general points are included here.

- Disposable surgical gloves should be used during sample collection to reduce the risk of infection spread. Open sores offer an entry point for microbial pathogens.
- Safe disposal of syringe and needles is vital. Needle stick injuries provide an excellent way of inoculating yourself with the patient's blood, which may contain an infective virus.
- Leaking specimens present a major and surprisingly frequent potential hazard, which can be prevented by the simple expedient of ensuring that sample bottles are not overfilled and tops are well secured. Most laboratories have a policy of discarding leaking specimens.
- Specimens should be transported in specially designed plastic bags which include a separate compartment for the accompanying pathology request form.
- Specimen spillages should be dealt with in accordance with local policy.
- The use of additional protection such as eye goggles or disposable gown should be considered when collecting samples from patients known to be infected with HIV, or other blood transmissible virus e.g. those which cause viral hepatitis. Specimens from such patients should be clearly identified in some way according to locally agreed policy.

Interpretation of laboratory results

The diversity of techniques used to examine patient samples results in many types of laboratory report. Anyone who has filed pathology reports in patient case notes will have noticed that test results may be expressed *quantitatively, semi-quantitatively or qualitatively*. All reports from the histopathology laboratory, for example, are qualitative; they take the form of highly technical written text, describing the appearance of tissue samples when viewed microscopically. The text will include a summary of the clinical significance of any deviations in appearance from that of normal tissue.

Microbiological reports tend to be either qualitative or semi-quantitative. Text describes which pathogenic micro-organisms have been isolated from the sample, but the sensitivity of these micro-organisms to antibiotics tested is reported semi-quantitatively. In contrast, most reports from clinical chemistry and haematology laboratories are quantitative; they take the form of numerical results. As with any other numerical measurement (e.g. body weight, temperature, pulse rate), all quantitative results reported by clinical laboratories are defined by the unit of measurement.

Table 2.2 Basic and derived SI units of measurement.

Basic SI unit	Measure of	Abbreviation or symbol
metre	length	m
kilogramme	mass (weight)*	kg
second	time	s
ampere	electric current	A
kelvin	temperature	K
mole	amount of a substance	mol
candela	luminous intensity	cd

* for the purposes of this text mass and weight are regarded as equivalent

Units of measurement used in clinical laboratories

Système International d'unités (SI units)

Since the 1970s, all units of scientific and clinical measurement in the UK have been based, wherever possible, on the SI system, devised in 1960. In the United States non-SI units continue to be used in the reporting of clinical laboratory results, so care must be taken when interpreting laboratory results reported in US medical and nursing journals. Of the seven basic SI units (Table 2.2), only three are relevant to clinical laboratories. They are:

- metre (m)
- kilogram (kg)
- mole (mol)

Although everyone is familiar with the metre as a unit of length and the kilogram as a unit of mass or weight, the mole requires some explanation.
What is the mole (mol)?
The mole is defined as the quantity of a substance whose mass in grams (g) is equal to its particle (i.e. molecular or atomic) weight. This is a useful measure because 1 mole of any substance contains the same number of particles, i.e. 6.023×10^{23}. This is known as Avogadro's number.

Examples
What is 1 mole of sodium (Na)?
Sodium is an element (single atom) whose atomic weight is 23.
Therefore 1 mole of sodium is 23 g of sodium.
What is 1 mole of water (H_2O)?
Water is a molecule, composed of 2 atoms of hydrogen and 1 atom of oxygen.
The atomic weight of hydrogen is 1.
The atomic weight of oxygen is 16.
Therefore the molecular weight of water is $(2 \times 1) + 16 = 18$.
Therefore 1 mole of water is 18 g of water.

What is 1 mole of glucose?

A molecule of glucose is composed of 6 carbon atoms, 12 hydrogen atoms and 6 oxygen atoms.

The molecular formula of glucose is written $C_6H_{12}O_6$.

The atomic weight of carbon is 12.

The atomic weight of hydrogen is 1.

The atomic weight of oxygen is 16.

Therefore the molecular weight of glucose is

$6 \times 12 =$	72	+
$12 \times 1 =$	12	+
$6 \times 16 =$	96	=
	180	

Therefore 1 mole of glucose is 180 g glucose.

Thus 23 g of sodium, 18 g of water and 180 g of glucose all contain 6.023×10^{23} particles, either atoms in the case of sodium or molecules in the case of water and glucose. Knowing the molecular formula of any substance allows the use of mole as a unit of amount. For some molecular complex chemicals present in blood, e.g. proteins, the precise molecular weight cannot be defined. The unit of amount (mole) cannot be used when measuring such substances.

Multiples and fractions of basic SI units

When the basic SI unit (metre, kilogram, or mole) is too large or too small for the measurement being made, it is convenient to use secondary units which are multiples or fractions of the basic unit. The SI system is decimal, so that SI secondary units are expressed as powers of ten of the basic unit. Table 2.3 describes the most commonly used secondary SI units of length, mass (weight) and amount used in clinical and laboratory medicine.

Units for measuring volume

Strictly speaking, the SI unit of volume should be based on the metre, i.e. cubic metre (m^3), cubic centimetre (cm^3), cubic millimetre (mm^3), etc.

However, when the SI system was adopted for clinical measurements, it was decided to retain the litre as a measure of fluid volume because it was already in use and is almost exactly the same as 1000 cm^3. In fact, 1 litre = 1000.028 cm^3.

So the litre (L or l) is the basic 'SI' unit of volume. From this are derived the following secondary units of volume used in clinical and laboratory medicine:

decilitre (dL or dl) = 1/10 (one tenth or 10^{-1}) of a litre
centilitre (cL or cl) = 1/100 (one hundredth or 10^{-2}) of a litre
millilitre (mL or ml) = 1/1000 (one thousandth or 10^{-3}) of a litre
microlitre (μL or μl) = 1/1 000 000 (one millionth or 10^{-6}) of a litre
Note: 1 ml = 1.028 cm³

Table 2.3 Secondary SI units of length, mass (weight) and amount used in laboratory medicine.

Basic unit of length – Metre (m)	
Secondary units	● **centimetre (cm)** is 1/100th (one hundredth i.e. 10^{-2}) of a metre 100 cm = 1 m ● **millimetre (mm)** is 1/1000th (one thousandth i.e. 10^{-3}) of a metre 1000 mm = 1 m 10 mm = 1 cm ● **micrometre (μm)** is 1/1 000 000 (one millionth i.e. 10^{-6}) of a metre 1 000 000 μm = 1 m 10 000 μm = 1 cm 1000 μm = 1 mm ● **nanometre (nm)** is 1/1 000 000 000 (one thousand millionth) of a metre 1 000 000 000 nm = 1 m 10 000 000 nm = 1 cm 1 000 000 nm = 1 mm 1000 nm = 1 μm

Basic unit of mass (weight) – Kilogram (kg)	
Secondary units	● **gram (g)** is 1000th (one thousandth i.e. 10^{-3}) of a kilogram 1000 g = 1 kg ● **milligram (mg)** is 1000th (one thousandth i.e. 10^{-3}) of a gram 1000 mg = 1 g 1 000 000 mg = 1 kg ● **microgram (μg)** is 1000th (one thousandth i.e. 10^{-3}) of a milligram 1000 μg = 1 mg 1 000 000 μg = 1 g 1 000 000 000 μg = 1 kg ● **nanogram (ng)** is 1000th (one thousandth i.e. 10^{-3}) of a microgram 1000 ng = 1 μg 1 000 000 ng = 1 mg 1 000 000 000 ng = 1 g 1 000 000 000 000 ng = 1 kg ● **picogram (pg)** is 1000th (one thousandth i.e. 10^{-3}) of a nanogram 1000 pg = 1 ng 1 000 000 pg = 1 μg 1 000 000 000 pg = 1 mg 1 000 000 000 000 pg = 1 g

Basic unit of amount – Mole (mol)	
Secondary units	● **millimole (mmol)** is 1000th (one thousandth i.e. 10^{-3}) of a mole 1000 mmol = 1 mol ● **micromole (μmol)** is 1000th (one thousandth i.e. 10^{-3}) of a millimole 1000 μmol = 1 mmol 1 000 000 μmol = 1 mol ● **nanomole (nmol)** is 1000th (one thousandth i.e. 10^{-3}) of a micromole 1000 nmol = 1 μmol 1 000 000 nmol = 1 mmol 1 000 000 000 nmol = 1 mol ● **picomole (pmol)** is 1000th (one thousandth i.e. 10^{-3}) of a nanomole 1000 pmol = 1 nmol 1 000 000 pmol = 1 μmol 1 000 000 000 pmol = 1 mmol

Units of concentration

Nearly all quantitative analysis of patient specimens involves determination of the concentration of a substance in blood or urine. Concentration is defined as the *amount or mass (weight)* of a substance that is contained in a specified *volume* of fluid. Units of concentration comprise two elements; the unit of amount or mass (weight) and the unit of volume. For example, if we weigh out 20 g (mass) of salt and dissolve it in 1 litre (volume) of water we have a solution of salt whose concentration is 20 grams per litre. In this case the unit of mass (weight) is the gram and the unit of volume is the litre and the SI unit of concentration is grams per litre or g/l. Where the molecular weight of the substance being measured is precisely defined, as it is for many of the blood-borne chemicals measured in clinical laboratories, the mole (unit of amount) is used.

Examples

The following 'real' examples demonstrate some of the variety of units used in the chemical analysis of blood.

What does the result 'plasma sodium 144 mmol/l' mean?
Every litre of blood plasma contains 144 mmol of sodium.
What does the result 'plasma albumin 23 g/l' mean?
There are 23 grams of albumin in every litre of blood plasma.
What does the result 'plasma iron 9 μmol/l' mean?
Every litre of blood plasma contains 9 micromoles of iron.
What does the result 'plasma B$_{12}$ 300 ng/l' mean?
There are 300 nanograms of vitamin B$_{12}$ in every litre of blood plasma.

Units of cell count

Much haematology testing involves counting the concentration of cells in blood. Here the unit of amount is the number of cells and the unit of volume is again the litre. Normally healthy individuals have between 4 500 000 000 000 (4.5 million million) and 6 500 000 000 000 (6.5 million million) red cells in every litre of blood. The unit of red cell count is the number of million million cells there are in one litre of blood, expressed in short notation as 10^{12} per litre or 10^{12}/l. This allows the use of manageable numbers, so in normal practice we might say a patient has a red cell count of 5.3. This does not of course mean the patient has only 5.3 red cells; rather in every litre of blood, the patient has 5.3 million million red cells. There are far fewer white cells than red cells in blood and this is reflected in the unit of the white cell count, which is 10^9/l or the number of thousand million cells in every litre of blood.

The reference (normal) range

When making any clinical measurement, for example weighing a patient or measuring pulse rate, results are interpreted by reference to what is normal. The same is true of tests performed on patient samples.

All quantitative tests have a reference range recorded alongside patient test results to aid interpretation. Biological variation determines that just as there is no clear cut demarcation between normal and abnormal height and weight, there is no clear cut demarcation between normal and abnormal concentration of any constituent of blood and urine. The use of the term reference range in preference to normal range is recognition of this limitation. Reference ranges are constructed

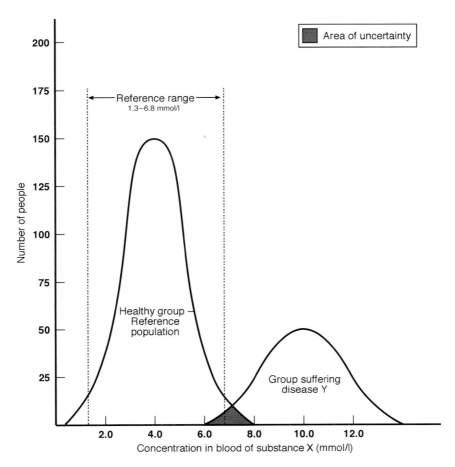

Figure 2.2 Demonstrating reference (normal) range for theoretical substance X and the overlap in blood concentration of X among healthy individuals and those suffering theoretical disease Y (see text for explanation).

by measuring the substance in question in a large population of apparently healthy 'normal' individuals.

The graph in Figure 2.2 describes the results of measuring the concentration of hypothetical substance X in the blood of a large population of apparently healthy individuals (the reference population), and those with a hypothetical disease Y.

Since the blood concentration of substance X is usually raised in those suffering disease Y, it is used as a blood test to confirm the diagnosis among those with symptoms of Y. From the graph it can be seen that the concentration of X among apparently healthy individuals ranges from 0.3 to 8.0 mmol/l. The chance that a particular result is normal diminishes the further that result is away from the average or mean result of the reference population, in this case 4.0 mmol/l. The extreme ends of the range *may* represent abnormality. To take account of this, all reference ranges are conventionally constructed by excluding the results of 2.5% of the reference population, whose results lie at either end of this 'normal' range. By definition, a reference range is the range in concentration of 95% of the reference (healthy) population. In this case, the reference range is 1.3–6.8 mmol/l. Using this reference range we can identify those who are suffering disease Y. Clearly, there is a high degree of certainty that patients with a blood X concentration of more than 8.0 mmol/l are suffering disease Y, and that those with a concentration of less than 6.0 mmol/l are not. However, there is a grey area of uncertainty for those whose blood levels lie between 6.0 and 8.0 mmol/l. The poor discriminating power near the limits of a reference range is very typical of quantitative laboratory tests and should always be taken into account when interpreting laboratory test results.

For example, supposing the local reference range for serum sodium is 135–145 mmol/l, there is no doubt that a sodium concentration of 125 mmol/l is abnormal and may require treatment. By contrast, an isolated sodium concentration of 134 mmol/l, although clearly outside the reference range, has no particular significance. Remember by definition 5% (i.e. 1 in 20) of the healthy population have a result outside the limits of a reference range.

Factors that affect the reference range

Various quite normal physiological factors may need to be taken into account when interpreting laboratory test results. Test results may be affected by:

- age of the patient
- sex of the patient
- pregnancy
- time of the day the sample was collected.

For example, blood urea concentration rises with age and blood hormone levels are different among adult males compared with adult females. Pregnancy can affect the results of laboratory tests of thyroid function. Blood glucose levels fluctuate throughout the day. Alcohol and many drugs can affect blood test results in a variety of ways. The precise nature and extent of these physiological and drug effects will be considered in more detail as each test is discussed.

Finally, reference ranges are dependent on the particular analytical techniques used by laboratories. When interpreting any individual patient result, it is important to use only the reference ranges constructed by the laboratory that produced the test result. Throughout this book the reference ranges quoted are a guide only but will approximate to the reference values for all laboratories, unless otherwise stated.

Sensitivity and specificity

The sensitivity and specificity of a diagnostic test defines just how reliable that test is in making or excluding the diagnosis it is intended for. The ideal diagnostic test is 100% sensitive and 100% specific. A test that is 100% sensitive identifies all those with the disease – there are no false negatives. One that is 100% specific is never positive in those without the disease – there are no false positives. To illustrate the concept, consider pregnancy testing. Suppose a pregnancy test has a quoted sensitivity of 99.5% and specificity of 99.7%. If 1000 pregnant women were submitted for the test, in 995 cases the results would be correctly positive but there would be five falsely negative results. If 1000 non-pregnant women were submitted for the test, 997 would be correctly negative but there would be three false positive results.

In practice, very few diagnostic tests are either 100% sensitive or 100% specific but of course the closer to this ideal, the more reliable is the test.

Critical values

When a patient test result lies outside the reference range, it is useful for nursing staff to know if the result warrants immediate clinical intervention. Should medical staff be informed urgently of this test result? The concept of critical values (inappropriately sometimes called 'panic' values) is intended to help with this area of decision-making. A critical value is defined as:

'a pathophysiological state at such variance with normal as to be life threatening, unless something is done promptly and for which some corrective action could be taken'.[1]

Not all tests warrant critical values but where appropriate throughout this book, suggested critical values for each test will be recorded alongside reference range values. As with reference ranges, critical values are determined by local laboratories; just as it is important to use locally constructed reference ranges in the interpretation of actual patient test results, so nurses should follow existing local protocol relating to critical values.

Difference between serum and plasma

Throughout this book, reference will be made to blood serum (or simply serum) and blood plasma (or simply plasma). Before leaving this introductory chapter it is important to clarify what these terms mean.

Blood is composed of cells (red cells, white cells and platelets) suspended in a liquid, which is essentially an aqueous (water) solution of many different inorganic and organic chemicals. It is this liquid which is analysed in most clinical chemistry and some haematological blood tests. The first step for all these tests is to separate and remove the liquid part from the cells. In physiology texts the liquid is called plasma. An alternative name is serum. The essential difference between serum and plasma is the sample tube into which blood is collected.

If blood is collected into a plain tube containing no additives, the blood clots and the liquid recovered is serum. By contrast, if blood is collected into a tube containing an anticoagulant the blood remains fluid (does not clot). The fluid that remains when cells have been removed from this sample is called plasma. With some important exceptions, most notably tests of blood coagulation, the results from testing either plasma or serum are virtually the same; in these circumstances it is a matter of local laboratory preference which is used.

Case history 1

On the second day following elective surgery, Alan Howard, a 46-year-old man, was feeling unwell. Blood was taken for a range of chemical tests and a full blood count (FBC). Among the results phoned back to the ward were the following:

Plasma sodium	135 mmol/l	(reference range 135–145)
Plasma potassium	8.0 mmol/l	(reference range 3.5–5.2)
Plasma bicarbonate	28 mmol/l	(reference range 25–35)
Plasma urea	5.5 mmol/l	(reference range 2.5–6.6)
Plasma calcium	1.1 mmol/l	(reference range 2.35–2.75)

The FBC results were normal. Realising that the potassium and calcium results were grossly abnormal, the patient's named nurse immediately informed the surgical house officer, who took a second sample. Twenty minutes later, the laboratory telephoned back with an entirely normal set of results. It transpired that the person who had taken the first sample had overfilled the full blood count bottle and tipped blood into the bottle for chemistry tests to bring the level in the full blood count bottle down to the right mark on the label. How did this cause the abnormal potassium and calcium results?

Discussion of case history

Blood for a full blood count must be prevented from clotting. This is achieved by the presence in the bottle of a chemical anticoagulant namely the potassium (K^+) salt of ethylenediaminetetraacetate (K^+–EDTA). This is an anticoagulant which works by chelating (effectively removing) calcium from blood. (Calcium is essential for the normal clotting process.) The addition of K^+–EDTA, while preventing blood from clotting, has two incidental effects: it raises the potassium concentration and reduces calcium concentration. The small volume of blood which was tipped into the bottle for urea and electrolytes contained sufficient K^+–EDTA to markedly reduce calcium concentration and increase potassium concentration. This case history demonstrates that a K^+–EDTA sample of blood is unsuitable for potassium and calcium estimation, and provides a graphic illustration of one of many ways in which poor sampling technique can adversely affect laboratory results. In this case, the abnormal results were actually incompatible with life and therefore easily identified. Less dramatic changes, which may remain undetected and therefore potentially more dangerous, can be caused by poor practice at the time of sample collection and transport.

Reference

1. Emancipator K (1997) Critical Values: ASCP Practice Parameter. *Am J Clin Pathol* **108**: 247–53.

Further reading

McCall RE & Tankersley CM (1998) *Phlebotomy Essentials* (2nd edn). Philadelphia: Lippincott.

Campbell J (1995) Making sense of the technique of venepuncture. *Nurs Times* **91**(31): 29–31.

Shah V & Tadido A (2005) Neonatal blood sampling. *www.bloodgas.org*

Ravel R (1995) Various factors affecting laboratory test interpretation. In *Clinical Laboratory Medicine* (6th edn). St Louis, Mosby. pp 1–8.

PART 2

Clinical biochemistry tests

Chapter 3
BLOOD GLUCOSE

The most significant reason for measurement of the concentration of glucose in blood is the diagnosis and monitoring of diabetes mellitus, a common chronic metabolic disease that can occur at any age. Current estimates suggest that in England alone 2.1 million (4.4% of the population) have diabetes,[1] this includes close to 1 million who are undiagnosed. The incidence of diabetes is increasing around the world.[2] Forecasts suggest that by 2010, 5.2% of the UK population will have diabetes.[1] As we shall see, abnormality in blood glucose concentration is not confined to those suffering diabetes.

Normal physiology

The carbohydrate present in the food we eat accounts for around 60% of our dietary requirement. In the gastrointestinal tract, complex food carbohydrates (starches) are digested by enzymes to simple molecules, for absorption to the blood stream. These simple molecules are the monosaccharides glucose, fructose and galactose. Of these, glucose is by far the most abundant, representing on average around 80% of absorbed monosaccharides. Once inside the body, most of the fructose and galactose is converted to glucose. Nearly all of our dietary carbohydrate is converted to glucose. Most cells in the body also have mechanisms for converting non-carbohydrates (fats and proteins) to glucose when demand for glucose is high and supply is low (starvation).

Why is glucose important?

Glucose can only function within cells, where it is the major source of energy. In every cell of the body this energy is realised by the metabolic oxidation of glucose to carbon dioxide and water. In the process, the energy contained within glucose is used to form the energy-rich compound adenosine triphosphate (ATP) from adenosine diphosphate (ADP). The energy contained within ATP in turn is used to drive the many chemical reactions within the cell that are needed for it to remain viable and fulfill its function (Figure 3.1).

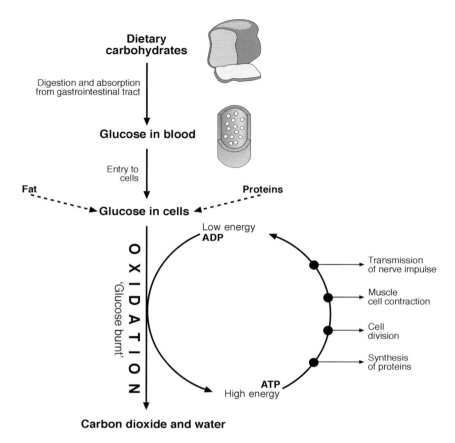

Figure 3.1 Glucose has central metabolic role within cells providing energy for the chemical reactions required for cells to function.

The oxidation of glucose, with resulting generation of energy-rich ATP, occurs in two major cellular metabolic pathways (Figure 3.2). They are the glycolytic pathway (sometimes called simply glycolysis or the Embden–Meyerhoff pathway after the scientists who first identified it) and the Krebs cycle (alternative name tri-carboxylic acid cycle). The process begins with the glycolytic pathway, in which glucose is converted (oxidised) via 13 separate enzymic reactions to the tri-carboxylic acid, pyruvate. The fate of pyruvate depends on the relative amount of tissue oxygen. In normally oxygenated tissue, pyruvate is converted to a substance called acetyl CoA which enters the Krebs cycle and joins (condenses) with another tri-carboxylic acid, oxaloacetic acid to form citric acid. In a further nine enzymic reactions, citric acid is converted back to oxaloacetic acid for condensation with more acetyl CoA generated by glycolysis.

Oxidation of 1 molecule of glucose in the glycolytic pathway yields 2 molecules of pyruvate and 8 molecules of ATP. Further oxidation of the two molecules of pyruvate generated by glycolytic pathway, in Krebs cycle yields a further 30 molecules

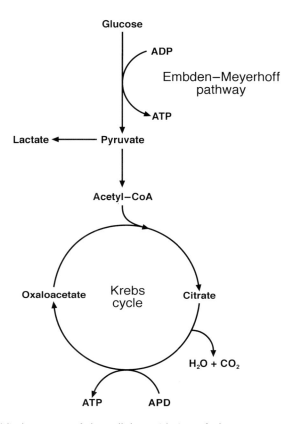

Figure 3.2 Simplified account of the cellular oxidation of glucose.

of ATP. So in total, oxidation of 1 molecule of glucose to CO_2 and H_2O yields 38 molecules of energy rich ATP.

In the absence of sufficient oxygen, glucose can be converted to pyruvate by the glycolytic pathway, but pyruvate cannot enter the Krebs cycle. Instead it is converted to lactate (lactic acid). Accumulation of lactic acid in the blood (lactic acidosis) is a cause of metabolic acidosis (Chapter 7), occurs in any pathological condition associated with poor tissue perfusion and therefore relative tissue hypoxia, and is a direct result of anaerobic glycolysis (i.e. glycolysis in tissues with relative oxygen deficiency).

Importance of maintaining normal blood glucose concentration

Unlike all other tissues, the brain is unable to manufacture or store glucose and is entirely dependent on a ready supply of glucose in blood for its energy requirements. The maintenance of a minimum amount of glucose in blood is essential for normal brain function. Blood glucose concentration above around 3.0 mmol/l ensures this function. It is equally important, however, to ensure that blood glucose concentration does not rise too high. Glucose is an osmotically active substance. This means that as the concentration of glucose in blood rises, its osmotic effect tends to draw water out of surrounding cells, leaving them relatively dehydrated.

In order to combat this potentially devastating effect on cells, the kidneys compensate by excreting glucose in urine when blood levels rise above a certain concentration called the renal threshold (usually around 10.0–11.0 mmol/l). However, in doing this, the valuable energy resource which glucose represents is lost from the body. For good health, blood glucose concentration must not rise above a maximum level, or the body's most significant energy resource will be lost in urine, but it must not fall too low either, or brain function will be threatened.

Glucose can be stored

Although all cells require glucose for energy, the demand may vary between cells and will vary at different times of the day. For example, muscle cell demand will be highest during exercise and lowest during sleep. Cellular demand for glucose does not always coincide with meals when glucose is available and there is therefore a need to store dietary glucose until it is required. Most cells in the body can store limited amounts of glucose, but three sorts of tissue mainly serve this function:

- liver
- muscle
- fat (adipose tissue).

The cells of these organs are able to remove glucose from blood and store it when demand is low or supply is high (immediately after meals). Between meals when glucose is in short supply glucose is mobilised from these stores.

Liver and muscle cells store glucose as the polymer molecule glycogen, which is effectively many glucose molecules joined together. The enzymic process by which glycogen is formed from glucose in these cells is called glycogenesis. The reverse process, called glycogenolysis, allows glucose to be recovered from this store and occurs in response to a falling blood glucose concentration. Glucose can be taken up by fat cells and converted by a process called lipogenesis to triglyceride, a fat, and stored in this form. Triglyceride can be mobilised from fat stores to provide energy by a process known as lipolysis, but this will only occur after glycogen stores are depleted. In this way glycogen provides short-term storage of glucose and fat provides long-term storage of glucose.

How is blood glucose concentration maintained within the normal range?

Despite the considerable variation in glucose intake and utilisation throughout the day, blood glucose concentration never usually rises above around 8.0 mmol/l or falls below around 3.5 mmol/l. Figure 3.3 describes typical normal daily fluctuation.

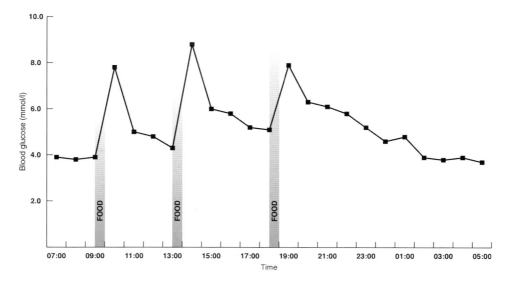

Figure 3.3 Typical variation of blood glucose concentration throughout the day.

Immediately after a meal, blood glucose concentration rises as glucose derived from food is absorbed from the gut. The cells of the body take up this glucose; some is utilised to satisfy current energy requirement and any excess is stored as glycogen in liver and muscle cells or as fat (triglyceride) in adipose tissue. As a consequence of this movement of glucose from blood to cells, blood glucose concentration falls between meals. However, in order to maintain minimum blood glucose concentration between meals, glucose is mobilised from hepatic glycogen stores. If necessary, glucose may also be manufactured within cells from non-carbohydrate sources such as protein, by a process called gluconeogenesis.

Both the uptake of glucose from blood by cells and the metabolic pathways involved in blood glucose regulation (glycogenesis, glycogenolysis, etc.) are under the overall control of hormones, the secretion of which are governed in turn by blood glucose concentration.

Hormonal control of blood glucose concentration

The pancreatic hormones insulin and glucagon are the most important for regulating blood glucose levels. Insulin has the effect of reducing blood glucose levels by:

- promoting uptake of glucose by cells from blood (the uptake of glucose by cells of the liver and central nervous system is independent of insulin)
- promoting the cellular metabolism (oxidation) of glucose to pyruvate (glycolysis)

- increasing formation of glycogen from glucose in liver and muscle (glyco-genesis)
- increasing formation of triglyceride from glucose in adipose cells (lipogenesis)
- inhibiting production of glucose from non-carbohydrate sources (gluconeo-genesis).

Insulin is synthesised in, and secreted by, the beta (β) cells of the pancreas in response to rising blood glucose concentration, and operates by binding to insulin receptors present on the surface of insulin sensitive cells. The normal hormonal response to rising blood glucose depends on:

- adequate amount of insulin and therefore normally functioning pancreatic β cells
- adequate and functioning insulin receptors on the surface of insulin sensitive cells.

Without either of these, blood glucose concentration continues to rise.

Glucagon is an insulin antagonist hormone synthesised in, and secreted from the alpha (α) cells of the pancreas in response to a falling blood glucose concentration. In direct contrast to the action of insulin, glucagon has the effect of raising blood glucose levels by:

- increasing hepatic production of glucose from glycogen (glycogenolysis)
- increasing production of glucose from non-carbohydrate sources (gluconeo-genesis).

To recap, rising blood glucose concentration stimulates the pancreas to secrete insulin. By its various effects, insulin reduces blood glucose concentration. Falling blood glucose levels induce glucagon secretion, which prevents further blood glucose reduction. Continuous synergy of these two opposing hormonal effects ensures that blood glucose concentration is maintained within normal limits.

Three further hormones are secreted in response to a low blood glucose concentration and also in response to stress. They are:

- cortisol, synthesised by the adrenal cortex
- adrenalin (epinephrine), synthesised by the adrenal medulla
- growth hormone, secreted by the anterior pituitary.

These all have the effect of increasing blood glucose concentration. Four hormones – glucagon, cortisol, adrenalin and growth hormone – prevent blood glucose concentration falling too low, but only insulin prevents blood glucose concentration from rising too high. This reflects the prime importance of maintaining adequate minimal level of glucose in blood for normal brain function. Table 3.1 provides a summary of the hormones involved in blood glucose regulation.

Table 3.1 Hormones involved in blood glucose regulation.

Hormone	Site of production and release	Released in response to	Overall effect on blood glucose concentration
Insulin	Pancreas (beta cells)	Raised blood glucose	Reduces blood glucose
Glucagon	Pancreas (alpha cells)	Reduced blood glucose	Increases blood glucose
Adrenalin (epinephrine)	Adrenal gland (medulla)	Stress	Increases blood glucose
Cortisol	Adrenal gland (cortex)	Reduced blood glucose and/or stress	Increases blood glucose
Growth hormone	Anterior pituitary gland	Reduced blood glucose and/or stress	Increases blood glucose

Laboratory measurement of blood or plasma glucose

Patient preparation

If the test is to determine fasting blood glucose, no food should be taken for at least 12 hours prior to blood sampling; otherwise no particular patient preparation is necessary.

Timing of sample

Blood glucose concentration varies throughout the day, highest at around one hour after the main meal of the day and lowest first thing in the morning before food; correct interpretation demands that the time be recorded on the specimen. Samples may be random (without reference to time of food), fasting (sample taken after an overnight 12-hour fast) or 2 hour post-prandial (sample taken two hours after a meal).

Sample requirement

Around 2 ml venous blood is collected into a special tube (most often grey or yellow top), containing the glucose preservative sodium fluoride and an anti-coagulant, potassium oxalate. Fluoride is an enzyme poison that effectively prevents continued red cell glycolysis, and therefore preserves glucose concentration. Anti-coagulant prevents the sample from clotting. The blood should be mixed with these chemicals by gentle inversion. Glucose may be measured directly on the whole blood sample, or on plasma.

Reference range

Fasting blood glucose	3.5–5.0 mmol/l
Random blood glucose	3.5–8.0 mmol/l
2 hr post-prandial glucose	At two hours after food, glucose levels should be falling towards normal fasting concentration.

(Note: Plasma glucose results are between 10–15% higher than those derived from whole blood.)

Terms used in interpretation of results

Normoglycaemia normal blood or plasma glucose concentration
Hyperglycaemia raised blood or plasma glucose concentration
Hypoglycaemia low blood or plasma glucose concentration

Critical values

Blood glucose < 2.2 mmol/l or > 25.0 mmol/l. Severe hypoglycaemia, particularly among neonates, is associated with the risk of convulsions, coma and permanent brain damage. Severe hyperglycaemia may signal ketoacidosis or hyperosmolal (non-ketotic) coma; these are acute life threatening complications of diabetes.

Causes of abnormal blood glucose

Abnormality of blood glucose concentration (either hyper- or hypoglycaemia) is almost always the result of too little or too much of one of the hormones required for normal regulation of blood glucose concentration. By far the most important cause of hyperglycaemia is diabetes mellitus.

Diabetes mellitus

Diabetes mellitus is the name given to a group of disorders that are characterised by hyperglycaemia, due to an absolute or relative deficiency of insulin. Glucose accumulates in blood for two main reasons. Firstly, glucose present in blood cannot enter cells (except those of the liver and brain) in the absence of an effective insulin response. Secondly, hepatic production of glucose from glycogen (glycogenolysis) is inappropriately increased by insulin deficiency.

Primary diabetes is classified on clinical and aetiological grounds to one of two types. Type 1 diabetes, which accounts for around 10–15% of the total diabetic population, results from selective autoimmune destruction of the insulin producing β cells of the pancreas. These people have an absolute insulin deficiency and require daily injections of exogenous insulin for survival. Type 2 diabetes is more common, accounting for around 85–90% of the diabetic population. Here the primary problem is not insulin deficiency but lack of insulin effect (sometimes called

Table 3.2 Major distinguishing features of type 1 and type 2 diabetes.

Type 1 Diabetes (insulin dependent diabetes mellitus IDDM)	Type 2 Diabetes (non-insulin dependent diabetes mellitus NIDDM)
Usually diagnosed in childhood	Usually diagnosed in adulthood
Little or no insulin reserves	Insulin production normal or may be raised
Less common (10–15% of total diabetic population	More common (around 85–90% of total diabetic population
Genetic factors less important as a cause	Genetic factors important – very often a family history
Patients typically not obese – may be thin	Obesity common
Ketoacidosis may be presenting feature; may also arise after diagnosis	Ketoacidosis extremely rare
Absolute need for insulin	No absolute requirement for insulin Treatment normally dietary manipulation and blood glucose lowering tablets

insulin resistance); the cellular response to normal physiological insulin levels is defective. Some of the distinguishing features of type 1 and type 2 diabetes are highlighted in Table 3.2.

Pregnancy is associated with many quite normal hormonal changes that predispose to hyperglycaemia and therefore diabetes. Depending on the population studied, as well as the criteria adopted for diagnosis, between 1 and 14% of women become temporarily diabetic during their pregnancy.[3] When diabetes is diagnosed during pregnancy it is called gestational diabetes. The diagnosis does not apply to those women with type 1 or type 2 diabetes who subsequently become pregnant. In most cases of gestational diabetes, the abnormality disappears at the end of the pregnancy as hormonal changes induced by pregnancy revert to non-pregnant values. However, up to 70% of women with a history of gestational diabetes eventually develop type 2 diabetes.[4]

In addition to type 1, type 2 and gestational diabetes, there is fourth group of diabetic patients whose diabetes is caused by some underlying, quite separate disease and by the action of some drugs (e.g. steroids). This very small subset of the total diabetic population is said to be suffering secondary diabetes. Successful treatment of the underlying disease or withdrawal of an offending drug cures diabetes in such cases. Causes of secondary diabetes are listed in Table 3.3.

Whether the disease is primary diabetes (i.e. type 1 or type 2), gestational diabetes or – much more rarely – secondary diabetes, all untreated diabetic patients have a raised blood glucose. A consistently normal blood glucose concentration excludes the diagnosis.

Signs and symptoms of diabetes

As long as blood glucose concentration remains within normal limits, urine contains no detectable glucose. However, as blood glucose concentration rises above

Table 3.3 Most common causes of secondary diabetes.

	Underlying pathology	Hormone affected	Effect on blood glucose
Acromegaly (gigantism)	Tumour of the pituitary gland	Increased cortisol production	Increased blood glucose
Phaeochromocytoma	Usually tumour of the adrenal medulla	Increased adrenalin production	Increased blood glucose
Cushing's Syndrome	Overactivity of adrenal cortex	Increased growth hormone production	Increased blood glucose
Haemochromatosis	Iron accumulation in pancreas – pancreatic damage	Decreased insulin production	Increased blood glucose
Chronic pancreatitis	Inflammation of pancreas – pancreatic damage	Decreased insulin production	Increased blood glucose

the renal threshold, which for most people (i.e. diabetics and non diabetics), is between 10 and 12 mmol/l, glucose begins to be lost in urine. By its strong osmotic effect, glucose draws water with it, causing polyuria (increased urine volume) and potential dehydration. This stimulates thirst centres in the brain to increase fluid intake. By these mechanisms severe hyperglycaemia causes five classical signs or symptoms of untreated diabetes:

- glucose excreted in urine (glycosuria)
- increased urination, often at night (polyuria, nocturia)
- thirst
- increased fluid intake (polydipsia)
- dehydration (only if compensatory increased fluid intake is not sufficient to replace fluid lost in urine).

Type 2 diabetes often has a long sub-clinical period during which hyperglycaemia is not sufficiently severe to cause symptoms, or perhaps mild symptoms may go unrecognised. A diagnosis is often made quite by chance when a raised blood glucose or glycosuria is discovered during a general health screen or investigation of some apparently unrelated medical problem. Diabetes is associated with increased risk of some bacterial and fungal infections, e.g. skin abscess or boils; urine tract infection; candida infection of the penis (balanitis) and female genital tract (vaginitis). Such infections may be the first sign of type 2 diabetes.

The damage to pancreatic cells that causes type 1 diabetes begins in the very early years and accumulates over several years until the resulting insulin deficiency is sufficient to cause clinical signs, usually in late childhood years or early adolescence. Onset is usually acute and the first evidence of diabetes among this group may be diabetic ketoacidosis, an acute and life threatening metabolic disturbance that results from severe insulin deficiency.

Diabetic ketoacidosis

In the absence of insulin, glucose cannot enter cells and an alternative energy source is required for cells to survive and function. Such an alternative is provided for by the stored fat (triglyceride) in adipose tissue. Many of the symptoms of diabetic ketoacidosis are a result of mobilisation of fat to provide energy in the absence of intracellular glucose. Incidentally, the mobilisation of fat as a source of energy is a quite normal physiological response to starvation, when dietary glucose is absent and glycogen stores are exhausted.

The first step in realising the potential energy in fat is enzymic splitting of triglyceride (lipolysis) to release constituent fatty acids. Fatty acids are transported from adipocytes via blood to all the cells of the body, where they are utilised as an energy source. In the liver, fatty acids are oxidised. The products of this oxidation are two keto-acids (acetoacetate and 3-hydroxybutyrate) and acetone, collectively called ketones. Normally these products of fat metabolism would be metabolised further. However, in diabetic ketoacidosis, the rate of their production outstrips the rate of their metabolism and they accumulate in blood and are excreted in urine. Some acetone is excreted by the lungs and can be smelt on the breath of a patient in ketoacidosis. Accumulation of keto-acids in blood overwhelms the normal homeostatic mechanisms that maintain normal blood pH, with development of metabolic acidosis (see Chapter 6).

Increased respiration (hyperventilation) to promote removal of carbon dioxide from the blood, thereby restoring normal blood pH, is a normal compensatory mechanism in metabolic acidosis. This is clinically evident as a deep sighing respiration (Kussmaul breathing) in patients with ketoacidosis. To summarise, in addition to symptoms already mentioned due to hyperglycaemia – glycosuria, polyuria, thirst, polydipsia and dehydration – patients in diabetic ketoacidosis also:

- have ketones in blood and urine (ketonaemia, ketouria)
- have the smell of acetone on their breath
- have a metabolic acidosis (low blood pH)
- hyperventilate (exhibit Kussmaul breathing)
- are usually hypotensive due to severe fluid and electrolyte loss in urine and vomit (vomiting is common in diabetic ketoacidosis)

Without treatment, patients have decreasing level of consciousness and can eventually lapse into coma. Low blood volume consequent on fluid loss threatens normal perfusion of the kidney, so acute renal failure may occur if blood volume is not restored immediately.

Laboratory diagnosis of diabetes

Criteria for laboratory diagnosis of diabetes are based on World Health Organization recommendations formulated in 1985[5] and revised in 1998 following recommendations by the American Diabetes Association.[6]

Diabetes is confirmed if a single fasting blood glucose is greater than 6.1 mmol/l (plasma glucose 7.0 mmol/l) or random blood glucose is greater than 10.0 mmol/l (plasma glucose 11.1 mmol/l) on at least two occasions. If a patient has symptoms strongly suggestive of diabetes but a fasting or random glucose concentration not sufficiently high to make the diagnosis, a glucose tolerance test (GTT) is indicated.

Glucose tolerance test

Principle
The GTT involves measuring blood glucose before and after ingestion of a stand-ard (75 g) glucose dose, on a fasted patient.

Patient preparation
For at least three days before the test, patients must be on a normal carbohydrate diet (i.e. > 150 g/day). The test is conducted in the morning following an overnight fast of at least 12 hours. The patient may have free access to water. Smoking on the morning of the test should be prohibited.

Test protocol
Blood is sampled for fasting glucose estimation and 75 g of glucose dissolved in 300 ml water administered by mouth (a more palatable alternative is 353 ml of Lucozade). Two hours later, a second blood sample is taken for glucose estimation.

Interpretation
The normal response to a glucose load is an initial increase in blood glucose, which stimulates insulin secretion. This in turn reduces blood glucose so that at two hours, glucose concentration has returned to near fasting levels. In both type 1 and 2 diabetes, blood glucose remains high. Table 3.4 describes how the results of a GTT are used to make or exclude a diagnosis of diabetes.

The term impaired glucose tolerance is reserved for those patients whose results do not indicate diabetes but which nevertheless are abnormal. Such patients are at increased risk of diabetes and should be retested annually.

Monitoring of diabetic treatment

Patients with type 1 diabetes have a lifelong need for daily insulin injections sup-plemented by dietary manipulation. For those with type 2 disease, a combination of dietary manipulation and oral hypoglycaemic (glucose lowering) tablets is usually sufficient, though some may require insulin injection eventually.

Whatever the treatment, a principal objective is to maintain blood glucose con-centration as close as is possible to that of the non-diabetic population. Norm-alisation of blood glucose concentration not only removes the acute symptoms and complications of diabetes such as dehydration, polyuria, thirst, ketoacidosis and hypoglycaemia, but also significantly reduces the risk of the devastating long-

Table 3.4 Interpretation of glucose tolerance test results.

	Fasting plasma glucose (mmol/l)	Plasma glucose at 2 hr after 75 g glucose
Diabetes mellitus unlikely	less than 5.5 (4.9)	less than 7.8 (6.7)
Impaired glucose tolerance	less than 7.0 (6.1)	7.8–11.1 (6.7–10.0)
Impaired fasting glycaemia	6.1–7.0 (5.3–6.1)	
Diabetes mellitus	Equal to or greater than 7.0 (6.1)	Equal to or greater than 11.1 (10.0)

Note: Figures in parentheses should be used for interpretation if blood glucose rather than plasma glucose is measured.

term complications of diabetes, kidney disease (diabetic nephropathy); loss of vision (diabetic retinopathy); nerve damage (diabetic neuropathy) and cardiovascular disease.[7,8,9] Striving to reduce blood glucose concentration to that of the non-diabetic population is associated with increasing risk of hypoglycaemia, an acute and dangerous consequence of diabetic over-treatment. A careful balance has to be maintained.

The target of ideal diabetic control for type 1 diabetes has been defined by the National Council for Clinical Excellence (NICE) as pre-prandial blood glucose concentration maintained in the range 4–8 mmol/l and post-prandial blood glucose concentration < 10.0 mmol/l for children and < 9.0 mmol/l for adults.[10] Diabetic patients, particularly those requiring insulin therapy, are encouraged to self-monitor their blood glucose concentration regularly.

Patient self monitoring – blood glucose

A range of handheld blood glucose meters designed for use by diabetic patients in their home is commercially available. All have a similar mode of operation and allow measurement of blood glucose concentration from a single drop of capillary blood within a minute or two. A drop of blood is placed on a reagent strip that is impregnated with dried reagents. The test strip is placed in the meter, which measures a colour change that results from reaction between reagents and glucose in blood. A digital readout of blood glucose concentration is displayed in a minute or two. If used strictly according to manufacturers' instructions, these systems provide results of sufficient accuracy and precision. However, poor technique can easily cause entirely erroneous results. An adequate training and continuing quality control programme is essential for results of optimum accuracy and precision. This requires co-operation between patients, diabetic nurse specialist and laboratory staff. The manufacturers of blood glucose monitors continue to refine their products, making them increasingly user friendly, but the following points still need to be borne in mind.

- Blood must be sampled from a clean, dry finger or ear lobe.
- Whatever the sampling device used for pricking the finger, it must result in free blood flow and not be dependent on squeezing the finger unduly, which can cause falsely low results. Warming the finger can increase blood flow.
- Blood must be dropped on (not smeared or spread) and must cover the entire reagent pad. False low results can occur if only part of the reagent pad is covered.
- Timing of the reaction, which begins as soon as the drop of blood makes contact with the reagent pad, is absolutely crucial.
- The reagent contained in strips can deteriorate so strips must be stored in accordance with manufacturers' instructions. They must not be used once the printed expiry date has passed.

Quality control is essential. Depending on the instrument, this may include calibration of the instrument using a glucose solution of known concentration. Some systems are internally calibrated. All systems should be tested at regular intervals using an external quality control solution of known blood glucose concentration. This confirms continuing reliability of both the glucose meter and the patient's analytical expertise.

Patient self-monitoring: urine testing

Before methods for the estimation of blood glucose concentration outside the laboratory were available, diabetic patients monitored blood glucose concentration by testing urine for the presence of glucose. The test is performed using one of several commercially available urine glucose test strips that are, in principle, similar to those used for measuring blood glucose. A colour change on dipping the strip in urine indicates the presence of glucose. The test is semi-quantitative, so increasing intensity of the colour change reflects increasing concentration of glucose in urine. A positive result indicates that at some time since the bladder was last emptied, blood glucose rose above the renal threshold, which is usually between 10 and 12 mmol/l.

Since the renal threshold varies and may be as low as 6.0 mmol/l, urine testing is a relatively crude indicator of blood glucose concentration. Furthermore, it is unable to distinguish hypoglycaemia from normoglycaemia; the test is negative in both instances. Despite these limitations, urine glucose testing continues to be used by diabetic patients to monitor blood glucose control. In fact current evidence assessed by the National Institute for Health and Clinical Excellence (NICE) suggests self-monitoring by blood testing is no more effective than urine testing at optimising blood glucose control among those with type 2 diabetes.[10]

Glycosylated haemoglobin (HbA1c)

This laboratory-based test is the most reliable way of assessing long-term blood glucose control, and current guidelines suggest all diabetic patients should be offered this test every 2–6 months.[10,11]

In health, around 5–8% of the haemoglobin that circulates in the red cells of blood has a glucose molecule attached and is said to be glycosylated. The actual amount of glycosylated haemoglobin (HbA1) is dependent on the concentration of blood glucose that red cells are exposed to during their 120-day life. At any one moment the percentage HbA1 reflects the mean (average) blood glucose concentration during the preceding two months, and provides the most reliable retrospective view of blood glucose control. HbA1c is composed of three fractions (HbA1a, HbA1b and HbA1c). Of these HbA1c is quantitatively the most significant, and this is the fraction measured in laboratories.

A 2.5 ml sample of venous blood collected into a bottle containing the anti-coagulant ethylene diamine tetra-acetic acid (EDTA) (usually purple top) is required. No particular patient preparation is necessary and the sample can be taken at any time of day.

Interpretation: *Approximate* reference range HbA1c 4.7–6.1%.

National guidelines[10,11] define target HbA1c < 7.5% for type 1 and type 2 diabetes. Those with type 2 diabetes who are also at higher than normal risk of cardiovascular disease benefit from tighter blood glucose control and have a target of < 6.5%. HbA1c above 7.5% represents increasingly poor blood glucose control and consequent increasing risk of suffering the long-term complications of diabetes.

Hyperglycaemia in the non-diabetic

Raised blood glucose does not necessarily indicate diabetes. A transient increase in blood glucose concentration often accompanies acute stress because adrenalin – a hormone produced in response to stress – is one of those that tend to increase blood glucose. An example of this mechanism is the transient hyperglycaemia that often accompanies myocardial infarction, but any severe stress, e.g. trauma or surgery, may be associated with raised blood glucose. For this reason, critically ill patients requiring intensive care represent a patient group particularly prone to hyper-glycaemia. What distinguishes these stress-related causes of hyperglycaemia from diabetes is their transitory nature. As the illness or trauma that precipitated the stress resolves, blood glucose concentration soon returns to normal.

Finally, administration of intravenous fluids containing glucose and a range of drugs (e.g. corticosteroids, phenytoin, thiazide and loop diuretics) may cause increase in blood glucose concentration.

Hypoglycaemia

Hypoglycaemia is defined as blood glucose concentration less than 2.2 mmol/l, although symptoms may occur above this concentration. Since the brain is dependent on an adequate supply of glucose in blood, low levels cause neuroglycopaenia, reduced glucose within the brain and throughout the central nervous system. Hypoglycaemia also stimulates synthesis and release of the adrenal hormone adrenalin to increase blood glucose. It is a combination of neuroglycopaenia and increased adrenalin secretion that causes symptoms of hypoglycaemia.

Signs and symptoms of hypoglycaemia

Those due to raised levels of circulating adrenalin may include:

- feeling of hunger
- palpitations
- sweating
- fainting
- tremor
- feeling of anxiety.

Those due to reduced glucose in cells of the brain (neuroglycopaenia) may include:

- lethargy
- headache
- confusion
- apparent drunkenness (unsteady gait, slurred speech)
- convulsions.

Untreated, severe hypoglycaemia results in coma and (rarely) permanent brain damage. The condition is potentially fatal.

Causes of hypoglycaemia

Inappropriately high level of insulin is usually the cause.

Accidental overdose of insulin among diabetic patient accounts for most cases of hypoglycaemia; for example failing to eat after an insulin injection may precipitate hypoglycaemia. Exercise tends to reduce blood glucose concentration; so less insulin is required. Excessive exercise without insulin dose reduction may precipitate a hypoglycaemia attack in the diabetic patient.

Hypoglycaemia among non-diabetics may be due to insulinoma (a rare tumour of the β cells of the pancreas) in which the normal control of insulin secretion is lost. The cells of the tumour continue to secrete insulin despite falling blood glucose.

A deficiency of any of the three hormones that increase blood glucose concentration and oppose the action of insulin may precipitate hypoglycaemia. For example, in Addison's disease, the cells of the adrenal gland that normally produce cortisol are destroyed, and the resulting cortisol deficiency may precipitate hypoglycaemia.

The liver plays a central role in regulating blood glucose levels; this function remains intact during mild to moderate liver disease but hypoglycaemia may be a feature of severe liver disease. Alcohol is metabolised in the liver and inhibits the process of liver gluconeogenesis, which provides glucose during starvation.

Alcoholics who are not eating adequately are particularly at risk of hypoglycaemia for this reason.

Hypoglycaemia may be a feature of the neonatal period, particularly among premature babies. Babies born to diabetic mothers are at increased risk during the hours following birth. However, there is often no identifiable cause. A very small minority of babies with hypoglycaemia, on further investigation, turn out to have an inherited (genetic) deficiency of one of the many enzymes involved in carbohydrate metabolism.

Case history 2

Mrs Bishop is a slightly anxious 25-year-old housewife whose older brother has recently been diagnosed as suffering type 2 diabetes. Mrs Bishop has read that diabetes runs in families and decides to test her urine for the presence of glucose, using her brother's urine test strips. A positive result convinces her that although she is well, she has diabetes. She goes to see her GP, who takes blood for glucose estimation. The random blood glucose result is well within the reference range at 6.2 mmol/l but despite attempts at reassurance, Mrs Bishop remains convinced she has diabetes. Her concern is fuelled by two subsequent urine tests that are also positive for glucose. Her GP suggests a glucose tolerance test. The results of this are:

Fasting plasma glucose	4.8 mmol/l
2 hour post glucose load, plasma glucose	7.5 mmol/l

Questions

(1) Is Mrs Bishop right to be concerned?
(2) Does she have diabetes?
(3) What is the significance of the positive urine test for glucose?

Discussion of case history

(1) Mrs Bishop is justified in her concern, it is possible to inherit a predisposition to diabetes; in around a third of type 2 diabetes cases there is a family history of the condition. Furthermore the presence of glucose in urine is a presenting feature of diabetes. The lack of symptoms is not an argument against the diagnosis. Many cases are discovered before symptoms develop, when blood or urine is tested for occupational or insurance health examinations.

(2) No. The results of Mrs Bishop's glucose tolerance test are entirely normal (see Table 3.4) and the diagnosis can be excluded on the basis of these results.

(3) Glycosuria, the presence of glucose in urine usually only occurs when blood glucose concentration is high and is therefore suggestive of diabetes. The renal threshold is the blood glucose concentration above which glucose is detectable in urine. Normally this is around 10–12 mmol/l. For some people however, the renal threshold is significantly lower and glucose may appear in urine at normal blood glucose concentration. Mrs Bishop is among this group. The term 'renal glycosuria' is used to describe this entirely benign defect of kidney function. Although the finding of glucose in urine should never be ignored, it does not necessarily indicate diabetes.

References

1. Diabetes Population Prevalence Model (DPPM) group (2005) Diabetes Population Prevalence Model – some key findings *www.diabetes.org.uk/infocentre/reports/prevalencemodel.doc*
2. King H, Aubert RE & Hermann WH (1998) Global burden of diabetes 1995–2025. Prevalence, numerical estimates and projections. *Diabetes Care* **21**(9): 1414–31.
3. Fischer U, Spinas G & Lehmann R (1999) Using fasting glucose concentrations to screen for gestational diabetes mellitus: prospective population based study. *Br Med J* **319**: 812–15.
4. Buchanan T & Xinag A (2005) Gestational diabetes mellitus. *J Clin Invest* **115**: 485–91.
5. World Health Organization Study Group: Diabetes mellitus (1985) *WHO Tech Rep Ser* **721**: 1–104.
6. Expert Committee on Diagnosis and Classification of Diabetes Mellitus (1997) Report of the expert committee on diagnosis and classification of diabetes mellitus. *Diabetes Care* **20**: 1057–58.
7. Diabetes Control and Complications Trial Research Group (DCCT) (1993) The effect of intensive treatment of diabetes on the development and progression of long term complications of diabetes. *New Eng J Med* **329**: 977–86.
8. UK Prospective Diabetes Study (UKPDS) group (1998) Intensive blood-glucose control with sulphonylureas or insulin compared with conventional treatment and risk of complication in patients with type 2 diabetes (UKPDS 33). *Lancet* **352**: 837–53.
9. Diabetes Control and Complications Trial Research Group (DCCT) (2005) Intensive Diabetes Treatment and Cardiovascular Disease in patients with Type 1 Diabetes. *New Eng J Med* **353**: 2643–53.
10. National Institute for Clinical Excellence NICE (2004) Type 1 diabetes: diagnosis and management of type 1 diabetes in children, young people and adults. *Clinical Guideline 15*. ISBN 1-84257-622-4 National Institute for Clinical Excellence.
11. McIntosh A, Hutchinson A *et al.* (2001) Clinical guidelines and evidence review for Type 2 diabetes: management of blood glucose. Sheffield: ScHARR, University of Sheffield.

Further reading

Chiasson J-L, Avis-Jilwan N *et al.* (2003) Diagnosis and treatment of diabetic ketoacidosis and the hyperglycemic hyperosmolar state. *CMAJ* **168**: 859–66.

Gallichan M (1997) Self monitoring of glucose by people with diabetes. *Br Med J* **314**: 964–68.

Hart SP & Frier B (1998) Causes, management and morbidity of acute hypoglycaemia in adults requiring hospital admission. *Q J Med* **91**: 505–10.

LeRoitt D & Smith DO (2005) Monitoring glycemic control – the cornerstone of diabetes care. *Clin Ther* **27**: 1489–99.

Mandrup-Poulsen T (1998) Diabetes. *Br Med J* **316**: 1221–25.

Useful website

www.diabetes.org.uk Diabetes UK – a wealth of information for diabetic patients and healthcare professionals with an interest in diabetes, along with links to other relevant sites.

Chapter 4

SERUM/PLASMA SODIUM AND POTASSIUM

The most frequently requested blood chemistry test is urea and electrolytes (U&E). This is not one, but five tests performed simultaneously on the serum or plasma recovered from one sample of blood. They are: serum or plasma concentration of sodium, potassium, bicarbonate, urea and creatinine. The first three are electrolytes, that is, positively or negatively charged ions in solution. This chapter focuses on the positively charged ions (cations), sodium (Na^+) and potassium (K^+). Bicarbonate, a negatively charged ion (anion) is considered in Chapter 7. Urea and creatinine are the subject of Chapter 5.

Normal physiology: sodium

Sodium is required for nerve cell conduction and bone formation but the principal function of sodium is maintenance of extracellular fluid volume. This function reflects the fact that sodium and water metabolism are inextricably linked. As will become clear, careful monitoring of water intake and output (fluid balance) is as important as measuring sodium concentration in elucidating the cause and monitoring treatment of electrolyte disturbances.

Distribution of body water

Around 60% of body weight is water; for an average adult weighing 70 kg this represents around 40 litres of water. Approximately 25 litres is contained within the cells of the body; this is called the intracellular fluid (ICF); and 14 litres is outside cells and called the extracellular fluid (ECF). The ECF comprises approximately 3.5 litres of plasma, the fluid part of the blood contained within the vascular system and 10.5 litres of interstitial (or extravascular) fluid, which fills the microscopical space between tissue cells (Figure 4.1).

It is vital for health that both the total amount of water in the body and its distribution between these compartments is constant. The passage of water across cell membranes, i.e. between the ECF and ICF, is dependent on the osmolarity on either side of the membrane; so long as this is equal, water will not pass and the volumes of each compartment are maintained.

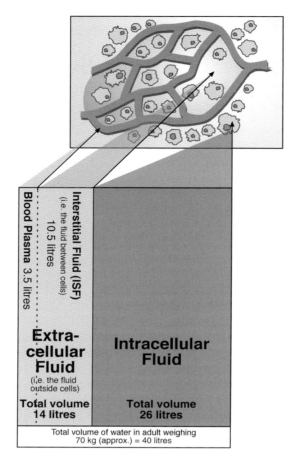

Figure 4.1 Distribution of water in adult (bodyweight approximately 70 kg).

How does sodium determine ECF volume?

The osmolarity of any solution is determined by the total concentration of dissolved solutes. Because they are present in relatively high concentrations in body fluids (i.e. ECF and ICF), compared with other solutes, electrolytes are the major determinants of osmolarity. Figure 4.2 describes the distribution of electrolytes between the ECF and ICF.

Within cells, the predominant cation is potassium; there is very little sodium within cells. By contrast, the ECF has a high concentration of sodium and very little potassium; these different electrolyte concentrations on either side of the cell membrane must be maintained by active transport. This active transport is achieved by the so-called sodium–potassium pump (Figure 4.3), an energy-requiring system present in the membrane of all cells; sodium is pumped out of cells in exchange for potassium.

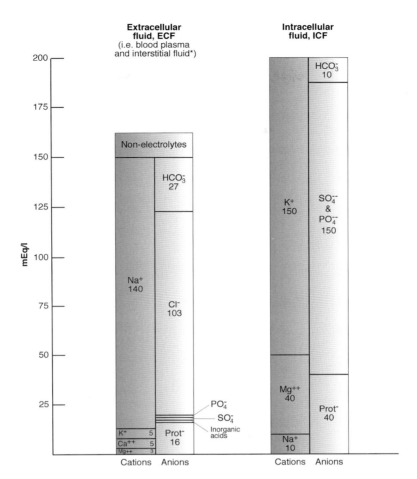

Figure 4.2 Comparison of the normal solute concentration in ECF and ICF.
NOTES: 1. mEq/l = mmol/l for monovalent ions (e.g. sodium, Na and Potassium, K but mEq/l must be divided by 2 to convert mmol/l for divalent ions (e.g. Calcium, Ca and Magnesium, Mg)
2. Figures for ECF refer specifically to blood plasma; interstitial fluid is very similar except that it has lower protein and higher chloride concentration

Without such active transport, sodium and potassium would diffuse passively across cell membranes until concentrations of ECF and ICF were equal. The active transport of sodium out of cells ensures its high concentration in the ECF, and therefore its predominant effect on overall osmolarity of the ECF. Since osmolarity determines the distribution of water between the ICF and ECF, sodium concentration determines ECF volume.

Control of water balance

To avoid dehydration or overhydration, water intake and output must be the same. A minimum urine volume (i.e. water loss) of 500 ml per day is required for

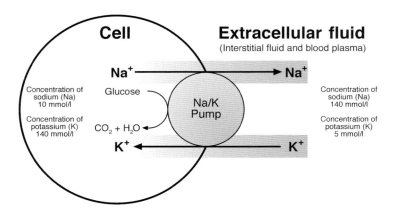

Figure 4.3 Maintenance of differential sodium and potassium concentration between cells and surrounding extracellular fluid.

excretion of the waste products of metabolism by the kidneys. To this must be added the water lost via the lungs in respired air (400 ml), via the skin in sweat (500 ml), and in faeces (100 ml). Thus a minimum of 1500 ml of water is lost from the body each day. Around 400 ml of water is produced by the body each day, a by-product of cellular metabolism. To maintain normal balance then, a minimum intake of around 1100 ml is required. In practice, fluid intake is greater than this minimum, but the kidneys are easily able to excrete an increased volume of water, to balance intake. In fact on average most people excrete between 1200–1500 ml of urine every day, and the kidneys have the capacity to produce a urine volume far in excess of this, if required.

Water intake and urine loss is controlled by plasma osmolarity. If for example water is being lost from the body without adequate replacement, the ECF volume decreases and osmolarity rises. This causes water to pass from cells into the ECF, restoring ECF volume and osmolarity to some extent. This internal movement of water can, however, only be a short term corrective as cells become relatively dehydrated. More water is required.

The normal response to this water deficit is described in Figure 4.4.

As blood with plasma of high osmolarity passes through the hypothalamus in the brain, special cells (osmoreceptors) respond to low osmolarity, with two simultaneous outcomes: the thirst response is invoked and the pituitary gland secretes antidiuretic hormone (ADH). Thirst induces increased water intake. ADH conserves body water by its action on the kidney. ADH increases water reabsorption to blood from the distal tubules and collecting ducts of the kidney; the result is excretion of concentrated urine of relatively low volume.

If too much water is ingested, ECF osmolarity falls. Osmoreceptors are not stimulated and the thirst stimulus and ADH secretion ceases. Dilute urine of relatively high volume is excreted, correcting the effective water overload. It must be remembered that around 8000 ml of water are secreted into the gastrointestinal tract each

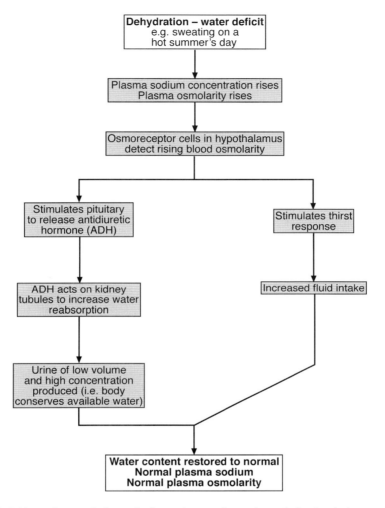

Figure 4.4 Normal water balance is dependent on intact hypothalamic-pituitary axis: adequate ADH, thirst response and renal function.

day as saliva, gastric juice, bile, pancreatic and intestinal juice. In health 99% of this water is reabsorbed and just 100 ml is lost in faeces. However, failure to conserve the water contained in these secretions can result in severe water imbalance. Maintenance of normal water balance is dependent on:

- an intact thirst response, which requires consciousness
- a normally functioning hypothalamus and pituitary gland
- a normally functioning kidney
- a normally functioning gastrointestinal tract.

Control of sodium balance

Just as health demands a balance between water intake and loss, the same is true of sodium. An adult normally contains around 3000 mmol of sodium, most of which, as we have seen, is present in the ECF (i.e. blood plasma and interstitial fluid) at a concentration of around 140 mmol/l.

A minimum of 10 mmol/day is lost in urine, sweat and faeces and this must be replaced to remain in balance. In fact, we ingest far more than this minimum: the average diet contains on average between 100 to 200 mmol per day, mostly as salt flavoring. Excess sodium is excreted by the kidneys, in urine. It is kidney regulation of sodium excretion that ensures normal sodium balance, despite wide variation in intake. Sodium excretion by the kidneys is dependent first on the glomerular filtration rate (GFR) (see Chapter 5). A relatively high GFR increases sodium excretion, and a low GFR increases sodium retention. Most (95–99%) of the sodium filtered at the glomerulus is actively reabsorbed to blood during passage through the proximal convoluted tubule. By the time the ultra-filtrate arrives in the distal convoluted tubule, just 1–5% of sodium filtered at the glomerulus remains. The fate of this sodium, that is whether it is excreted in urine or reabsorbed to blood, is largely dependent on the blood concentration of the adrenal hormone, aldosterone. This hormone acts on the cells of the distal tubule to enhance sodium reabsorption in exchange for potassium or hydrogen ions. Thus in the presence of high levels of aldosterone, most of the remaining sodium in the distal tubule is reabsorbed; if aldosterone concentration is low, no more is reabsorbed and urine of relatively high sodium concentration is excreted.

Aldosterone secretion by the adrenal cortex is controlled by the renin-angiotensin system (Figure 4.5). Renin is an enzyme produced by and secreted from the cells of the juxtaglomerulus of the kidney when blood flow through the glomerulus falls. Since the rate of blood flow through the kidneys (indeed any organ) is dependent on blood volume and therefore sodium concentration, it follows that renin is secreted from the kidneys when plasma sodium is relatively low.

Renin enzymically splits a protein known as renin substrate which circulates in the blood; one of the products of this enzymic action is a small peptide of ten amino acids called angiotensin I. A second enzyme produced predominantly in the lung, called angiotensin converting enzyme (ACE) then splits two amino acids from angiotensin I. The remaining eight amino-acid peptide is the hormone angiotensin II. This hormone has two important effects.

- It causes capillary blood vessels to narrow (a process called vasoconstriction), increasing blood pressure, and thereby increasing renal blood flow.
- It stimulates the cells of the adrenal cortex to synthesise and secrete aldosterone, the effect of which as described above is reabsorption of sodium, and thereby restoration of normal blood volume and renal blood flow.

An additional hormone, atrial natriuretic peptide (ANP), released by the atrial cells of the heart in response to rising blood pressure and volume, has an antagonistic effect to that of aldosterone. The effect of rising blood levels of ANP is

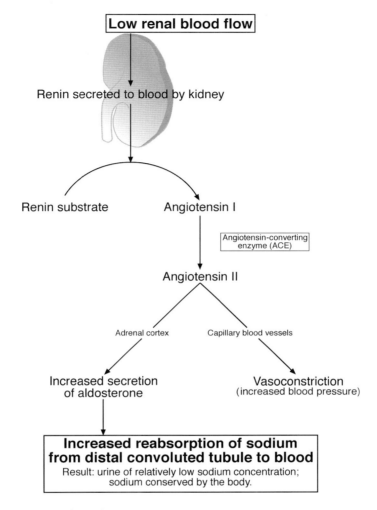

Figure 4.5 Renin-angiotensin system.

reduced sodium reabsorption from the distal tubule and excretion of urine with relatively high sodium concentration.

Around 1500 mmol of sodium is excreted into the gastrointestinal tract along with water every day (see above). Normally all, save around 10 mmol which is excreted in faeces, is reabsorbed to blood. Failure of gastrointestinal sodium reabsorption inevitably leads to potential sodium deficit, which becomes real if renal compensation is incomplete.

To summarise, sodium balance is chiefly dependent on:

- normal kidney function
- appropriate secretion of aldosterone by the adrenal cortex gland (which in turn is dependent on an intact renin-angiotensin axis)
- normal gastrointestinal function

Normal physiology: potassium

Potassium is required for the action of many metabolic enzymes, electrical transmission of nerve impulses and muscle contraction. Virtually all of the body's 3000 mmol of potassium is contained within cells. Just 0.4% is in plasma where it can be measured, so plasma potassium is a poor indicator of total body potassium. The maintenance of normal plasma potassium concentration, which is essential for health, depends on maintaining overall potassium balance.

Normal control of potassium balance

A minimum of around 40 mmol of potassium is lost from the body every day in urine, faeces and sweat. This must be replaced in order to maintain balance. Normal dietary intake is of the order of 100 mmol/day, obtained from citrus fruits, leafy vegetables, potatoes and bread. The kidneys ensure that sufficient potassium is excreted in urine to match that ingested. As with sodium, most of the potassium filtered at the glomerulus of the kidney is reabsorbed in the first (proximal) part of the kidney tubule. Fine regulation occurs in the distal part of the tubule and collecting ducts. Potassium can be either secreted from blood into the tubule in exchange for sodium ions, or reabsorbed at this point. As has already been made clear, sodium-potassium exchange is enhanced by the renin-angiotensin-aldosterone axis, so that under the influence of aldosterone, as sodium is reabsorbed, potassium is lost in urine.

The amount of potassium lost in urine is also affected by the kidneys' role in maintaining the pH of blood within normal limits. One of the mechanisms for preventing blood becoming too acidic is renal excretion of excess hydrogen ions in urine. This hydrogen ion excretion occurs by exchange with sodium ions in the distal tubule. This means that in acidosis less sodium is available for exchange with potassium and consequently relatively less potassium is excreted in urine. As we shall see, there are other ways in which potassium balance is affected by acid-base balance.

Around 60 mmol of potassium is normally secreted into the gastrointestinal tract every day but most is reabsorbed; just 10 mmol/day is lost in faeces. Potassium deficit can occur if this gastrointestinal reabsorption is defective.

Movement of potassium across cell membranes

The high concentration of ICF potassium and low concentration of ECF (plasma) potassium is maintained by the sodium-potassium pump. Increased and decreased activity of this pump can have profound effect on the plasma potassium level, as potassium shifts between the ECF and ICF. In addition, since hydrogen ions compete with potassium for exchange across the cell membranes, disturbances of acid-base balance may affect the plasma potassium concentration. An abnormal increase or decrease in plasma potassium concentration does not necessarily mean an overall body deficit or excess, it may simply reflect a shift of potassium into or out of cells.

Maintenance of a normal plasma potassium level is thus dependent on:

- adequate dietary intake of potassium
- normal renal function
- normal gastrointestinal tract function
- normal production of aldosterone by adrenal glands
- maintenance of normal acid-base balance
- normal action of the sodium-potassium pump.

Laboratory measurement of sodium and potassium

Patient preparation

No particular patient preparation is necessary. Sodium and potassium are frequently requested on patients receiving fluids intravenously. Sampling blood from an arm into which intravenous fluid is being administered may cause errors and should be avoided.

Timing of sample

Blood may be sampled at any time for sodium and potassium but as these estimations may be made more than once a day on the same patient, it is important to record the time the sample was collected.

Sample requirements

Around 5 ml of venous blood is required. Measurement may be made on the serum or plasma recovered from a blood sample. If local policy is to use serum, then blood must be collected into a collection tube without anticoagulant. Plasma estimation requires collection into a tube containing the anticoagulant lithium heparin. No other anticoagulant is suitable for sodium and potassium estimation.

Poor technique during blood collection may cause damage to the membrane of blood cells (haemolysis), resulting in erroneously high potassium concentration. This is because potassium is present in such high concentration within cells compared with plasma (Figure 4.2); damage to (red and white) cells results in a massive influx of potassium (and other cell contents) from cells into plasma. Haemolysis has relatively little effect on serum/plasma sodium concentration because its concentration in cells is low, compared with that of plasma. Haemoglobin released from haemolysed red cells changes the colour of serum/plasma from straw-coloured to red, providing laboratory staff with a means of identifying haemolysed samples. Haemolysis may occur if blood is forced at pressure through syringe needles, if blood is shaken violently or frozen. It is a frequent occurrence if there has been any difficulty in collecting blood. Haemolysed samples are unsuitable for potassium analysis.

Some sodium and potassium analysers, including those sited in intensive care units or recovery rooms, allow immediate analysis on whole blood without the need to separate serum or plasma. Blood must be collected into a syringe or bottle containing the anticoagulant lithium heparin. There is no way of knowing if such samples are haemolysed.

Effects of storage

When blood is removed from the body, the available energy source, glucose required for normal maintenance of the sodium pump is soon used up and the sodium-potassium pump begins to fail. At this point potassium begins to leak from cells into plasma and sodium passes from plasma into cells. As with haemolysis, the effects are greater for potassium and erroneously high serum/plasma potassium concentrations are seen in samples left for more than a few hours. Blood for potassium estimation must be transported to the laboratory within an hour or so. Samples are best left at room temperature during any delay in transport. Blood left for more than three hours before transport to the laboratory is unsuitable for potassium analysis.

Interpretation of results

Reference range

Serum/plasma sodium 135–145 mmol/l
Serum potassium 3.5–5.2 mmol/l
(plasma potassium is slightly lower than serum potassium)

Critical values

Serum/plasma sodium < 120 mmol/l or > 160 mmol/l
Serum/plasma potassium < 2.5 mmol/l or > 6.0 mmol/l

Terms used in interpretation

Hyponatraemia reduced plasma/serum sodium concentration, i.e. sodium < 135 mmol/l

Hypernatraemia raised plasma/serum sodium concentration, i.e. sodium > 145 mmol/l

Hypokalaemia reduced plasma/serum potassium concentration, i.e. potassium < 3.5 mmol/l

Hyperkalaemia raised plasma/serum potassium concentration, i.e. potassium > 5.2 mmol/l

Causes of hyponatraemia

As we have seen, sodium and water metabolism are inextricably linked. Serum/plasma sodium concentration is dependent on two variables; the amount of sodium in the ECF and the amount of water in the ECF, i.e. ECF volume. Hyponatraemia, the most common electrolyte abnormality occurring in 14% of hospitalised patients,[1] may develop if sodium is lost from the body in excess of water (sodium depletion) or if there is an abnormal excess of ECF water relative to sodium (sodium dilution). It is important to remember that serum sodium concentration is a poor indicator of total body sodium; hyponatraemia can be present if total body sodium is normal, raised or decreased.

Sodium depletion

Abnormal losses of both sodium and water via the gastrointestinal tract occur during protracted vomiting and diarrhoea, from skin during profuse sweating or as a result of burns. Haemorrhage represents a loss of both sodium and water. The effect that these losses have on serum sodium concentration depends on the concentration of the fluid lost compared with that of plasma. Excessive vomiting, diarrhoea, or sweating are generally associated with predominant water deficiency and therefore a tendency for serum sodium to rise. However if these conditions are treated with fluid relatively deficient of sodium (i.e. hypotonic solutions), hyponatraemia will develop. This is a common cause of hyponatraemia.

Fluid lost during extensive burns and during haemorrhage has the same concentration as that of serum and in these cases, despite being sodium depleted, patients have a near normal sodium concentration. However, hyponatraemia will again develop if the fluid used to replace losses is relatively deficient of sodium.

Excessive loss of sodium in urine is the cause of the hyponatraemia that often accompanies diuretic therapy and contributes to the hyponatraemia seen in renal failure. The hormone aldosterone regulates sodium loss in urine. A deficiency of the hormone results in increased inappropriate losses of sodium in urine. Addison's disease is characterised by destruction of the adrenal gland; the resulting deficiency of aldosterone causes hyponatraemia.

Excess ECF water

Mild hyponatraemia is a frequent finding among any population suffering disease (the mean sodium concentration of hospital inpatients is 3–5 mmol lower than a control population in good health). The sick cell syndrome is thought to be the cause of this non-specific mild hyponatraemia frequently seen in generalised illness. The sick cell is one in which reduced cellular energy causes an abnormal increase in cell membrane permeability. This allows a slight abnormal shift of water from the ICF to the ECF, effectively diluting plasma sodium. This transient slight fall in serum sodium concentration usually requires no treatment and resolves as the underlying illness is treated.

Untreated diabetes mellitus is often associated with hyponatraemia. Glucose is an osmotically active substance. If, as is the case in diabetes, its concentration in blood rises, water flows from cells into the ECF to correct the rising ECF osmolality. The increased ECF volume that results from this shift of water effectively dilutes sodium. This tendency to hyponatraemia in diabetes is compounded by the sodium loss in urine that accompanies the osmotic diuresis, as excess glucose is excreted in urine.

The importance of antidiuretic hormone (ADH) for renal regulation of water loss has already been discussed. The syndrome of inappropriate antidiuretic hormone (SIADH) results in abnormal retention of water, with dilution of sodium and therefore hyponatraemia. SIADH may complicate the course of many serious pathologies including some lung cancers, infectious disease of the lungs, head injury, brain tumours and Guillain–Barré syndrome. Some drugs can also precipitate SIADH.

Water and sodium excess is a feature of oedema, accumulation of fluid in the interstitial space. Such fluid accumulation occurs in liver disease (cirrhosis), cardiac failure and renal failure. Despite increased total body sodium, water excess usually predominates in oedema with resulting hyponatraemia. Sodium replacement therapy is, of course, not indicated for this subset of hyponatraemic patients who have more than sufficient sodium but are retaining abnormal amounts of water. The causes of hyponatraemia are summarised in Table 4.1.

Causes of hypernatraemia

Hypernatraemia is much less common than hyponatraemia. Although excess sodium can cause hypernatraemia, relative water depletion is more often the cause.

Excess sodium

Hypernatraemia may occur during over-vigorous sodium replacement therapy among patients with sodium depletion.

Uncontrolled secretion of aldosterone by a tumour of the adrenal gland is the cause of sodium retention of Conn's syndrome (primary hyperaldosteronism). The kidneys respond to high plasma sodium by excreting less water; this tends to restore plasma sodium concentration towards normal but is usually insufficient and slight hypernatraemia is a common finding in Conn's syndrome.

Excess cortisol (another hormone which affects renal loss of sodium), a feature of Cushing's syndrome has a similar effect.

Water deficit

Despite maintenance of normal amounts of sodium, hypernatraemia will develop if water output in urine, sweat, faeces and expired air exceeds water intake. Inability of the kidneys to retain water may cause hypernatraemia in chronic renal failure. Abnormal loss of fluid of relatively low sodium concentration is a feature of protracted vomiting, diarrhoea and sweating. All result in hypernatraemia if fluid intake is not increased to replace losses.

The thirst response is essential for adequate intake. A minimum loss of water from the body each day is inevitable. Under normal circumstances the thirst response

Table 4.1 Summary of some significant causes of abnormal serum sodium and potassium.

Causes of low serum sodium

- Heart failure
- Cirrhosis
- Diabetic ketoacidosis
- Acute renal failure
- SIADH
- Addison's disease
- Diuretic therapy
- Fluid replacement therapy for vomiting, diarrhoea, burns, etc.

Causes of raised serum sodium

- Protracted vomiting or diarrhoea
- Chronic renal failure
- Failure of thirst response (e.g. unconciousness, head trauma)
- Diabetes insipidus
- Conn's syndrome
- Cushing's syndrome
- Overvigorous sodium replacement therapy
- Lithium therapy

Causes of low serum potassium

- Inadequate intake (chronic starvation)
- Diuretic therapy
- Severe or chronic diarrhoea or vomiting
- During treatment of diabetic ketoacidosis
- Pyloric stenosis
- Alkalosis
- Conn's syndrome
- Bartter's syndrome
- Liquorice and purgative abuse

Causes of raised serum potassium

- Renal failure
- Excessive potassium administration
- Severe tissue damage (trauma major surgery)
- Acidosis including diabetic ketoacidosis
- Addison's disease
- Poor specimen handling (e.g. blood cells haemolysed, delayed transport to the laboratory)

ensures that we take sufficient water to replace these losses. Unconscious patients, and those who have sustained head injury involving damage to hypothalamic thirst centres within the brain are at increased risk of water depletion and therefore hypernatraemia, because they are unable to respond to thirst.

The ability of the kidneys to conserve water when necessary by excreting urine of low volume and high concentration is dependent on adequate amounts of ADH (see Figure 4.4). A deficiency of ADH or in some cases, lack of ADH effect on the kidney tubules, is the cause of diabetes insipidus. This syndrome results in water depletion as urine of inappropriately high volume and low concentration is excreted. Failure of the pituitary to secrete ADH can be due to damage to the hypothalamus or the pituitary (e.g. head injury, neurosurgery). Some rather rare invasive tumours of the hypothalamus and pituitary can cause diabetes insipidus. Infections of the central nervous system (meningitis and encephalitis) sometimes precipitate diabetes insipidus.

In some cases of diabetes insipidus, ADH production and secretion are normal, but the kidney tubules are unable to respond normally. This so called nephrogenic diabetes insipidus can be inherited, or precipitated by the action of some drugs (lithium, used in the treatment of manic depressive disorders is the most widely documented).

The causes of hypernatraemia are summarised in Table 4.1.

Causes of hypokalaemia

Inadequate intake rarely causes hypokalaemia but may be a feature of chronic starvation, for example in anorexia nervosa. Most cases are the result of increased losses from the body. Increased loss of potassium in urine is an unwanted side effect of some diuretic drugs. (e.g. frusemide, Lasix). Diuretic therapy is probably the most common cause of hypokalaemia. Potassium supplements may need to be prescribed for patients receiving diuretic therapy.

The adrenal cortex hormone aldosterone regulates potassium excretion in urine. Excess aldosterone causes abnormally high urinary losses of potassium with resulting hypokalaemia and is a feature of Conn's syndrome, in which there is excessive aldosterone secretion by an adrenal tumour. Raised levels of aldosterone in part accounts for the severe hypokalaemia that occurs in those with the very rare Bartter's syndrome and in a similar condition precipitated by liquorice abuse!

Like sodium, potassium can be lost in abnormally high amounts from the gastro-intestinal tract; for example severe acute diarrhoea and the chronic diarrhoea associated with purgative abuse can result in sufficient potassium to be lost from the body to cause hypokalaemia. Vomiting is not usually associated with significant potassium depletion except in the specific case of pyloric stenosis, in which the projectile vomiting of acid contents of the stomach causes alkalosis.

Hypokalaemia may be caused not by loss of potassium from the body but by a shift of potassium from the ECF into cells. Such an abnormal shift occurs for one of two reasons: increased activity of the sodium–potassium pump or if there is a hydrogen ion deficit, i.e. raised blood pH (alkalosis). In the first case, potassium passes into cells in exchange for sodium; in the second, potassium passes into cells in exchange for hydrogen ions (to correct ECF pH). The pancreatic hormone insulin increases the activity of the sodium-potassium pump, so a shift of potassium from ECF to cells occurs during insulin therapy for diabetic ketoacidosis. This contributes to the hypokalaemia that often occurs as diabetic ketoacidosis is treated.

Incidentally, this action of insulin is used therapeutically to reduce plasma potassium in those with severe hyperkalaemia, whatever the cause.

The passage of potassium from ECF to cells in exchange for hydrogen ions is a feature of alkalosis and is the reason for the hypokalaemia of pyloric stenosis. This tendency to hypokalaemia during alkalosis is potentiated by increased renal excretion of potassium as hydrogen ions are conserved to in an attempt to raise blood pH. Other causes of alkalosis that may be associated with hypokalaemia are considered in Chapter 6.

The causes of hypokalaemia are summarised in Table 4.1.

Causes of hyperkalaemia

Excessive intake of potassium during treatment with potassium supplements to correct potassium depletion may cause hyperkalaemia but most cases of hyperkalaemia are the result of reduced potassium excretion by the kidneys. As kidneys fail, they lose the ability to excrete potassium in urine; chronic renal failure is the most common cause of hyperkalaemia.

Autoimmune destruction of the adrenal glands, i.e. Addison's disease, results in a deficiency of aldosterone, the hormone which regulates renal excretion of potassium. The hormone deficiency results in reduced potassium excretion and therefore hyperkalaemia.

Most of the body's potassium is contained within cells; widespread damage to cells results in release of potassium into the ECF. For example, severe trauma may result in hyperkalaemia, as may the massive cell destruction associated with cytotoxic therapy for the treatment of leukaemia. This tendency to hyperkalaemia due to tissue destruction will be potentiated by any degree of renal dysfunction.

Potassium passes from cells into the ECF in exchange for hydrogen ions if blood is abnormally acidic. For this reason, acidosis is often associated with hyperkalaemia. The causes of acidosis are outlined in Chapter 6. Special mention, however, is made here of the acidosis associated with untreated diabetes.

Untreated diabetic ketoacidosis is usually associated with hyperkalaemia, although whole body potassium is depleted. Potassium depletion occurs due to increased urinary losses of potassium during the osmotic diuresis caused by urinary excretion of glucose. This potassium depletion is masked, however, by movement of potassium out of cells into the ECF, due to acidosis, and dehydration consequent on the massive amounts of water lost during the osmotic diuresis. Although severely depleted of potassium, serum levels are normal or high. The potassium depletion soon becomes apparent as the acidosis and dehydration are corrected; hypokalaemia develops as potassium returns to cells and rehydration is effected.

It is as well to emphasise the possibility that a raised potassium level might be due solely or partially to poor practice during collection, storage and transport of specimens (see sample collection, page 59). This so-called 'pseudo' hyperkalaemia is quite a common finding and must be considered as a possible cause in all cases of hyperkalaemia.

The causes of hyperkalaemia are summarised in Table 4.1.

Consequence of abnormal serum/plasma sodium and potassium concentration

Signs and symptoms of hyponatraemia

The clinical effect of low serum sodium depends on the cause, the magnitude of the abnormality, and rapidity of onset. Mild hyponatraemia (130–135 mmol/l), is not usually associated with symptoms, but most patients with a plasma sodium of less than 125 mmol/l will experience some symptoms; these will be more severe if the decrease is rapid. As we have seen, most cases of severe hyponatraemia are due to relative water excess. Symptoms result from overhydration of cells; the cells of the brain are particularly sensitive to this water excess and neurologic symptoms predominate. Headache, lethargy, mental depression and confusion may develop. Severe hyponatraemia (plasma sodium < 115 mmol/l), particularly of rapid onset, is associated with convulsions and coma; if left untreated severe hyponatraemia can be fatal.

If hyponatraemia is due to both sodium and water depletion as in, say, late Addison's disease, symptoms of low ECF volume (circulatory shock) predominate; these include reduced blood pressure, tachycardia and dizziness. If, on the other hand, hyponatraemia is associated with sodium and water excess, symptoms associated with increased ECF volume predominate; these include weight gain, oedema, hypertension and breathlessness on exertion (pulmonary oedema).

Signs and symptoms of hypernatraemia

Most cases of hypernatraemia result from a water deficit of both the ECF and ICF. Rapidity of changes increases the severity of symptoms, which are essentially those of dehydration: thirst, dry mouth, difficulty in swallowing and red swollen tongue. Cerebral cell dehydration causes neurological symptoms including confusion and lethargy, increased neuromuscular activity (twitching) and eventually coma. Like hyponatraemia, severe hypernatraemia can be fatal.

Signs and symptoms of hypokalaemia

Symptoms of hypokalaemia do not usually arise until potassium concentration falls below 3.0 mmol/l, but when they do arise are related to the function of potassium in transmission of nerve impulses to muscle.

Muscular weakness associated with general lethargy is the most common symptom. Constipation due to impaired muscle tone of the gastrointestinal tract may be a problem. In severe potassium depletion muscular paralysis may occur.

Cardiac muscle is frequently affected resulting in cardiac arrhythmias including tachycardia and sinus bradycardia. Typical electrocardiogram (ECG) changes which can be used to diagnose hypokalaemia include prolongation of the P–R interval and depression of the S–T segment. The toxic effects of digoxin therapy on cardiac muscle are potentiated by hypokalaemia. Metabolic alkalosis (Chapter 7), which often accompanies hypokalaemia, may result in symptoms of tetany.

Signs and symptoms of hyperkalaemia

Hyperkalaemia may be accompanied by vague feelings of muscle weakness, not as pronounced as those that are characteristic of hypokalaemia. Affected patients may be apathetic or even confused. Slurred speech is occasionally evident. The most significant effect of hyperkalaemia however, is life-threatening changes in cardiac muscle contraction. As serum potassium rises above 7.0 mmol/l there is a real risk of cardiac arrest and sudden death. Characteristic changes in an ECG trace during severe hyperkalaemia include tall, peaked T waves, low or missing P waves and broadening of the QRS complex. Urgent potassium-lowering therapy is required for patients with severe hyperkalaemia.

Case history 3

Mark Andrews is a healthy 22-year-old athlete who represents his US college at a high level in intercollegiate American-style football. After a particularly intense training session, he reported to the team doctor complaining of muscle cramps. The doctor diagnosed dehydration and ordered intravenous (IV) fluid replacement therapy. Over a period of five hours Mark received five litres of hypotonic saline in 5% dextrose; a further 3 litres of fluid was taken by mouth. Within an hour or so of receiving the IV fluids, Mark appeared acutely ill and was admitted to the emergency room at his local hospital in a confused and disoriented state, unable to follow the simplest of instructions. He was having trouble breathing. Blood was taken for U&E; among the results the laboratory reported was serum sodium 121 mmol/l.

Questions

(1) Is the serum sodium low, normal or raised?
(2) Could the sodium result explain Mark's clinical state?
(3) Why were IV fluids administered?
(4) What would be the principle of treatment in this case?

Discussion of case history

(1) The serum sodium is significantly reduced. Mark was hyponatraemic on admission.

(2) Yes. Most cases of hyponatraemia including the one under discussion are due not to a deficit of sodium but to fluid (water) excess. Because the sodium is effectively diluted in this water excess, this form of hyponatraemia is referred to as 'dilutional hyponatraemia'. The excess water in the ECF results in a shift of water from ECF across cell membranes so that cells become relatively overhydrated or water logged.

   The cells of the brain are particularly sensitive to this excess water; the symptoms of confusion and lack of mental agility are due to the excess water in the cells of Mark's brain. Accumulation of water in the lungs results in pulmonary oedema, the cause of Mark's breathlessness.

(3) Hypotonic saline (i.e. a salt solution with a sodium concentration less than that of plasma) was administered to correct the fluid deficit (dehydration) that was assumed to have occurred during training. The fluid replacement was clearly over-vigorous in this case.

(4) When Mark was admitted he simply had too much water in his body. The principle of treatment is water restriction and diuretic therapy to increase the rate of water loss via the kidneys, i.e. increase urine volume.

References

1. Smith D, McKenna K & Thompson C (2000) Hyponatraemia. *Clin Endocrinol* 52: 667–78.

Further reading

Evans K & Greenberg A (2005) Hyperkalemia: a review. *J Intensive Care Med* 20: 272–90.

Harrington L (2005) Potassium protocols: in search of evidence. *Clin Nurse Spec* 19: 137–41.

Lin M, Liu S, & Lim I (2005) Disorders of water imbalance. *Emerg Med Clin North Am* 23: 749–70.

Marshall W & Bangert S (2004) Water, sodium and potassium. In: *Clinical Chemistry (5th edition)* pp 13–39. Edinburgh: Mosby. ISBN: 0-7234-3328-3.

Schaefer T & Wolford R (2005) Disorders of potassium. *Emerg Med Clin North Am* 23: 723–747.

Yeates K, Singer M & Morton A (2004) Salt and water: a simple approach to hyponatremia. *CMAJ* 170: 365–369.

Chapter 5

SERUM/PLASMA UREA AND CREATININE AND CREATININE CLEARANCE

Measurements of the serum or plasma concentration of urea and creatinine are included in the most commonly requested profile of blood chemistry, 'urea and electrolytes' (U&E). They are both tests of kidney function. Creatinine clearance is not included in a U&E profile, but is another test of kidney function; it involves measuring the creatinine concentration of a 24-hour urine collection as well as the plasma or serum concentration of creatinine.

Normal physiology

Formation of urine by the kidneys: what is GFR?

The kidneys are sophisticated blood filters, ridding the body of unwanted products of metabolism (including urea and creatinine), along with other substances surplus to the body's immediate needs. Urine, the product of kidney filtration, is an aqueous solution of these unwanted chemicals. By their ability to vary both the volume and composition of urine, the kidneys play a major role in maintaining the constancy of both blood plasma and the interstitial fluid surrounding all the cells of the body. This constant internal environment is essential for normal cell function; life depends upon it.

The functional unit of the kidney is the nephron (Figure 5.1), which consists of the glomerulus, and the kidney tubule.

There are around 1 million nephrons in each kidney. Formation of urine begins at the glomeruli where blood is presented at the rate of around 1.25 litres every minute. The net filtration pressure within the capillary bed enables the passage of water and all other substances of medium and low molecular weight present in blood (including urea and creatinine) to pass from the blood into the Bowman's capsule. The so-called glomerular filtrate formed is essentially protein-free blood plasma (the protein and cells of blood are too large to pass through the filter).

The rate at which this filtrate is formed is called the glomerular filtration rate (GFR). In health the GFR is around 125 ml/minute or 180 litres per day. If there

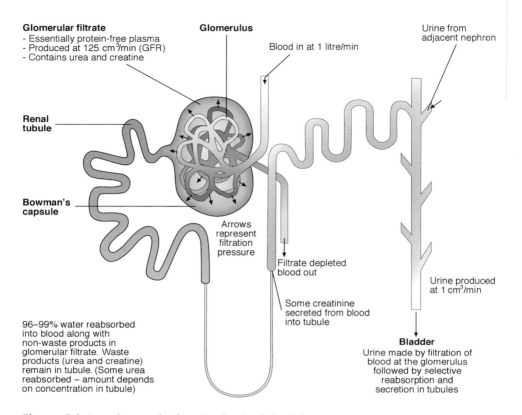

Glomerular filtrate
- Essentially protein-free plasma
- Produced at 125 cm^3/min (GFR)
- Contains urea and creatine

Glomerulus

Blood in at 1 litre/min

Urine from adjacent nephron

Renal tubule

Bowman's capsule

Arrows represent filtration pressure

Filtrate depleted blood out

Urine produced at 1 cm^3/min

Some creatinine secreted from blood into tubule

96–99% water reabsorbed into blood along with non-waste products in glomerular filtrate. Waste products (urea and creatine) remain in tubule. (Some urea reabsorbed – amount depends on concentration in tubule)

Bladder
Urine made by filtration of blood at the glomerulus followed by selective reabsorption and secretion in tubules

Figure 5.1 A nephron – the functional unit of the kidney.

were no way of reabsorbing the product of glomerular filtration, the whole of the blood volume would be lost within a few hours! In fact, the composition and volume of the glomerular filtrate is greatly modified as it passes through the tubule. Around 99% of the filtered water and essential constituents of blood, e.g. electrolytes, amino acids, glucose, etc. are reabsorbed back into the blood. There is capacity in the kidney for a few substances to be secreted from the blood into the tubule during final regulation of urine composition. The exact amount of water and nutrients reabsorbed depends upon the body's requirement at the time, but urine, the final product of first filtration, then tubular reabsorption and secretion, is produced at the rate of around 1 ml per minute, i.e. 1.5 l/day.

The glomerular filtration rate (GFR) is a parameter of prime importance to nephrologists because it defines renal function. All those with loss of kidney function, whatever its cause, have reduced GFR. There is good correlation between GFR and severity of kidney disease and GFR begins to fall very early in development of kidney disease, long before symptoms are evident. Renal disease may be acute (developing over a period of hours or days) or chronic (slowly progressive

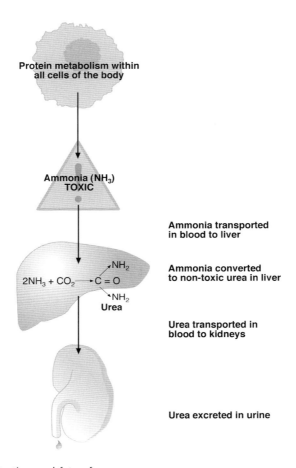

Figure 5.2 Production and fate of urea.

developing over a period of years). The rapidity at which GFR decreases distinguishes acute from chronic renal disease.

What are urea and creatinine?

Normal cellular metabolism of proteins and amino acids results in production of ammonia (NH_3). This toxic by-product of metabolism is transported in the blood to the liver where it is safely converted to urea by a series of enzyme mediated reactions known as the urea cycle. (Figure 5.2)

Urea itself has no metabolic function; as a waste product of normal metabolism, it must be eliminated from the body. Once synthesised in the liver it is transported via the blood to the kidney where it is excreted in urine.

Creatinine has a similar fate; like urea, it is a waste product of metabolism, more precisely muscle metabolism; it is released to blood from muscle cells and transported to the kidneys where it is excreted in urine along with urea. If the ability of the kidneys to excrete urea and creatinine is compromised, they accumulate in blood; the serum concentration of both rises.

Renal handling of urea and creatinine

Both urea and creatinine are filtered from blood at the glomerulus. Since both are waste products of metabolism there is no reason for either to be reabsorbed. However, a proportion of filtered urea is reabsorbed and this tendency to reabsorption is greater if the urea concentration of the filtrate is particularly high. No creatinine is reabsorbed, but a small amount is normally secreted from blood into the tubule. Notwithstanding these two minimal effects, the amount of urea and creatinine excreted in urine is dependent on the glomerular filtration rate; as GFR falls, so does urea and creatinine excretion. As excretion falls, blood levels rise.

Creatinine clearance: a measure of GFR

Although plasma concentration of urea and creatinine concentration are affected by and are a reflection of the GFR, neither is a direct measure. No increase in concentration of either occurs until around 50% of kidney function is lost (that is GFR is reduced by 50%) so they are poor indicators of early renal disease. Although the test has shortcomings, the creatinine clearance is currently the most widely used measure of GFR. In essence, creatinine clearance measures the volume of blood plasma that is cleared of creatinine during passage through the kidneys in one minute. The higher the clearance, the more effective are the kidneys at removing creatinine from blood and excreting it in urine.

Laboratory measurement of serum/plasma urea and creatinine

Patient preparation

No particular patient preparation is necessary.

Timing of sample

Blood may be sampled at any time of the day unless the blood is being sampled for creatinine clearance (see below).

Sample requirements

These two tests are usually performed as part of the U&E screen. Around 5 ml of venous blood is required for U&E. Measurement may be made on either the serum or plasma recovered from a blood sample. If local policy is to use serum, then blood must be collected into a collection tube without anticoagulant. Plasma estimation requires collection into a collection tube containing the anticoagulant lithium heparin.

Effects of storage

Unlike the other parameters measured in a U&E screen, urea and creatinine concentration remains stable when blood is stored for up to 24 hours at room temperature.

Laboratory measurement of creatinine clearance

Creatinine clearance involves measurement of the concentration of creatinine in blood and an aliquot recovered from a well-mixed 24-hour urine collection. Measurement of the total 24-hour urine volume is also required. From these measurements the clearance is calculated using the formula:

Creatinine clearance (ml/min) = (UV/P) × (1.73/X)

where U = urine creatinine concentration (mmol/l)
      V = urine flow (ml per minute)
      P = plasma/serum creatinine concentration (μmol/l)
      X = patient's body surface area (m^2) calculated from height and weight

Gross inaccuracies can occur if the 24-hour urine collection is not complete.

Patient preparation

Some laboratories recommend that patients should be on a meat-free diet to minimise dietary related changes in serum/plasma creatinine concentration. Since serum/plasma creatinine concentration and therefore creatinine clearance is affected by muscle mass, it is usual practice to make a correction to the creatinine clearance result that takes account of muscle mass. This correction requires that patient's height and weight be recorded on the request card.

Sample requirements

- a 24-hour urine collection (Table 5.1). Some laboratories require that urine for creatinine clearance be collected into a bottle containing an acid preservative
- 5 ml venous blood sample for serum/plasma creatinine estimation.

Timing of sampling

The 24-hour urine collection may be started at any time of the day but it is essential that *all* urine passed during the 24-hour period be collected. Blood must also be collected at some time during that 24-hour period, preferably just before a meal.

Table 5.1 Protocol for collection of 24-hour urine.

Clinical diagnosis and monitoring are occasionally aided by measurement of the rate of urinary excretion of a substance normally present in urine. This requires collection of a timed (usually a 24-hour) urine sample.

The validity of the results derived from a 24-hour urine collection depends crucially on an accurately timed sample. The object is to collect *all* the urine passed during a 24-hour period.

- Obtain a 24-hour urine container for the test requested from the laboratory. Some tests require a container with an acid preservative. This may be a corrosive acid, e.g. concentrated hydrochloric acid, so care must be taken.
- Label the bottle with patient details and the date and time of the start of the urine collection.
- Explain to the patient that all the urine passed during the 24-hour collection period must be saved.
- At a convenient time (usually 9.00 am) any urine in the bladder is voided and discarded.
- *All* the urine passed after 9.00 am must be collected into the container.
- At 9.00 am on the following day the bladder is again emptied. This last sample must be added to the collection. No urine passed after 9.00 am on the second day should be included.
- The urine collection, along with relevant test request form should be transported to the laboratory as soon as possible.

Notes
Sometimes the 24-hour urine volume exceeds the 2 litre capacity of the collection container. If this is the case a second urine container must be obtained to complete the collection. *All* the urine passed *must* be collected.

If the patient inadvertently discards some urine during the collection period, all the urine collected to that point must be discarded, a new bottle obtained from the laboratory and collection restarted.

The urine container should be stored in the sample fridge during the collection period.

Interpretation of results

Approximate reference ranges

Serum/plasma urea concentration	2.5–6.5 mmol/l
Serum/plasma creatinine concentration	55–105 µmol/l
Creatinine clearance	70–130 ml/minute

Critical values

Serum/plasma urea	> 28.0 mmol/l
Serum/plasma creatinine	> 400 µmol/l

Old age is associated with gradual deterioration in renal function, so urea increases with increasing age. The tendency for creatinine concentration to increase due to reduced renal excretion in old age is off set by decreased production due to age-related reduction in muscle mass. Creatinine clearance gradually decreases with increasing age.

The concentration of urea in blood is a reflection of the balance between rate of liver synthesis and the rate of renal excretion. The concentration of creatinine in blood is a reflection of the balance between production by muscle cells and the rate of renal excretion. If synthesis/production increases and/or excretion decreases, blood plasma concentration rises. If synthesis/production decreases and/or excretion increases, blood plasma concentration falls.

Causes of reduced plasma/serum urea concentration

Pregnancy
Pregnancy is normally associated with an increased GFR and therefore increased rate of urea excretion; pregnant women typically have lower plasma/serum urea concentration than non-pregnant women.

Low protein diet
Urea synthesis is a function of amino acid and protein metabolism which in turn is affected by dietary intake of proteins. Those on a low protein diet synthesise less urea than those on a normal diet.

Liver disease
Urea synthesis occurs in the liver. Although this function is not usually affected in mild to moderate liver disease, liver failure is associated with decreased urea synthesis and accumulation in blood of toxic ammonia.

Causes of a reduced plasma/serum creatinine

Pregnancy
Pregnancy is associated with increased excretion of creatinine.

Muscle mass decrease
Creatinine is produced by muscle cells. Any disease associated with significant decrease in muscle mass (e.g. muscular dystrophy, severe malnutrition) may result in abnormally low plasma creatinine concentration.

Causes of an increased plasma/serum urea and creatinine concentration

Renal causes
Both urea and creatinine concentration of blood are raised if glomerular filtration rate (GFR), that is renal function, is significantly reduced. The glomerulus is analogous to any other filtration system where the rate of filtration depends on three factors:

- the rate at which the liquid (blood in this case) to be filtered is presented to the filter

- the patency of the filter (a 'blocked' filter will result in a slower filtration rate
- any opposing pressure on the other side of the filter, reducing filtration rate

Extending this analogy to the many causes of renal disease allows a simplified classification of renal disease to prerenal (reduced blood flow to kidneys), renal (damage to the filter itself) and post-renal (obstruction to urine flow) renal disease. Table 5.2 describes such an approach, emphasising that a low GFR and therefore raised concentration of urea and creatinine can be a feature of all causes of renal dysfunction. These tests provide no information about the cause of renal dysfunction.

However, they are good markers of renal disease progression, because as renal function (GFR) falls, urea and creatinine concentration rises.

It is important to emphasise that a normal urea and creatinine concentration does not exclude early renal disease; concentrations only begin to rise reliably after considerable loss of renal function. Figure 5.3 illustrates this point; plasma urea and creatinine concentrations do not rise above normal until the GFR has fallen to around 40 ml/min, less than 50% of its normal value.

Although a marked increase in urea concentration (i.e. a level greater than around 10.0 mmol/l) always indicates renal damage, a slight to moderate increase in urea (from around 6.5 to around 10.0 mmol/l) may be the result of some other pathology.

Table 5.2 Low GFR and therefore raised serum urea and creatinine is a feature of all renal dysfunction.

Pre-renal (renal) disease	Renal disease	Post-renal renal disease
Low GFR due to reduced blood volume being presented to the glomerulus for filtration. Kidneys structurally normal but functionally compromised.	Low GFR due to damage to filter (glomerulus) i.e. 'blocked filter'. Kidney structurally abnormal and therefore functionally compromised	Low GFR due to blockage on the distal side of the glomerulus opposing filtration pressure.
Principal causes	**Principal causes**	**Principal causes**
• Any condition which results in low blood volume (hypovolaemia) i.e. hypovolaemic shock • Major haemorrhage (e.g. trauma, major surgery) • Significant salt and water depletion (e.g. severe diarrhoea and vomiting, extensive burns) • Septic shock • Cardiogenic shock i.e. reduction in cardiac output due to myocardial infarction, heart failure.	• Glomerulonephritis due to inflammation or infection • Diabetic nephropathy (a complication of long-standing diabetes) • Polycystic kidney disease • Gout • Toxic damage (drugs, heavy metals)	Any condition which results in urine retention: • renal or ureteric stores • tumours that obstruct urine flow (e.g. carcinoma of the bladder, prostate)

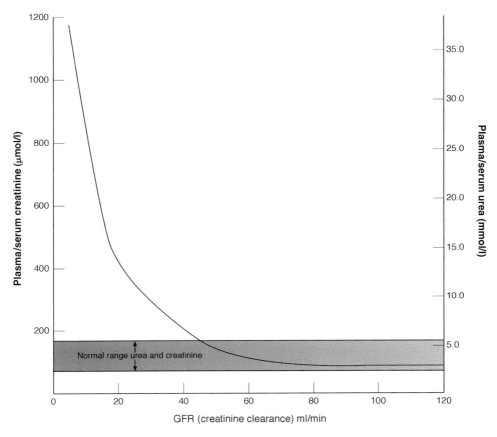

Figure 5.3 Relationship between glomerular filtration rate (GFR) and plasma concentration of urea and creatinine.
Note: plasma concentration of urea and creatinine remains normal until GFR is reduced by more than 50%.

In these cases, creatinine levels remain normal. A marginally raised urea accompanied by a normal plasma creatinine concentration result is likely to be due to non-renal causes. A marginally raised urea accompanied by an equivalent rise in creatinine indicates renal dysfunction.

Non-renal causes of raised urea

High protein diet

• Urea synthesis is increased among those on a high protein diet.

Chronic starvation

Chronic starvation is accompanied by increased protein catabolism as the body uses its energy reserves for survival; increased protein catabolism results in increased urea synthesis.

Gastrointestinal bleeding

Gastrointestinal bleeding from ulcers, malignancy etc., is associated with increased protein absorption (blood within the gut is effectively a protein rich meal!) and therefore increased urea synthesis.

Dehydration

The amount of urea reabsorbed into the blood by the kidney tubules after glomerular filtration is increased in those who are dehydrated.

Causes of a reduced creatinine clearance

Since creatinine clearance is a direct measure of GFR, its value decreases as GFR falls. A reduction in creatinine clearance indicates renal damage. The actual level provides an estimate of the extent of that damage, but provides no information about its cause since a reduced GFR may be a feature of all causes of renal failure. Creatinine clearance is a more sensitive indicator of early renal disease than either plasma urea or plasma creatinine measurement. The accuracy of creatinine clearance results depends crucially on the accuracy of the 24-hour urine collection.

Effects of increased plasma and urea creatinine concentration

Although it is clear that advanced renal disease, whatever the cause, is associated with abnormal amounts of urea and creatinine in blood and that the actual levels provide useful clinical information about severity, there is no evidence that the symptoms of renal disease are a direct result of either a raised plasma urea or creatinine concentration. However, those with a raised plasma urea and creatinine concentration may suffer any of the following major signs and symptoms of renal disease:

- renal pain, i.e. low back pain
- failure to maintain normal urine flow of 1000–2000 ml/day
  - anuria no urine flow
  - oliguria < 500 ml/day
  - polyuria > 2000 ml/day
- raised blood pressure (hypertension)
- accumulation of fluid in tissues (oedema)
- presence of blood and/or protein in urine (haematuria/proteinuria).

Uraemic syndrome

Uraemic syndrome is the constellation of signs and symptoms that arise in those who have established renal failure with GFR < 15 ml/min. This degree of renal dysfunction is of course always associated with marked increase in plasma urea concentration and it was once thought that the symptoms were due to a toxic effect of urea, hence the name. However it has become clear that this is not the case, rather a range of toxic substances accumulate in blood contributing to the signs and symptoms associated with uraemic syndrome. These include:

- progressive fatigue, confusion fits and eventually coma
- loss of appetite, nausea, vomiting, diarrhoea
- itching
- anaemia and resulting breathlessness
- electrolyte, water and acid-base disturbances.

Estimating GFR from plasma creatinine

One of several limitations of the creatinine clearance test is that it requires accurate collection of 24-hour urine. This is not only time consuming and unpleasant for both patient and nursing staff but prone to error, due to poor timing of specimen collection or inadvertently not collecting all the urine passed in the 24-hour period. Errors in collection can lead to gross overestimates or underestimates of creatinine clearance.

It is possible to estimate creatinine clearance – and thereby GFR – from plasma creatinine concentration, without the need for urine collection. One of the most widely used formulae for this estimation was devised by Cockcroft and Gault in 1976.[1] The Cockcroft–Gault equation predicts creatinine clearance from plasma creatinine, age, weight, height, sex and ethnicity thus:

$$\text{creatinine clearance (ml/min)} = \frac{(140 - \text{age in years}) \times \text{weight (kg)}}{\text{serum/plasma creatinine (}\mu\text{mol/l)}}$$

for males, multiply result by 1.2
for females, multiply result by 1.04
for those of Black African origin, multiply result by 1.18

Recently published national guidelines[2] for the identification and monitoring of patients with chronic renal disease advise the use of a refined version of the Cockcroft–Gault equation in preference to creatinine clearance for estimation of GFR. The recommended formula, which does not require the patient's weight or height is:

$$\text{GFR} = 186 \times \{[\text{serum/plasma creatinine} \div 88.4]^{-1.154}\}$$
$$\times \text{age}^{-0.0203} \times 0.0742 \text{ (if female)} \times 1.21 \text{ (if African black)}$$

Units of measurement

GFR	ml/min
Serum/plasma creatinine	μmol/l
Age	years

The guidelines advise that plasma creatinine should be measured and estimated GFR calculated every 3–12 months for all those with established chronic renal

Table 5.3 Recommendations for annual serum creatinine testing.

Annual measurement of serum creatinine is advised for the following adult patient groups who are at risk of chronic kidney disease.

Those with:

- Diabetes
- Coronary heart disease or any other condition associated with atherosclerosis
- Heart failure
- Hypertension
- Systemic lupus erythematosus
- Rheumatoid arthritis
- Myeloma
- Urine stone disease
- Persistent proteinuria
- Unexplained haematuria
- A long-term prescription for any potentially nephrotoxic drug

disease (frequency depending on severity of disease). In addition, they advise annual measurement in those at high risk of developing renal disease (Table 5.3).

Case history 4

Jane Redbridge, a 48-year-old housewife, was brought by ambulance to the local accident and emergency department, having collapsed while out shopping. She reported feeling very tired recently, and was concerned that she had been passing black stools, a sign (called melaena) that indicates the presence of blood in the gastrointestinal tract. On examination she appeared clinically anaemic and hypotensive; a provisional diagnosis of gastrointestinal bleed of unknown cause was made. Blood was sampled for full blood count (FBC) and urea and electrolytes (U&E). The following results were obtained:

Sodium	139 mmol/l
Potassium	4.1 mmol/l
Bicarbonate	24 mmol/l
Urea	9.2 mmol/l
Creatinine	78 µmol/l

Questions

(1) Are the urea and creatinine results normal?
(2) Do the urea and creatinine results indicate renal disease?
(3) Do the results support the provisional diagnosis?
(4) Are there other conditions that might be suggested by this pattern of urea and creatinine results?
(5) Would you expect Mrs Redbridge to have a normal creatinine clearance?

Discussion of case history

(1) Mrs Redbridge's plasma urea concentration is raised but her creatinine is well within the reference range.

(2) A urea concentration of 9.2 mmol/l is consistent with considerable loss of renal function. Tiredness and anaemia incidentally may also be a feature of chronic kidney disease. However, a normal creatinine level suggests that Mrs Redbridge's kidneys are functioning normally, and therefore consideration should be given to non-renal causes of raised urea.

(3) Yes. Bleeding into the gut results in a marked increase in protein absorption as the blood is 'digested' by gut enzymes. Such a high protein intake increases urea production. If urea production exceeds urinary excretion, urea accumulates in blood. Creatinine is produced by contracting muscle cells and blood levels are unaffected by increased protein intake. The combination of raised urea and normal creatinine supports the provisional diagnosis.

(4) While a raised plasma creatinine concentration nearly always indicates renal disease, there are several non-renal causes including gastrointestinal bleeding for a marginally raised plasma urea concentration. Chronic starvation, dehydration and a very high protein diet may result in a similar pattern of urea and creatinine levels exhibited by Mrs Redbridge.

(5) If, as seems likely from laboratory results, Mrs Redbridge has normally functioning kidneys, then her creatinine clearance would be normal.

References

1. Cockcroft D & Gault M (1976) Prediction of creatinine clearance from serum creatinine. *Nephron* **16**: 31–41.
2. Royal College of Physicians (2005) *Chronic kidney disease in adults: UK guidelines for identification, management and referral.* London: RCP.

Further reading

Lameire N, Van Biesen W & Vanholder R (2005) Acute renal failure. *Lancet* **365**: 417–430.
Manjunath G, Sarnak M & Levey A (2001) Estimating glomerular filtration rate. Dos and don'ts for assessing kidney function. *Postgrad Med* **110**: 55–62.
Parmer M (2002) Chronic renal disease. *Br Med J* **325**: 85–90.

Chapter 6

SERUM/PLASMA CALCIUM AND PHOSPHATE

Most of the calcium and phosphate in the body is present in bone, but a small and vital fraction of each is present in blood. The two tests that are the focus of this chapter, measurement of serum/plasma concentration of calcium and phosphate, are often requested together with two other blood tests considered in Chapter 10: albumin and alkaline phosphatase. The four tests, together known as a bone profile, are used in the first line investigation of patients who are suspected of suffering metabolic bone disease. The origins of bone disease often lie in distant organs (parathyroid glands, kidneys and gastrointestinal tract) that are involved in the regulation of plasma calcium and phosphate concentration. Measurement of calcium and phosphate is thus often appropriate in investigation of patients suffering disease of these organs. Three other broad groups of patients in whom plasma calcium is often measured are those suffering malignant disease, the critically ill and preterm babies.

Point of care testing in intensive care units often includes the measurement of plasma calcium. In these circumstances, nursing staff may be responsible for the analytical process.

Normal physiology

Dietary source of calcium and phosphorus

A normal western diet contains on average around 1000 mg calcium/day. Recommended minimum intake for adults is 700 mg/day. The most common source is milk and dairy products; alternative sources include green leafy vegetables, soybean and nuts. Flour and some breakfast cereals are fortified with calcium, and in some areas, tap water is a significant source of calcium. Less than a half of ingested calcium is normally absorbed from the gastrointestinal tract, predominantly at the duodenum; the rest is excreted in faeces. The actual amount that is absorbed is under hormonal control and so is adjusted to suit requirements at the time.

Most foods contain some phosphorus and a normal diet contains around 1000 mg/day, predominantly from meat and dairy foods.

Body distribution of calcium and phosphate

The adult body contains around 1 kg of calcium (Ca) and 600 g of phosphorus (P), the latter combined with oxygen and present as phosphate (PO_4). Almost all (99%) of this calcium and 85% of phosphate is contained in bone as crystals of hydroxyapatite, which has the chemical formula $Ca_{10}(PO_4)_6OH_2$. Together with the protein collagen, hydroxyapatite crystals are the major structural components of bone and teeth; calcium and phosphate together comprise 65% of bone weight. A small amount (< 1%) of the calcium in bone is exchangeable with calcium in blood; this allows movement of calcium into bone when blood concentration is high and in the reverse direction when blood calcium is low.

Just 350 mg (8.7 mmol) of calcium circulates in blood plasma at a concentration of around 2.5 mmol/l. Half of this is bound to the protein albumin and the rest circulates as 'free' ionised calcium (Ca^{++}). Only the ionised fraction is physiologically functional. Finally, a very tiny but physiologically vital fraction of total body calcium resides in all cells. The concentration of calcium in cells is of the order of nanomols/l, one-thousandth of the concentration in blood plasma.

The 15% of phosphate that is not present in bone is divided between tissue cells and the extracellular compartment, which includes blood plasma. Around 1% of the body's phosphate is present in blood plasma at a concentration of around 1.0 mmol/l.

Function of calcium and phosphate

Both calcium and phosphate have significant roles other than the one they share as major structural component of bones and teeth. The ionised calcium that circulates in blood plasma is an essential cofactor for the enzymes involved in blood coagulation. It is also a source for the calcium required for many cellular processes, including electrical conductance of nerve impulses, cardiac and skeletal muscle contraction, and the signalling between nerve and muscle cells (neuromuscular transmission). Calcium signalling is an essential part of the process by which many hormones affect target tissue cells. Thus the function of many hormones is dependent on ionised calcium. There are, in fact, few physiologic functions that can proceed in the absence of minute quantities of intracellular ionised calcium.

Phosphate is an integral part of many key biological molecules. These include the nucleic acids DNA and RNA, phospholipids (structural components of all cell membranes) and many other substances of intermediary cell metabolism, including adenosine triphosphate (ATP), the most significant source of chemical energy for cell metabolism. Inorganic phosphate, i.e. the phosphate which is not integrated into larger biological molecules, acts as a buffer in blood and urine, and is thus involved in the vital process of maintaining normal blood pH.

The many functions of calcium and phosphate depend on the maintenance of their plasma concentrations within narrow limits. The next section describes the mechanisms that maintain normal plasma calcium concentration. Disturbance of one or more of these mechanisms is often the cause of abnormal plasma calcium and/or phosphate results.

Normal control of plasma calcium concentration

The concentration of calcium in plasma reflects a balance between dietary derived calcium absorbed via the gastrointestinal tract and that lost from the body in urine. In addition, as outlined above, calcium can move between plasma and bone. These routes of calcium movement, and thereby plasma calcium concentration, are under the control of two hormones: parathormone (PTH) and the vitamin D-derived hormone, calcitriol. These hormones also have effect on plasma phosphate concentration.

Source, secretion and effect of PTH

Parathormone (PTH) is the calcium regulating hormone produced and secreted by the four tiny (rice grain-sized) parathyroid glands, sited close to, or embedded in the surface of the thyroid gland. Parathyroid cells sense the plasma-ionised calcium concentration of blood flowing through the gland. Reduction in concentration of plasma-ionised calcium stimulates parathyroid gland production and secretion of PTH (Figure 6.1). The PTH is transported in blood to its two target organs: kidneys and bone. The effect of PTH is to release calcium from bone to blood and decrease renal excretion of calcium in urine. The net result is restoration of normal plasma calcium concentration. As plasma calcium concentration rises, PTH secretion diminishes. PTH also has a plasma phosphate-lowering effect through its action on the kidney, where it increases urine excretion of phosphate. Overall, then, the effect of PTH is to raise plasma calcium and lower plasma phosphate.

Source, secretion and effect of calcitriol

Calcitriol (alternative name 1,25 dihydroxycholecalciferol), the other main calcium-regulating hormone, is derived from vitamin D and released from the kidneys. Although diet is a source of vitamin D, it is also synthesised in the skin by the action of sunlight on a cholesterol-like substance (7-dehydrocholesterol) present in skin cells. By a two-step process, vitamin D derived from diet, as well as that synthesised in skin, is converted to calcitriol (Figure 6.2). The first step occurs in the liver and the second in the kidneys. The second step, which results in release of calcitriol to blood from kidney, is under the control of PTH. When plasma calcium is low and therefore PTH levels are high, renal production and secretion of calcitriol is also high. Production and secretion of calcitriol is like that of PTH promoted by reduced plasma-ionised calcium and inhibited by rising plasma-ionised calcium concentration as well as rising plasma phosphate concentration.

The principal action of calcitriol is on the gastrointestinal tract where it promotes absorption of dietary calcium and phosphate. The net effect is a rise in plasma calcium and phosphate concentrations. By the integrated action of PTH and calcitriol, plasma calcium and phosphate concentrations are maintained within normal limits.

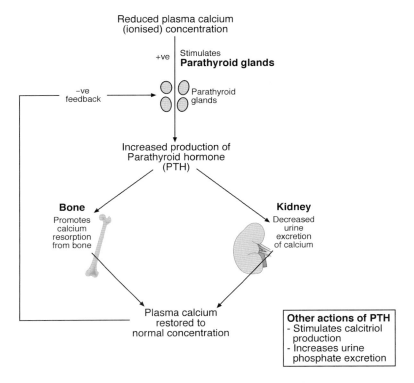

Figure 6.1 Parathormone control of plasma calcium concentration.

To summarise, the maintenance of normal plasma calcium and phosphate concentration depends on:

- normal diet containing adequate calcium, phosphorus and vitamin D
- normal gastrointestinal function for dietary absorption of all three
- exposure to sunlight for adequate endogenous production of vitamin D
- normal parathyroid function, for appropriate secretion of PTH
- normal liver and renal function, for conversion of vitamin D to calcitriol
- normal renal function, for secretion of calcitriol and appropriate adjustment of calcium and phosphate loss in urine
- normal bone metabolism for appropriate movement of calcium (and phosphate) between blood and bone.

The preservation of normal plasma ionised calcium concentration is more important for survival than preserving normal amounts of calcium in bone and if calcium is in short supply, the body sacrifices bone mineralisation in order to maintain plasma calcium concentration.

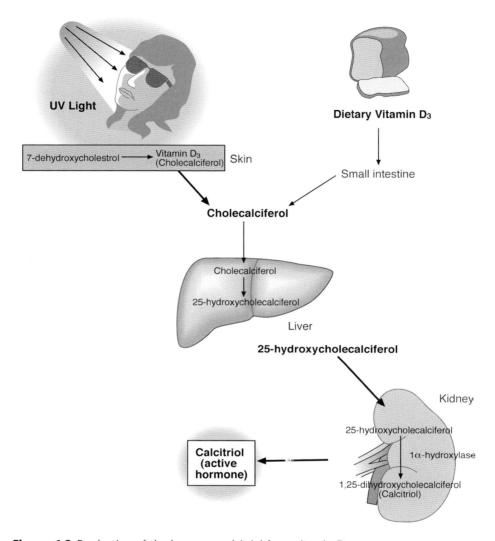

Figure 6.2 Production of the hormone calcitriol from vitamin D.

Measurement of calcium and phosphate

In the laboratory total plasma calcium (i.e. ionised calcium plus calcium bound to albumin) is measured. Point of care calcium measuring analysers sited in intensive care and emergency departments measure only the physiologically active ionised fraction of total calcium. This has important implications for sample collection and interpretation of results (see below).

Patient preparation

No particular patient preparation is necessary.

Timing of sample

Blood for both calcium and phosphate can be collected at any time of day.

Sample requirements

For laboratory measurement of total plasma calcium

Around 5 ml of venous blood is sufficient for laboratory estimation of calcium and phosphate. Measurement may be made on either plasma or serum recovered from a blood sample. If local policy is to use serum then blood must be collected into a plain collection tube that does not contain anticoagulant. Plasma estimation requires collection into a tube containing the anticoagulant lithium heparin. No other anticoagulant is suitable for calcium and phosphate analysis.

Use of a tourniquet can affect calcium results. Blood for calcium estimation should be collected without the use of a tourniquet. Poor technique during blood collection can cause damage to the membrane of blood cells and resulting haemolysis (see page 59). Phosphate is present at much higher concentration in the cells of blood than plasma, and damage to cells causes release of phosphate to plasma and a falsely raised result. Haemolysed samples are thus unsuitable for phosphate estimation.

For reasons discussed below the concentration of albumin is required to interpret calcium results. Therefore, unless a recent albumin result is available, a request for albumin estimation should accompany request for calcium.

For point of care measurement of ionised calcium

Modern blood gas analysers sited in intensive care units, recovery rooms and emergency departments often have incorporated technology for calcium measurement at the same time, and with the same anticoagulated arterial blood specimen used for blood gas analysis. (see Chapter 7). These instruments measure the physiologically active ionised fraction of total calcium. The same specialised attention to collection and sampling of blood for blood gases (pages 106–107) is necessary if only ionised calcium estimation is required.

Ionised calcium can be measured on venous as well as arterial blood, provided it is processed in the same way that arterial blood is processed for blood gas analysis. Interpretation of ionised calcium does not require albumin estimation. Phosphate cannot be measured at the point of care – only laboratory-based methods are available.

Interpretation of results

The concentration of plasma albumin and the pH of blood must be taken into account when interpreting calcium results.

Effect of albumin on calcium

For accurate interpretation of laboratory derived plasma or serum calcium results, a correction has to be made if serum/plasma albumin concentration is abnormal. Various formulae have been devised to make the correction – this is one of the most commonly used:

> If plasma albumin is greater than 45 g/l
> 'corrected' Ca (mmol/l) = measured Ca (mmol/l) − [0.02 × albumin (g/l) − 45]
> If plasma albumin is less than 40 g/l
> 'corrected' Ca (mmol/l) = measured Ca (mmol/l) + [0.02 × (40 − albumin g/l)]

As ionised calcium is unaffected by albumin concentration, no correction is necessary for results derived from methods (usually point of care methods) which measure the ionised calcium fraction only.

Effect of blood pH on calcium

The proportion of total calcium in blood that is in the ionised 'free' state is affected by the pH of blood. High blood pH (alkalosis) results in less calcium being in the ionised state and low blood pH (acidosis) results in more calcium being in the ionised state. The clinical implication of this effect of blood pH on plasma calcium is demonstrated in Case history 6 (page 115) but the general point to be made here is that interpretation of calcium results is a little more complicated if the patient has a condition in which acid-base is disturbed.

Approximate reference (normal) ranges

Serum/plasma calcium ('corrected' total)	2.20–2.60 mmol/l
Plasma calcium (ionised)	1.15–1.30 mmol/l
Serum/plasma phosphate	0.80–1.40 mmol/l

Critical values

Serum/plasma calcium ('corrected' total)	< 1.50 mmol/l > 3.30 mmol/l
Plasma calcium (ionised)	< 0.80 mmol/l > 1.60 mmol/l

Terms used in interpretation

Hypercalcaemia   serum/plasma calcium ('corrected' total) > 2.60 mmol/l or plasma ionised calcium > 1.30 mmol/l

Hypocalcaemia	serum/plasma calcium ('corrected' total) < 2.20 mmol/l or plasma ionised calcium < 1.15 mmol/l
Hyperphosphataemia	serum/plasma phosphate > 1.40 mmol/l
Hypophosphataemia	serum/plasma phosphate < 0.80 mmol/l

Causes of raised plasma/serum calcium

The two most common causes of hypercalcaemia are malignant disease (cancer) and primary hyperparathyroidism.

Hypercalcaemia and malignant disease

Excessive production by tumour cells of a protein called parathormone-related polypeptide (PTHrP) is thought to be the main cause of the hypercalcaemia which can affect cancer patients.[1] As its name implies, PTHrP is structurally and functionally similar to the calcium-regulating hormone parathormone (PTH) produced by the parathyroid glands. The action of PTHrP is like that of PTH to promote calcium movement from bone to blood, with a consequent rise in plasma calcium concentration. However, whereas PTH production is controlled by plasma calcium concentration – i.e. promoted by reduced calcium concentration and inhibited by increased concentration – PTHrP production by tumour cells is under no such control. The inevitable consequence of the uncontrolled PTHrP production by tumour cells is abnormal loss of calcium from bone and increasing blood calcium concentration.

Although hypercalcaemia can occur in all cancer types, it is more common in some than others, so cancers of the lung, breast, head, throat and oesophagus are more likely to be associated with hypercalcaemia than those of the kidney, bowel and stomach.

Multiple myeloma, a haematological malignancy of the bone marrow, is the malignant disease most commonly associated with hypercalcaemia; nearly a half of all myeloma patients are affected. In this case, hypercalcaemia is not due to PTHrP, but to the bone destruction (and consequent release of calcium) that results from infiltrating tumour cells.

Generally speaking, hypercalcaemia develops late in the evolution of solid tumour cancers, when disease is at an advanced stage and spread beyond the primary site particularly to bone; it is therefore a poor prognostic sign. It is still important to detect because treatment is invariably successful in normalising plasma calcium, and relief from symptoms of hypercalcaemia can improve the quality of life of cancer patients.[2]

Primary hyperparathyroidism

Persistently raised plasma calcium in the absence of malignant disease is most likely due to primary hyperparathyroidism, the second most common cause of hypercalcaemia among hospitalised patients and the most common cause among the general population. Although this condition can occur at any age and in both sexes, it most commonly affects postmenopausal women.[3] Excessive, uncontrolled secretion of PTH by a benign tumour called an adenoma in one of the four parathyroid glands is the cause of the hypercalcaemia in nearly all cases of primary hyperparathyroidism. In a minority of patients, increased PTH is a result of an abnormal increase in size (hyperplasia) of all parathyroid glands.

Many cases are discovered by chance when biochemical screening for investigation of apparently unrelated symptoms reveals raised plasma calcium concentration. Non-specific symptoms of hypercalcaemia (e.g. depression, constipation) may have been present for years before diagnosis and some patients (usually those with only very mild hypercalcaemia, 2.60–2.80 mmol/l) are asymptomatic. If left untreated, primary hyperparathyroidism can cause bone demineralisation (due to the uncontrolled effect of PTH on bone), deposition of calcium in kidney and consequent renal disease, urinary calcium stones, and in rare cases, hypercalcaemia of such severity that life is threatened.[4] Surgical removal of the offending adenoma is the only curative treatment.

Rare causes
The two causes outlined above account for close to 80% of hypercalcaemia cases. Relatively common conditions that are only rarely associated with hypercalcaemia include chronic renal failure and thyrotoxicosis. Around 10% of patients suffering sarcoidois, a rare chronic disease predominantly affecting the lungs, are hypercalcaemic because of abnormal increase in calcitriol production and consequent increased absorption of dietary calcium. The same mechanism accounts for the hypercalcaemia that affects those with tuberculosis (TB) and those who have taken excessive doses of vitamin D. Finally some drugs, notably thiazide diuretics and lithium, can cause hypercalcaemia. Occasionally no cause can be identified for hypercalcaemia.

The main causes of increased plasma/serum calcium are summarised in Table 6.1.

Causes of reduced plasma/serum calcium

Hypocalcaemia is less common than hypercalcaemia. Since the action of the calcium-regulating hormones PTH and calcitriol is to raise plasma calcium, it is to be expected that deficiency or reduced action of either hormone may lead to hypocalcaemia.

Hypoparathyroidism: reduced production of PTH
Hypoparathyroidism is rare, most cases being the result of damage to parathyroid glands during surgery. The anatomical intimacy of parathyroid and thyroid render the parathyroid glands and/or their blood supply particularly vulnerable to unintended damage during thyroid surgery. The small size and variable anatomy of parathyroid glands contributes to this vulnerability. The same mechanism accounts for the hypocalcaemia that may develop after surgical removal of parathyroid adenoma, to cure primary hyperparathyroidism.

Around 14% of patients undergoing total thyroidectomy develop temporary hypoparathyroidism. Permanent hypoparathyroidism is much less common,

Table 6.1 Principal causes of abnormal plasma calcium and phosphate.

Causes of raised plasma calcium (hypercalcaemia)

- Malignancy (common cause)
- Hyperparathyroidism (common cause)
- Chronic renal failure
- Thyrotoxicosis
- Sarcoidosis
- Drugs (e.g. lithium, thiazide diuretics)

Causes of reduced plasma calcium (hypocalcaemia)

- Hypothyroidism (due to parathyroid/thyroid surgery)
- Hypothyroidism (autoimmune destruction, congenital absence of parathyroid gland)
- Vitamin D deficiency due to
  - dietary deficiency
  - lifestyle that reduces exposure to sun
  - malabsorption due to gastrointestinal/pancreatic disease
- Critical illness
- Chronic renal failure
- Chronic liver disease
- Neonatal period (immature parathyroid gland)

Causes of raised plasma phosphate (hyperphosphataemia)

- Renal failure
- Marked tissue/cell destruction (e.g. rhabdomyolysis/chemotherapy)
- Hypoparathyroidism

Causes of reduced plasma phosphate (hypophosphataemia)

- Primary hyperparathyroidism
- Poor nutrition
- Malabsorption due to gastrointestinal disease
- Vitamin D deficiency
- Diabetic ketoacidosis

occurring in just 2% of patients.[5] The risk of hypoparathyroidism and consequent hypocalcaemia is reduced by less radical surgery[6] but the postoperative management of all patients recovering from thyroid and parathyroid surgery includes careful monitoring of plasma calcium.

Rarer causes of hypoparathyroidism and consequent hypocalcaemia include damage to the parathyroid as a result of autoimmune disease and congenital absence or reduced development of the parathyroid glands.

Reduced production of calcitriol

Hypocalcaemia is a feature of the childhood bone disease rickets and its adult equivalent osteomalacia. In both cases, hypocalcaemia is due to deficiency of vitamin D, the substance from which calcitriol is synthesised. Hypocalcaemia develops because in the absence of adequate calcitriol, normal amounts of dietary calcium and phosphate cannot be absorbed. Deficiency of vitamin D that leads to hypocalcaemia can arise in a number of ways. It may simply be because the diet contains insufficient vitamin D or because disease of the gastrointestinal tract (e.g. coeliac, Crohn's disease) or pancreas (chronic pancreatitis) prevents normal amounts of vitamin D being absorbed from food. Lack of exposure to sunshine and consequent reduced synthesis of vitamin D can also cause vitamin D deficiency

The normal physiological response to reduced plasma calcium whatever its cause, is increased production of PTH and resulting movement of calcium from bone to blood. If vitamin D deficiency remains uncorrected, PTH secretion remains high. The loss of calcium from bone induced by PTH leads to the bone-deforming features of rickets in children and bone demineralisation of osteomalacia in adults.

Hypocalcaemia is a common feature of chronic renal failure and a less common feature of some chronic liver disorders and primary biliary cirrhosis. This reflects the key role that both kidney and liver play in conversion of vitamin D to calcitriol, as well as the specific role that the kidneys play in minimising calcium loss in urine. The hypocalcaemia associated with chronic liver disease is potentiated by vitamin D deficiency, consequent on reduced bile production by the liver (bile acids are required for absorption of vitamin D). Some anticonvulsant drugs, which are metabolised in the liver, reduce vitamin D metabolism in the liver and thereby calcitriol production. Patients taking these drugs are at long-term risk of hypocalcaemia and consequent bone demineralisation.

Hypocalcaemia in the critically ill
Hypocalcaemia is a common feature of critical illness. Up to 85% of patients being cared for in intensive care units develop hypocalcaemia.[7] Only methods that measure ionised calcium should be used to assess calcium status among intensive care patients. This is because the mathematical corrections used to correct total calcium for abnormal albumin (see above) have been shown to be inaccurate in this patient group.[8] The conditions that are most often associated with hypocalcaemia among intensive care patients include: acute renal failure, alkalosis, sepsis, acute pancreatitis, severe burns, and rhabdomyolysis. Massive blood transfusion may cause hypocalcaemia.

Neonatal hypocalcaemia
Hypocalcaemia is not uncommon during the first day or two of life. Fetal bone development requires a relatively high plasma calcium concentration *in utero*. The physiological transition from an intrauterine environment to neonatal independence includes a rapid reduction in plasma calcium during the first 24–48 hours of life. Transient hypocalcaemia during this early period is thought to be an exaggeration of this physiological response due to an insufficient PTH response from immature parathyroid glands (transient hypoparathyroidism). Premature and low birthweight babies being cared for in intensive care are at particular risk of this hypocalcaemic mechanism, as are babies born to diabetic mothers.

Late onset neonatal hypocalcaemia, occurring during the second week after birth, is thought be the result of inadequate renal response to PTH due to immature kidneys. Vitamin D deficiency, as a result of maternal deficiency during pregnancy, may also manifest as hypocalcaemia during this early period of life.

The main causes of reduced plasma/serum calcium are summarised in Table 6.1.

Causes of raised plasma/serum phosphate

By regulating the amount of phosphate that is lost from the body in urine, the kidneys have a central role in maintaining normal blood levels. The most common cause of raised serum/plasma phosphate is renal failure (both acute and chronic). A failing kidney is unable to excrete excess phosphate as efficiently as normal, so blood concentration rises.

Excessive intake of phosphate is a rare cause of hyperphosphataemia. This may occur in patients who are being fed parenterally. Vitamin D enhances absorption of dietary phosphate, so increased serum phosphate may occur in cases of vitamin D intoxication.

The very high concentration of phosphate within tissue cells as compared with that of extracellular fluid (blood) means that in cases of severe tissue destruction (e.g. rhabdomyolysis) there is an increase in blood levels as phosphate leaks from damaged cells to blood. Any illness or treatment (e.g. cancer chemotherapy) that is associated with marked tissue catabolism can result in raised plasma phosphate.

As already discussed, PTH has an important role in regulating plasma phosphate levels – it increases renal excretion of phosphate. This explains the raised plasma phosphate that is evident in those with PTH deficiency (hypoparathyroidism).

The main causes of increased serum/plasma phosphate are summarised in Table 6.1.

Causes of reduced plasma/serum phosphate

Hypophosphataemia develops as a result of three main mechanisms: reduced phosphate entering the body, increased phosphate losses (in urine) from the body, and movement of phosphate from blood plasma into cells.

The presence of phosphate in almost all foodstuffs makes inadequate dietary intake a rare cause of hypophosphataemia but it can occur if poor nutrition is long-standing, for example in alcoholism and eating disorders such as anorexia nervosa. Inadequate absorption of phosphate may lead to hypophosphataemia in patients with chronic gastrointestinal conditions such as Crohn's disease and coeliac disease; this being part of a wider malabsorption syndrome involving many dietary nutrients. Calcitriol, the hormone derived from vitamin D, is essential for adequate absorption of dietary phosphate so vitamin D deficiency leads to hypophosphataemia.

One of the actions of PTH is to increase phosphate excretion in urine. It is to be expected, then, that PTH excess (hyperparathyroidism) is associated with excessive losses of phosphate in urine and consequent hypophosphataemia.

Hypophosphataemia caused by movement of phosphate from blood into tissue cells is a feature of diabetic ketoacidosis (page 43) and respiratory alkalosis (page 110).

The main causes of reduced plasma/serum phosphate are summarised in Table 6.1.

Consequences of abnormal serum/plasma calcium and phosphate

Many of the clinical consequences of abnormal plasma calcium can be related to the central role that calcium plays in transmission of signals between nerve cells (neural transmission) and between nerve and muscle cells (neuromuscular transmission). The function of central nervous system, skeletal muscle, heart and gastrointestinal tract are particularly dependent on this calcium mediated signalling and any or all of these organ systems may be affected if plasma calcium is abnormal.

Signs, symptoms and consequences of raised calcium
In general, the range and severity of symptoms reflect the degree of hypercalcaemia. So many patients with mild hypercalcaemia, usually defined as plasma/serum calcium between 2.60 and 3.00 mmol/l are asymptomatic, while those with calcium greater than 3.50 mmol/l almost always manifest a range of signs and symptoms, some of which threaten survival.

Common gastrointestinal symptoms include nausea, vomiting and constipation. Central nervous system involvement can result in neuropsychiatric symptoms including lethargy, depression and confusion; psychosis, seizures and coma may occur. Muscular weakness and fatigue are common. Cardiac involvement includes arrhythmias with characteristic ECG changes. Cardiac arrest can be precipitated by severe hypercalcaemia, so a plasma calcium concentration greater than 3.5 mmol/l constitutes a clinical emergency, warranting immediate calcium lowering therapy.

Inability of the kidneys to concentrate urine effectively is a common feature of moderately severe hypercalcaemia; this is manifest as polyuria (increased urine volume) and resulting polydipsia (thirst). Long standing hypercalcaemia, even if it is mild, can lead to deposition of calcium in kidneys and tendency to form renal stones; increasing loss of renal function consequent on either of these can lead in the long term to renal failure.

Signs, symptoms and consequences of reduced calcium
Mild hypocalcaemia, roughly defined as total corrected plasma calcium in the range 1.80–2.20 mmol/l may occur without symptoms, but more severe hypocalcaemia is invariably associated with symptoms of tetany that result from increased neuromuscular excitability. These include loss of nerve sensation, tingling sensation, painful muscular spasms, twitching and in severe cases, convulsions and seizures. Laryngeal spasm restricts normal respiration and can be a life threatening effect of severe hypocalcaemia.

Cardiac arrhythmias with characteristic ECG changes may be a feature.

Central nervous system involvement may result in neuropsychiatric symptoms such as anxiety depression and psychosis among those with long standing hypocalcaemia. Long-standing hypocalcaemia is associated with higher than normal risk of cataracts and heart failure.

Signs, symptoms and consequences of raised phosphate

There are no symptoms directly attributable to a raised plasma phosphate but by the combined action of several mechanisms, raised phosphate causes a reduction in serum/plasma calcium. For this reason, many patients with hyperphosphataemia may be suffering symptoms of hypocalcaemia (outlined above). In the long term, hyperphosphataemia can lead to the precipitation of calcium phosphate in tissues, a pathological process known as calcification.

One important aspect of this is that calcification of arteries is involved in the process of atherosclerosis, which leads to coronary heart disease and strokes. It is now suspected that the high risk of a cardiovascular death in patients with chronic renal failure is due, at least in part, to the hyperphosphataemia and resulting calcification of arteries that so often occurs in this patient group.[9]

Signs, symptoms and consequences of reduced phosphate

Most patients with hypophosphataemia have plasma phosphate in the range 0.5–0.8 mmol/l. Such a mild reduction is not associated with symptoms and is of little clinical significance. However, severe hypophosphataemia, usually defined as serum/plasma phosphate < 0.3 mmol/l, has important clinical consequences. Symptoms include muscle weakness. This may affect muscles involved in respiration, causing respiratory difficulties. Severe muscle destruction (rhabdomyolysis), consequent on reduced ATP can occur. Reduced phosphate in erythrocytes can cause increased red cell destruction and resulting anaemia. Central nervous system symptoms include confusion, seizures and, rarely, coma.

Case history 5

Mrs Riddle, a 42-year-old woman, attended her GP surgery on two occasions over a period of a month, complaining of constipation. Physical examination was normal and Mrs Riddle considered herself to be in good health, apart from the constipation. On her second visit when she reported no real resolution of the constipation, blood was taken for a full biochemical profile. The laboratory report included the following results:

Plasma calcium	2.68 mmol/l
Plasma albumin	32 g/l
Plasma phosphate	0.8 mmol/l

Questions

(1) What is Mrs Riddle's 'corrected' plasma calcium?
(2) Which of the following do the results indicate: normocalcaemia, hypocalcaemia, or hypercalcaemia?

(3) What are the most likely diagnosis and cause of constipation?

(4) What blood test would help to confirm this diagnosis?

Discussion of case history

(1) The corrected plasma calcium is 2.84 mmol/l (see calculation, page 88).

(2) Both uncorrected and corrected plasma calcium are greater than 2.60 mmol/l, indicating raised plasma calcium, that is hypercalcaemia. The severity of the increase as indicated by the laboratory result 2.68 mmol/l is masked by a slightly reduced albumin. Only by correcting for this low albumin can the true severity (2.84 mmol/l) be revealed.

(3) Although there are many rare causes of hypercalcaemia, most (80%) are due to either malignant disease (cancer) or hyperparathyroidism (excess parathormone, PTH). In most cases of hypercalcaemia due to malignancy, cancer is in an advanced state and already diagnosed. Since Mrs Riddle is relatively young, feels generally fit and well – apart from her complaint of constipation – advanced cancer seems an unlikely cause of her hypercalcaemia. The most likely diagnosis is hyperparathyroidism. Constipation is a common symptom of hypercalcaemia. The absence of other symptoms of hyperparathyroidism is not unusual – many patients with the condition are asymptomatic at the time of diagnosis.

(4) The diagnosis of hyperparathyroidism depends on demonstrating increased PTH in blood – a request for plasma PTH is indicated.

References

1. Takai E, Yano T, Iguchi H *et al.* (1996) Tumor-induced hypercalcemia and parathyroid hormone-related protein in lung carcinoma. *Cancer* **78**: 1384–87.
2. Lamy O, Jenzer-Closuit A & Burckhardt P (2001) Hypercalcaemia of malignancy: an undiagnosed and undertreated disease. *J Intern Med* **250**: 73–79.
3. Birkenhager JC & Bouillon R (1996) Asymptomatic primary hyperparathyoidism. *Postgrad Med J* **72**: 323–26.
4. Wong P, Carmeci C *et al.* (2001) Parathyroid crisis in a 20 year old – an unusual cause of hypercalcaemic crisis. *Postgrad Med J* **77**: 468–70.
5. Bron LP & O'Brien C (2004) Total thyroidectomy for clinically benign disease of the thyroid. *Br J Surg* **91**(5): 569–74.
6. Ozbas S, Kocak S *et al.* (2005) Comparison of the complications of subtotal, near total and total thyroidectomy in the surgical management of mulitnodular goitre. *Endocr J* **52**: 199–205.
7. Hastbacka J & Pettila V (2003) Prevalance and predictive value of ionized hypocalcaemia among critically ill patients. *Acta Anaesthesiol Scand* **47**: 1264–69.
8. Dickerson R, Alexander KH *et al.* (2003) Accuracy of method to estimate ionized and 'corrected' serum calcium concentrations in critically ill multiple trauma patients receiving specialised nutrition support. *J Parenter Enteral Nutr* **28**(3): 133–41.
9. Fatica R & Dennis V (2002) Cardiovascular mortality in chronic renal failure: hyperphosphatemia, coronary calcification, and the role of phosphate binders. *Cleve Clin J Med* **69**(Suppl 3): S21–27.

Chapter 7
BLOOD GASES

The use of the term blood gases does not fully describe this test because although it includes measurement of the two physiologically important gases present in blood, oxygen (O_2) and carbon dioxide (CO_2), it also includes measurement of the pH of blood, along with several other parameters of acid-base balance. The test is most frequently used for monitoring two patient groups: the critically ill and those with chronic respiratory disease. Clinically significant changes in the measured parameters of blood gases can occur over very short periods of time in the critically ill, so that they may require blood gas measurement every few hours. For this reason, blood gas analysers are often sited where critically ill patients are being cared for, in intensive care units, emergency departments and recovery rooms. In these circumstances, responsibility for analysis of blood gases frequently falls upon nursing staff. It is the only blood test that requires sampling of arterial blood; all other blood tests are performed on venous blood.

Normal physiology

Normal cellular metabolism is associated with continuous production of carbon dioxide (CO_2) and hydrogen ions (H^+), as oxygen (O_2) is consumed. The rates of production and consumption vary according to the level of metabolic activity. Health demands that despite this variation in production and consumption, the blood content of all three be maintained within narrow limits. The mechanisms which maintain the three parameters within normal limits are a complex synergy of action involving chemical buffers in blood, the red cells (erythrocytes) which circulate in blood and the function of three organs: lungs, kidney and brain. Blood gases is a test that monitors the ability of the body to maintain these mechanisms. An understanding of test results then depends on a basic knowledge of respiratory physiology and normal acid-base balance. Although interrelated, these two topics are treated separately here for convenience only.

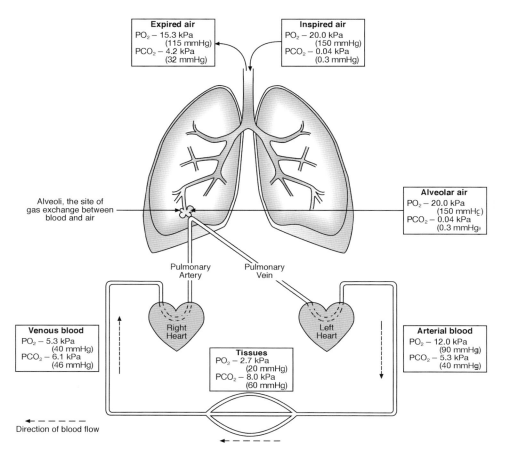

Figure 7.1 Oxygen and carbon dioxide content of air within lungs, systemic blood (venous and arterial) and tissues.

Respiratory physiology

The object of respiration is to supply oxygen, present in inspired air, to every tissue cell and eliminate carbon dioxide, a waste product of tissue metabolism, in expired air. Venous blood returning from the tissues is low in oxygen and loaded with carbon dioxide (see Figure 7.1). It is mixed in the right side of the heart and pumped to the lungs via the pulmonary artery. In the lungs, carbon dioxide passes from blood in exchange for oxygen. The blood, now with less carbon dioxide, but loaded with oxygen is pumped back to the heart via the pulmonary vein and out, via the aorta through the arterial system, for delivery of oxygen to the tissues.

Basic principles of gases in biological systems: units of measurement and diffusion

The amount of a gas present in systems, including biological systems, is defined by the pressure it exerts, traditionally measured as the height in millimetres of a column of mercury (Hg). For example, the pressure of atmospheric air (i.e. baro-metric pressure) at sea level is 760 mmHg. This means that at sea level, the gases contained in the air we breath have a combined pressure sufficient to support a column of mercury 760 mm high. In a mixture of gases, as air is, the total pressure is simply the sum of the partial pressures (represented by the symbol P) of each gas. Since air comprises 21% oxygen, 0.03% carbon dioxide and 78% nitrogen, the partial pressure of oxygen (PO_2) in inspired air at sea level is equal to 21% of total atmospheric pressure (i.e. $21/100 \times 760$) or 150 mmHg and par-tial pressure of carbon dioxide (PCO_2) = $0.03/100 \times 760$ or 0.2 mmHg.

In clinical laboratories, the Système Internationale (SI) unit of pressure, the kilo-Pascal (kPa) has replaced mm Hg as the unit of choice when measuring partial pressures of gases. Pressure is defined as force per unit area. The SI unit of force is the Newton (N) and the SI unit of area is the square metre (m^2). Thus the derived SI unit of pressure, the Pascal (named after the 17th century physicist), is defined as 1 Newton per square metre ($1 N/m^2$). The kilo-Pascal (kPa) is one thousand Pascals (i.e. $1000 N/m^2$). Some physiology texts continue to express the partial pressure of gases in blood in mmHg. To convert mmHg to kPa, simply multiply by 0.133.

Figure 7.1 describes the PO_2 and PCO_2 of inspired air, alveolar air (the air deep within the lungs), venous blood, arterial blood, and tissues.

The rate of diffusion of a gas across a physiological membrane is determined by the partial pressure of that gas on either side of the membrane. Gas diffuses from high partial pressure to low partial pressure. The greater the difference on either side of the membrane, the faster gas diffuses. The significance of this simple prin-ciple will become apparent as the exchange of gases between blood and lungs, and between blood and tissues, is examined more closely.

Gas exchange at the lungs

The site of gas exchange between blood and lungs is the alveolar membrane, the thin lining of the microscopic cul-de-sacs of lung structure, called alveoli. The millions of alveoli provide a massive alveolar membrane surface area for gas exchange: 80 square metres in the adult lung. On one side of the membrane is alveolar air. On the other are blood capillaries so small that only one blood cell can pass through. Gases diffuse across this membrane in an attempt to equalise the amount of each gas on either side of the membrane. So oxygen diffuses from the alveoli (PO_2 13.3 kPa) to the blood (PO_2 5.3 KPa) and carbon dioxide dif-fuses from the blood (PCO_2 6.1 KPa) to alveoli (PCO_2 4.8 KPa).

Successful gas exchange between the lungs and blood is dependent on:

- adequate alveolar ventilation by the lungs – this is the mechanical process, due to the elastic recoil of lungs, that ensures movement of air in and out of alveoli
- normal numbers of functioning alveoli
- sufficient blood flow through the pulmonary capillaries (i.e. adequate perfusion).

Transport of oxygen in blood

Oxygen passes across the alveolar membrane into the blood flowing through pulmonary capillaries. In the blood, a small proportion of the oxygen is dissolved in blood plasma, but most is transported bound to the protein haemoglobin contained within red blood cells. The haemoglobin molecule has four oxygen binding sites, allowing a maximum of four molecules of oxygen to combine with each molecule of haemoglobin. The product is oxyhaemoglobin. The oxygen delivery function of haemoglobin, that is its ability to 'pick up' oxygen at the lungs and 'release' it to tissue cells is made possible by a reversible conformational change in the quaternary structure (shape) of the haemoglobin molecule that alters its affinity for oxygen. In the deoxy state, haemoglobin has low affinity for oxygen and in the oxy state it has high affinity for oxygen. A range of environmental factors determines the haemoglobin state (oxy or deoxy). The most significant of these is PO_2. Haemoglobin present in blood with relatively high PO_2 has much greater affinity for oxygen than the haemoglobin present in blood with relatively low PO_2. The oxygen dissociation curve (Figure 7.2) describes this relationship graphically.

It is clear from the graph that at the high PO_2 that prevails in arterial blood, haemoglobin is almost 100% saturated with oxygen. By contrast at low PO_2 (in venous blood and tissues) haemoglobin has lower affinity and % haemoglobin saturation is consequently much lower. This is crucial for maximum loading of oxygen onto haemoglobin in the arterial blood at the alveoli of the lungs and unloading of oxygen from haemoglobin at the tissues. The tissue release of oxygen from oxyhaemoglobin induced by low PO_2 is potentiated by the relatively high PCO_2 and low pH that prevails in the tissues.

For adequate oxygenation of tissues:

- blood must contain sufficient haemoglobin
- that haemoglobin must be > 95% saturated with oxygen in arterial blood
- to achieve > 95% oxygen saturation, arterial blood PO_2 must be > 10 kPa (Figure 7.2)
- maintenance of arterial PO_2 above 10 KPa is dependent on the factors required for normal gas exchange between lungs and blood (see above).

Acid-base balance: the maintenance of normal blood pH

Normal cellular metabolism requires that blood pH be maintained within the range 7.35–7.45 despite continuous production of hydrogen ions, which tend to reduce

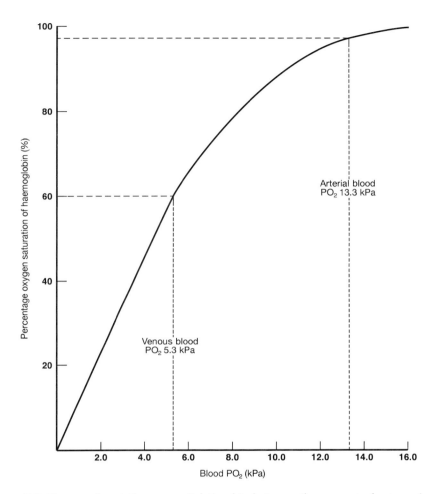

Figure 7.2 Oxygen dissociation curve. Relationship between the amount of oxygen in blood PO_2 and the amount of oxygen carried by haemoglobin (% Hb saturation).

pH. Even slight excursions outside this range have deleterious effects and a pH of less than 6.8 or greater than 7.8 is considered incompatible with life. A brief review of some basic concepts is required for an understanding of acid-base balance in the body.

What is pH?

pH is a logarithmic scale (0 to 14) of acidity and alkalinity. Pure water has a pH of 7 and by convention neutral (i.e. neither acidic nor alkaline). pH above 7 is alkaline and pH less than 7 is acidic. The term pH is an abbreviation of *puissance de hydrogen* (*puissance* is French for power). It is thus a measure of hydrogen ion activity or concentration. pH is defined as the negative log to the base 10 (i.e. $\log_{10}$) of the hydrogen ion concentration in moles per litre or:

$$pH = -\log_{10}[H^+] \qquad \text{(Equation 1)}$$

where $[H^+]$ = hydrogen ion concentration in mol/l
  From this equation:

pH 7.4 = H^+ concentration of 40 nmol/l
pH 7.0 = H^+ concentration of 100 nmol/l
pH 6.0 = H^+ concentration of 1000 nmol/l

  It is evident that:

- the two parameters change inversely – as hydrogen ion concentration increases, pH falls
- due to the logarithmic nature of the pH scale, an apparently small change in pH is in fact a large change in hydrogen ion concentration – doubling hydrogen ion concentration, for example, results in a fall of only 0.3 of a pH unit.

Some laboratories report hydrogen ion concentration (reported as nmol/l) in preference to pH.

What are acids and bases?

An acid is a substance that dissociates in solution to *release* hydrogen ions. A base *accepts* hydrogen ions.
  For example, hydrochloric acid (HCl) dissociates to hydrogen ions and chlorine ions:

$$HCl \rightarrow H^+ + Cl^- \qquad \text{(Equation 2)}$$

whereas bicarbonate (HCO_3^-), a base, accepts hydrogen ions to form carbonic acid:

$$HCO_3^- + H^+ \rightarrow H_2CO_3 \qquad \text{(Equation 3)}$$

  A strong acid like hydrochloric acid dissociates easily, yielding many hydrogen ions; it therefore has a very low pH.
  A weak acid, by contrast, dissociates less easily, yielding fewer hydrogen ions and therefore a relatively higher pH than a strong acid.

What is a buffer?

Chemical buffers are compounds in solution which resist change in pH caused by addition of an acid, by 'mopping up' hydrogen ions resulting from acid dissociation.
  A buffer is the conjugate base of any weak acid. Because of its prime physiological importance for the maintenance of blood pH, the bicarbonate buffer system will be used as an example (there are several other buffer systems in blood). The buffer in this instance is bicarbonate, the conjugate base of the weak acid, carbonic acid. When a strong acid, e.g. hydrochloric acid is added to a solution of

sodium bicarbonate (the buffer), the hydrogen ions from the strongly dissociating hydrochloric acid are incorporated into carbonic acid, a weakly dissociating acid:

$$H^+Cl^- \quad + \quad NaHCO_3 \quad \rightarrow \quad H_2CO_3 \quad + \quad NaCl$$

Hydrochloric acid   Sodium bicarbonate   Carbonic acid   Sodium chloride   (Equation 4)

a strong acid   the buffer   a weak acid

The important point here is that because the hydrogen ions from hydrochloric acid have been incorporated into a weak acid, which does not dissociate readily, the total number of hydrogen ions in solution and therefore the pH does not change as much as would have occurred in the absence of the buffer. Although a buffer minimises changes in pH, due to addition of hydrogen ions, it cannot entirely eliminate them because even weak acids dissociate to some extent. A very useful (if at first sight daunting!) equation defines the pH of all buffer systems in terms of the concentrations of their weak acid and conjugate base, it is called the Henderson–Hasselbalch equation. For the bicarbonate buffer system this equation is:

$$pH = 6.1 + \log\frac{[HCO_3]}{[H_2CO_3]} \qquad\qquad \text{(Equation 5)}$$

Where $[HCO_3]$ is the concentration of the conjugate base, bicarbonate and $[H_2CO_3]$ is the concentration of the weak acid, carbonic acid.

This equation reveals that pH is governed by the ratio of the concentration of base (HCO_3^-) to concentration of acid (H_2CO_3).

As hydrogen ions are added to bicarbonate (the buffer), the concentration of bicarbonate falls (as it is converted to carbonic acid), and the concentration of carbonic acid rises (*equation 3*). If acid (hydrogen ions) continue to be added to the system bicarbonate would eventually be consumed (all would be converted to carbonic acid). At this point, there would be no buffering capacity and pH would fall sharply with addition of more acid. However, if carbonic acid could be continuously removed from the system as it was generated, and bicarbonate continuously replenished, then buffering capacity and therefore pH could be maintained, despite continued addition of hydrogen ions.

As will become clear with more detail of the physiology of acid-base balance, that is, in effect, what happens in the body. The lungs ensure removal of carbonic acid (as carbon dioxide) and the kidneys ensure continuous regeneration of bicarbonate. The role of the lungs in maintenance of normal blood pH thus depends on a singular characteristic of the bicarbonate buffering system, the conversion of carbonic acid to carbon dioxide and water. The following equation outlines the relationship of all elements of the bicarbonate buffering system as it operates in the body:

$$H^+ \quad + \quad HCO_3^- \leftrightarrow \quad H_2CO_3 \quad \leftrightarrow H_2O + \quad CO_2$$

Hydrogen ions   Bicarbonate   Carbonic acid   Water   Carbon dioxide

It is important to note that the reactions are reversible. Direction is dependent on the relative concentration of each element. For example, a rise in carbon dioxide forces reaction to the left with increased production of carbonic acid and ultimately hydrogen ions. This explains the acidic potential of carbon dioxide and brings us to the important contribution that the lungs play in preserving normal blood pH.

Lungs and maintenance of normal blood pH

The main contribution of the lungs to the maintenance of a normal pH is regulation of the amount of carbon dioxide in blood. The actual amount of carbon dioxide in blood reflects a balance between that produced by cellular metabolism and that eliminated by the lungs in expired air, during respiration. Respiratory chemoreceptors in the brain detect changes in the carbon dioxide content of blood, increasing respiration if carbon dioxide is high and reducing respiratory rate if low. Thus respiratory rate is the main determinant of carbon dioxide excretion by the lungs and therefore the amount of carbon dioxide in blood.

The sequence of events from CO_2 production in the tissues to elimination in expired air is described in Figure 7.3.

Carbon dioxide diffuses out of tissue cells to surrounding capillary blood. A small proportion dissolves in blood plasma and is transported to the lungs unchanged. However, most diffuses into red cells, where an enzyme called carbonic anhydrase facilitates its combination with water to form carbonic acid. The acid dissociates, with production of hydrogen ions and bicarbonate. Hydrogen ions combine with deoxygenated haemoglobin (haemoglobin is acting as a buffer here) preventing a dangerous fall in cellular pH, and bicarbonate diffuses along a concentration gradient from red cell to plasma. Thus most of the carbon dioxide produced in the tissues is transported to the lungs as bicarbonate in blood plasma.

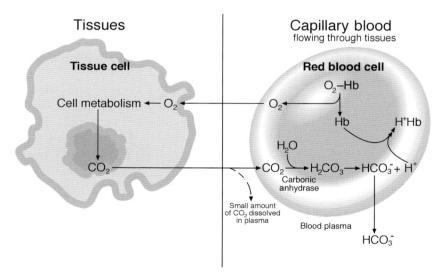

Figure 7.3a Delivery of oxygen (O_2) to tissues and first step in the elimination of carbon dioxide (CO_2).

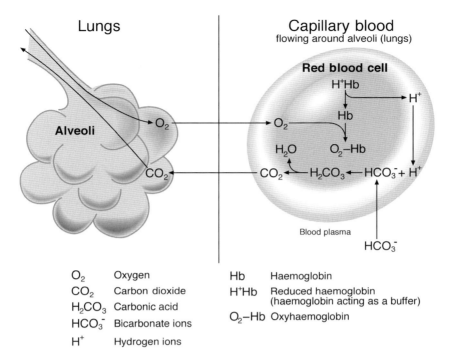

Figure 7.3b At the lung alveoli bicarbonate is converted back to carbon dioxide (CO_2), which is eliminated by the lungs in expired air.

A small proportion of the carbon dioxide that diffuses into red cells is transported bound to haemoglobin.

At the alveoli in the lungs, the process is reversed (Figure 7.3b). Hydrogen ions are displaced from haemoglobin as it takes up oxygen from inspired air. The hydrogen ions are now buffered by bicarbonate, which diffuses from plasma back into red cell, and carbonic acid is formed. As the concentration of this rises, it is converted to water and carbon dioxide. Finally, carbon dioxide diffuses down a concentration gradient from red cell to alveoli for excretion in expired air.

Kidneys and maintenance of normal blood pH

Normal cellular metabolism results in continuous production of hydrogen ions. We have seen that by combining with these hydrogen ions the buffers in blood minimise their effect. However, buffering does not remove hydrogen ions from the body and maintenance of normal blood pH depends ultimately on the ability of the body to eliminate hydrogen ions. At the same time, it is important to continuously replenish the bicarbonate used in buffering. These two tasks, elimination of hydrogen ions and regeneration of bicarbonate, are accomplished by the kidneys, specifically the renal tubule cells. These cells are rich in the enzyme carbonic anhydrase, which facilitates the formation of carbonic acid from carbon dioxide and water. The carbonic acid dissociates to hydrogen ions and bicarbonate. The bicarbonate is reabsorbed to blood and hydrogen ions pass into the lumen of the tubule and are eliminated from the body in urine. This urine elimination of hydrogen ions depends on the presence in urine of buffers, principally phosphate and ammonia ions.

Summary

Maintenance of normal blood pH is dependent on:

- adequate blood buffering capacity
- normally functioning respiratory chemoreceptors in the brain
- normally functioning lungs (elimination of carbon dioxide)
- normally functioning kidneys (elimination of hydrogen ions and regeneration of bicarbonate).

Measurement of blood gases

Patient preparation

Many patients who require blood gas analysis may be receiving oxygen therapy or artificial ventilation. Changes in oxygen and mechanical ventilation therapy will affect results. It is preferable to allow the effects of these changes to stabilise for 30 minutes before sampling blood. The patient should be well rested and warned that arterial sampling may be more painful than venepuncture.

Timing of sampling

Apart from the advice provided above, the timing of sampling is not important. Some laboratories prefer to be informed by phone before sampling to ensure that analysis is performed immediately the sample arrives. Blood gases are frequently ordered more than once daily on the same patient, so it is important to record the time of blood sampling on the accompanying request card.

Sample requirements

Around 2 ml of heparinised arterial blood is required. An arterial puncture (Table 7.1) is potentially more hazardous and usually more painful than venepuncture. Blood must be collected into a syringe that contains heparin to prevent the blood from clotting. Small clots, preventing analysis, can form if blood is not mixed adequately with the heparin. The metabolic activity of blood cells continues after blood sampling with consumption of oxygen and production of carbon dioxide. For this reason, blood for blood gases should be analysed immediately it is sampled. If there is to be any delay (more than 10 minutes), the syringe must be packed in

Table 7.1 Collection of arterial blood sample.

Arterial blood is routinely sampled from the radial artery in the wrist, the femoral artery in the groin or the brachial artery in the arm.

The syringe must be loaded with the 0.5 to 1 ml lithium or sodium heparin solution (1000 units per ml) to prevent blood from clotting in the syringe. Pre-heparinised syringe packs specifically for arterial blood collection are usually used.

The procedure is more painful than venepuncture so local anaesthetic is sometimes injected prior to arterial puncture.

Aseptic technique including gloved hands is required to prevent infection.

- Locate the injection site by feeling for pulsating artery.
- Prepare the site by cleaning first with alcohol and then iodine antiseptic solution. Allow to dry.
- Inject local anaesthetic to the site (optional).
- Hold the blood gas syringe with needle attached between forefinger and thumb (like holding a dart) and with other hand relocate artery.
- Warn patient before inserting the needle bevel side uppermost into the skin at an angle of 45 degrees (90 degrees in the case of a femoral artery stab) just behind the finger locating the artery.
- Advance the needle in the direction of the artery.
- When the artery is punctured, blood will automatically flow into syringe due to arterial pressure.
- When sufficient blood has been collected withdraw the needle and immediately place a sterile gauze pad over the injection site. Firm finger pressure must be appled for a minimum of five minutes.
- Eject any air from syringe containing sample and discard needle to sharps disposable box.
- Cap syringe and invert syringe several times to ensure adequate mixing of blood with heparin solution.
- Immerse barrel of syringe in packed ice and arrange *immediate* transport to laboratory.

ice to inhibit blood cell metabolism. Any air present in the syringe after blood collection will equilibrate with blood giving falsely raised blood PO_2. It is important to expel all air from the syringe after blood collection.

Arterial blood may be sampled from an indwelling arterial line. Capillary blood obtained from a finger prick, earlobe or heel stab may be used if arterial blood collection poses a problem, for example in neonates. The same principles apply; blood sample must be heparinised, contain no air bubbles and be analysed immediately.

Analysis

Blood is injected directly from the syringe into the blood gas analyser. Inside the analyser, three separate electrodes measure pH, PCO_2 and PO_2. Using pH and PCO_2, the machine calculates several other parameters, the most frequently used in practice are bicarbonate and base excess. The machine prints the measured and calculated parameters within a minute or so after injection of the sample.

Interpretation of blood gas results

Reference ranges: adults

pH   7.35–7.45
(hydrogen ion (H^+) concentration 35–45 nmol/l)
PCO_2 4.7–6.0 kPa (35–45 mm Hg)
PO_2 10.6–13.3 kPa (80–100 mm Hg)
Bicarbonate   22–28 mmol/l
Base excess/deficit   −2 to +2 mmol/l

Reference range: neonates[1]

pH   7.31–7.47
PCO_2 3.8–6.5 kPa (28–49 mmHg)
PO_2 4.3–8.1 kPa (32–61 mmHg)
Bicarbonate   15–25 mmol/l

Critical values: adults

pH   < 7.2 or > 7.6
PCO_2 < 2.7 kPa or > 9.3 kPa
PO_2 < 5.3 kPa
Bicarbonate   < 10 mmol/l or > 40 mmol/l

Terms used in blood gas interpretation

Acidosis/acidaemia   pH < 7.35 or H^+ concentration > 45 nmol/l
Alkalosis/alkalaemia   pH > 7.45 or H^+ concentration < 35 nmol/l
Hypercapnia PCO_2 > 6.0 kPa
Hypocapnia PCO_2 < 4.7 kPa
Hypoxaemia PO_2 < 10.6 kPa
Hypoxia   Reduced oxygen tension in tissues, tissues poorly
                      oxygenated

Clinical disturbances of acid-base balance

Most disturbances of acid-base balance can be attributed to one of three broad causes:

- disease or damage to organs (kidney, lungs, brain) whose normal function is necessary for acid-base homeostasis
- disease that causes abnormally increased production of metabolic acids such that homeostatic mechanisms are overwhelmed
- medical intervention (e.g. mechanical ventilation, some drugs).

To understand how blood gas results (pH, PCO_2 and bicarbonate) can be used to identify the cause and monitor disturbances of acid-base balance we must return to the Henderson–Hasselbalch equation

$$pH = 6.1 + \log \frac{[HCO_3]}{[H_2CO_3]}$$

Where $[HCO_3]$ is the concentration of the conjugate base, bicarbonate and $[H_2CO_3]$ is the concentration of the weak acid, carbonic acid.

Bicarbonate (HCO_3^-) is calculated during blood gas measurement but carbonic acid (H_2CO_3) is not. However, there is a relationship between carbonic acid concentration and PCO_2, a measured parameter of blood gases, which allows restatement of the Henderson–Hasselbalch equation in terms of the three measured parameters of blood gas analysis, pH, PCO_2 and bicarbonate:

$$pH = 6.1 + \log \frac{[HCO_3^-]}{PCO_2 \times 0.23}$$

Removing all constants from this equation, we can state that:

$$pH \propto \frac{[HCO_3^-]}{PCO_2}$$

This simple relationship, crucial for an understanding of all that follows concerning acid-base disturbances, states that blood pH is proportional to the ratio of bicarbonate concentration to PCO_2. It allows the following deductions.

- pH remains normal so long as the ratio $[HCO_3] : PCO_2$ remains normal.
- pH increases (i.e. alkalosis occurs) if *either* $[HCO_3]$ increases *or* PCO_2 decreases.
- pH decreases (i.e. acidosis occurs) if *either* $[HCO_3]$ decreases *or* PCO_2 increases.
- If *both* PCO_2 *and* $[HCO_3]$ are increased by relatively the same amount, the ratio and therefore the pH are normal.
- If both PCO_2 *and* $[HCO_3]$ are decreased by relatively the same amount, the ratio and therefore the pH are normal.

Classification of acid-base disturbances

All acid-base disturbances are by convention classified to one of four groups, depending on whether the primary abnormality is in PCO_2 or bicarbonate concentration. Primary disturbance of PCO_2 is referred to as a respiratory disturbance (reflecting the role that the respiratory system plays in regulating PCO_2) and primary disturbance of bicarbonate is called metabolic.

- If the primary disturbance is raised PCO_2 (which causes acidosis, see above) the condition is called *respiratory acidosis*.

- If the primary disturbance is reduced PCO_2 (which causes alkalosis, see above) the condition is called *respiratory alkalosis.*
- If the primary disturbance is reduced bicarbonate (which results in acidosis, see above) the condition is called *metabolic acidosis.*
- If the primary disturbance is raised bicarbonate (which results in alkalosis, see above) the condition is called *metabolic alkalosis.*

Causes of the four acid-base disorders

Respiratory acidosis
(primary increase in PCO$_2$, reduced pH)
Respiratory acidosis is characterised by increased PCO_2 due to inadequate ventilation (hypoventilation) and consequent reduced elimination of CO_2 from the blood. Respiratory disease such as bronchopneumonia, asthma, chronic obstructive pulmonary disease (emphysema, chronic bronchitis) may all be associated with hypoventilation sufficient to cause respiratory acidosis. Some drugs (e.g. morphine and barbiturates) and head injury can cause respiratory acidosis by depressing or damaging the respiratory centre in the brain that regulates respiration. Damage or trauma to the chest wall and the musculature involved in the mechanics of respiration may reduce ventilation rate. This explains the respiratory acidosis that can complicate the course of diseases such as poliomyelitis, Guillain–Barré syndrome and recovery from severe chest trauma. Respiratory acidosis can be classified as acute (i.e. rapid onset, for example during an acute asthmatic attack) or chronic (for example in chronic respiratory diseases such as emphysema between acute exacerbations). PCO_2 greater than 7.0 kPa is defined as respiratory failure.

Respiratory alkalosis
(reduced PCO$_2$, increased pH)
By contrast, respiratory alkalosis is characterised by reduced PCO_2 due to excessive alveolar ventilation and resulting excessive elimination of CO_2 from blood. Reduced oxygen in blood (hypoxaemia) can stimulate increased ventilation sufficiently to cause respiratory alkalosis. Conditions in which this mechanism might operate to cause respiratory alkalosis include severe anaemia, pulmonary embolism and adult respiratory distress syndrome. Stress-related hyperventilation sufficient to cause respiratory alkalosis is often a feature of anxiety attacks and response to severe pain. One of the less welcome properties of salicylate (aspirin) is its stimulatory effect on the respiratory centre. This effect accounts for the respiratory alkalosis that occurs following salicylate overdose. Finally, overenthusiastic mechanical ventilation can cause respiratory alkalosis.

Metabolic acidosis
(reduced bicarbonate, reduced pH)
Reduced bicarbonate is always a feature of metabolic acidosis. This occurs for one of two reasons: increased consumption of bicarbonate in buffering an abnormal acid load or increased loss of bicarbonate from the body. Diabetic ketoacidosis (page 43) and lactic acidosis (page 35) are two conditions characterised by

overproduction of metabolic acids and consequent exhaustion of bicarbonate. In the first case, abnormally high blood concentrations of keto-acids (β-hydroxybutyric acid and acetoacetic acid) reflect the severe metabolic derangements that result from insulin deficiency.

All cells produce lactic acid if they are deficient of oxygen, so increased lactic acid production and resulting metabolic acidosis occurs in any condition in which oxygen delivery to the tissues is severely compromised. Examples include cardiac arrest, and any condition associated with hypovolaemic shock (e.g. massive fluid loss). The liver plays a major role in removing the small amount of lactic acid that is produced during normal cell metabolism, so that lactic acidosis can be a feature of liver failure.

Abnormal loss of bicarbonate from the body can occur during severe diarrhoea. If unchecked, this can lead to metabolic acidosis. Failure to regenerate bicarbonate and excrete hydrogen ions explains the metabolic acidosis that occurs in renal failure.

Metabolic alkalosis
(increased bicarbonate, increased pH)
Bicarbonate is always raised in metabolic alkalosis. Rarely, excessive intravenous administration of bicarbonate or ingestion of bicarbonate in antacid preparation can cause metabolic alkalosis, but this is usually transient. Abnormal loss of hydrogen ions from the body can be the primary problem; bicarbonate, which would otherwise be consumed in buffering these lost hydrogen ions, consequently accumulates in blood. Gastric juice is acidic and gastric aspiration or any disease process in which gastric contents are lost from the body represents a loss of hydrogen ions. The projectile vomiting of gastric juice, for example, explains the metabolic alkalosis that can occur in patients with pyloric stenosis. Severe potassium depletion can cause metabolic alkalosis due to the reciprocal relationship between hydrogen and potassium ions.

Consequence of acid-base disturbances: compensation

Because of the prime importance of maintaining a normal blood pH, the body will always attempt to return an abnormal pH to normal. This process is called compensation. To understand compensation, it is important to recall that pH is governed by the ratio $[HCO_3] : PCO_2$. So long as the ratio is normal, pH will be normal. Primary respiratory disturbances of acid-base, in which PCO_2 is abnormal, are compensated for by adjustment of the metabolic component bicarbonate (HCO_3). Conversely, a primary disturbance of bicarbonate is compensated for by adjustment of the respiratory component, PCO_2.

Consider the patient with metabolic acidosis whose pH is low because bicarbonate concentration $[HCO_3]$ is low. To compensate for the low $[HCO_3]$ and restore the all-important ratio towards normal, the patient must lower their PCO_2. Chemoreceptors respond to rising hydrogen ion concentration (low pH) causing increased ventilation (hyperventilation) and thereby increased elimination of carbon dioxide; the PCO_2 falls and the ratio $[HCO_3] : PCO_2$ returns towards normal.

Compensation for metabolic alkalosis, in which $[HCO_3]$ is high by contrast, involves depression of respiration and thereby retention of carbon dioxide so that the PCO_2 rises to match the increase in $[HCO_3]$. However, depression of respiration has the unwelcome side effect of threatening adequate oxygenation of tissues. For this reason, respiratory compensation of metabolic alkalosis is limited.

Primary disturbances of PCO_2 (respiratory acidosis and alkalosis) are compensated for by renal adjustments which result in changes in bicarbonate concentration. Thus the renal compensation for respiratory acidosis (raised PCO_2) involves increased renal reabsorption of bicarbonate and compensation for respiratory alkalosis (reduced PCO_2) involves reduced bicarbonate reabsorption.

If the compensatory mechanism is sufficient to return the pH to normal, the patient is said to be fully compensated. If the compensatory mechanism is sufficient to return the pH towards normal, but insufficient to actually achieve normality, the patient is said to be partially compensated. The concept of an 'acid-base balance' allows the process of compensation to be conveyed visually (Figure 7.4).

It must be remembered that compensation whether partial or complete is not a state of normality; the ratio $[HCO_3]$: PCO_2 and therefore the pH may be normal, but both $[HCO_3]$ and PCO_2 are abnormal. Only successful treatment of the primary disturbance can return PCO_2 and $[HCO_3]$ to normal. Table 7.2 summarises blood gas results before, during and after compensation of acid-base disorders.

Renal compensation of respiratory disorders is much slower than respiratory compensation of metabolic disorders. In the first case, compensation occurs over a period of days or weeks but in the second, evidence of compensation is seen within hours.

Consequences of acid-base disturbances: clinical signs and symptoms

Whatever the cause, acid-base disturbances themselves result in signs and symptoms. Raised PCO_2 (hypercapnia) has non-specific effects on the central nervous system which may include confusion, headache and hand tremor. Coma may ensue if levels are particularly high. Reduced PCO_2 results in symptoms of lightheadedness or dizziness. Acidosis can cause hyperkalaemia; patients affected may have characteristic symptoms and ECG changes (page 67). Alkalosis decreases plasma concentration of ionised calcium; this causes symptoms of tetany, which include painful muscle cramps and spasm, pins and needles and paraesthesia. As we have seen, potassium depletion is an important cause of metabolic alkalosis, but alkalosis can itself cause hypokalaemia so that symptoms and signs of hypokalaemia (page 66) often accompany alkalosis, whatever the cause. Compensation for metabolic acidosis involves deep and rapid respiration to eliminate CO_2.

Mixed acid-base disturbances

Thus far, it has been assumed that any particular patient with a disturbance of acid-base balance suffers only one of the four categories of acid-base imbalance discussed. While this may well be the case, patients can present with a mixture

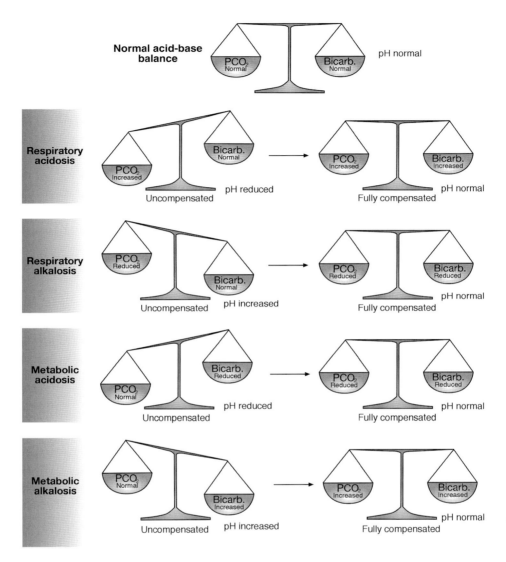

Figure 7.4 The 'acid-base balance': compensation restores normal pH.

of two or even three disturbances making interpretation of blood gas results more complex. As an example of a mixed disturbance, consider a patient with a chronic respiratory disease such as emphysema who has a heart attack and suffers cardiac arrest. Before the arrest, the patient has a partially compensated respiratory acidosis due to long-standing emphysema. The cardiac arrest causes metabolic acidosis. Results of blood gas analysis within a few hours after the arrest will reflect the combined effect of both respiratory and metabolic acidosis. Having regard to the causes of single acid-base disturbances, it is not difficult to imagine many other clinical situations in which a patient might be suffering more than one type of acid-base disturbance.

Table 7.2 Blood gas results in disturbances of acid-base balance.

Primary disturbance	Common causes	Compensatory mechanism	Initial blood gas results (uncompensated)	Blood gas results after partial compensation	Blood gas results after full compensation
Respiratory acidosis *primary increase in PCO$_2$*	Hypoventilation Respiratory failure Lung disease Depression of brain respiratory centre	RENAL & RBC increase bicarbonate	pH decreased PCO$_2$ increased Bicarb. normal	pH decreased but closer to normal PCO$_2$ increased Bicarb. increased	pH normal PCO$_2$ increased Bicarb. increased
Respiratory alkalosis *primary decrease in PCO$_2$*	Hyperventilation Anxiety attacks Stimulation of brain respiratory centre	RENAL & RBC decrease bicarbonate	pH increased PCO$_2$ decreased Bicarb. normal	pH increased but closer to normal PCO$_2$ decreased Bicarb. marginally decreased	pH normal PCO$_2$ decreased Bicarb. decreased
Metabolic acidosis *primary decrease in bicarbonate*	Renal failure Diabetic ketoacidosis Circulatory failure – clinical shock	RESPIRATORY decrease PCO$_2$	pH decreased PCO$_2$ normal Bicarb. decreased	pH decreased but closer to normal PCO$_2$ marginally decreased Bicarb. decreased	pH normal PCO$_2$ decreased Bicarb. decreased
Metabolic alkalosis *primary increase in bicarbonate*	Bicarbonate administration Potassium depletion	RESPIRATORY but very little compensation in metabolic alkalosis	pH increased PCO$_2$ normal Bicarb. increased	Very little compensation in metabolic alkalosis	

Causes and consequences of a low arterial blood PO$_2$

(hypoxaemia)
Breathing air which has relatively low PO$_2$ (e.g. atmospheric air at high altitude) will result in a low arterial blood PO$_2$, but clinically the most important causes are those in which gas exchange with blood across the alveolar membrane is compromised due to respiratory disease. Reduced PO$_2$ may thus occur in any condition that causes respiratory acidosis (p 110). However, hypoxaemia can occur in the absence of respiratory acidosis for example in pulmonary oedema. In the early stages of respiratory disease the hypoxic drive induced by low PO$_2$ increases respiration (and therefore CO$_2$ elimination) sufficient to maintain a normal or even low PCO$_2$. Respiratory acidosis develops late on in the disease process when even the hypoxic drive is insufficient to prevent CO$_2$ retention.

Finally, inadvertent sampling of venous blood rather than arterial blood causes falsely low results and this explanation should be considered if there is no clinical reason for a low PO$_2$.

From Figure 7.2 it can be seen that reduction in PO$_2$ reduces oxygen saturation of haemoglobin and therefore oxygen delivery to the tissues. Respiratory failure (defined in adults as a PO$_2$ of less than 8.0 kPa) causes breathlessness, confusion, sweating, tachycardia and cyanosis. In patients with accompanying respiratory acidosis, the symptoms of hypercapnia (page 112) may also be present.

Case history 6

When Mr Bridges, a 70-year-old man with a 10-year history of emphysema experienced sudden worsening of his symptoms, his wife called their GP who arranged immediate transfer to hospital. On arrival he was breathless, even while lying still. He was drowsy and confused. Arterial blood was sampled for blood gases. The laboratory reported the following results:

pH	7.28
PCO$_2$	8.8 kPa
Bicarbonate	35 mmol/l
PO$_2$	5.4 kPa

On admission to intensive care, he was mechanically ventilated and given oxygen. After 30 minutes' ventilation the patient showed signs of tetany. Results of blood gases at this time were:

pH	7.59
PCO$_2$	3.4 kPa
Bicarbonate	33 mmol/l
PO$_2$	10.9 kPa

Questions

(1) What was Mr Bridges acid-base and oxygen status on arrival at hospital?
(2) How does emphysema result in such an acid-base disturbance?
(3) Explain the relationship between symptoms and blood gas results.
(4) What is the acid-base and oxygen status after mechanical ventilation? Explain the marked change.
(5) What are the symptoms of tetany? Why did Mr Bridges have such symptoms?

Discussion of case history

(1) On arrival at hospital, Mr Bridges was acidotic (low pH). Acidosis may be respiratory (due to raised PCO_2) or metabolic (due to reduced bicarbonate). In this case, the acidosis is clearly of respiratory origin. A marked reduction in PO_2, consistent with respiratory failure and the medical history, substantiate this. Raised bicarbonate indicates some degree of compensation, emphasising the long-standing (chronic) nature of his condition. However, since the pH remains abnormal, compensation is incomplete. At the time of admission, then, Mr Bridges was suffering severe partially compensated respiratory acidosis and severe hypoxaemia.

(2) Emphysema is a chronic disease of the lungs in which the normal elasticity of the air sacs (alveoli) is progressively lost due to the destructive action of enzymes released from dead and dying phagocytic cells, recruited to the lungs to fight infection and inflammation. In the normal lung, these enzymes would be inactivated by specific blood-borne proteins, but in the emphysema patient, the balance between destructive enzyme production and inactivating protein production is lost. The consequence of the disease process is reduced alveolar area for exchange of oxygen and carbon dioxide between the environment and blood: PO_2 falls and PCO_2 rises. The rising PCO_2 in blood results in reduced blood pH (acidosis). To compensate and return pH towards normal, the kidneys regenerate more bicarbonate than usual and bicarbonate concentration increases.

(3) The cardinal symptom of emphysema is progressively worsening breathlessness due to hypoxaemia. Eventually, as in the case of Mr Bridges, the PO_2 drops so low that even at rest the patient is literally gasping for air. Severe hypercapnia may account for the confusion and drowsiness experienced by Mr Bridges.

(4) After 30 minutes of mechanical ventilation, Mr Bridges had a raised pH (alkalosis) which may be respiratory (reduced PCO_2) or metabolic (increased bicarbonate) in origin. Since the bicarbonate level remained unchanged, it must be the marked reduction in PCO_2 – brought about by mechanical ventilation – that caused the alkalosis. As a result of overenthusiastic ventilation, Mr Bridges then suffered respiratory alkalosis. The normal renal compensation for respiratory alkalosis is to decrease bicarbonate by renal mechanisms involving increased elimination in urine and decreased regeneration of bicarbonate. But this is a relatively slow process occurring over days rather than minutes, so in this case there was no evidence of compensation. Respiratory alkalosis due to overenthusiastic mechanical ventilation can be quickly corrected by reducing the rate of mechanical ventilation.

(5) The symptoms of tetany, which include 'pins and needles' sensation, muscular spasms, and – rarely – convulsions are due to a reduction of ionised plasma calcium, a substance required for normal neuromuscular transmission. Calcium in blood is present in two almost equal fractions: half is bound to the protein albumin and is physiologically inactive, and the other half is 'free' physiologically active, ionised calcium. The proportion of total calcium which is in the ionised state is determined in part by the pH of blood; if the pH of blood is high (i.e. alkalotic) then less calcium than normal is in the ionised physiologically active form and more is present bound to albumin and therefore physiologically inactive. Patients who have a raised blood pH, no matter what the cause, often have tetany. The symptoms of tetany disappear as the alkalosis is corrected and blood pH returns to normal.

Reference

1. Cousineau J, Anctil S *et al.* (2005) Neonate capillary blood gas reference values. *Clin Biochem* **38**: 905–907.

Further reading

Courtney S, Weber K *et al.* (1990) Capillary blood gases in the neonate: a reassessment and review of the literature. *Am J Dis Child* **144**: 168–72.

Crawford A (2004) An audit of the patient's experience of arterial blood gas testing. *Br J Nurs* **13**: 529–32.

Kellum J (2000) Determinants of blood pH in health and disease. *Crit Care* **4**: 6–14.

Kirskey K, Holt-Ashley M & Goodroad BK (2001) An easy method for interpreting results of blood gas analysis. *Crit Care Nurse* **21**: 49–54.

Sassoon C & Arruda J (eds) (2001) Acid base physiology and disorders: A special issue. *Respir Care* **46**: 328–403.

Thomson W, Adams J & Cowan R (1997) *Clinical Acid-Base Balance*. Oxford: Oxford Medical Publications.

Woodrow P (2004) Arterial blood gas analysis. *Nurs Stand* **18**(21): 45–52.

Chapter 8

SERUM/PLASMA CHOLESTEROL AND TRIGLYCERIDES

The principal use of this blood test is to help assess an individual's overall risk of the cardiovascular diseases that result from atherosclerosis. The most significant of these is coronary heart disease (CHD), which affects an estimated 2.6 million in the UK and is second only to cancer (all types) as the leading cause of death in the UK.[1] There is overwhelming evidence that too much cholesterol and/or triglyceride in the blood increases the risk of CHD and other related cardiovascular disease. The higher the level, the greater is this risk. The test is also used to monitor the effectiveness of therapy (drugs and dietary manipulation) aimed at reducing the amount of cholesterol and triglyceride in blood.

Normal physiology

What are cholesterol and triglycerides?

Apart from inorganic elements such as sodium, potassium, calcium etc., there are four broad classes of chemical present in the human body and the food we eat. They are: proteins, carbohydrates, nucleic acids and lipids (or fats). Although structurally dissimilar (Figure 8.1), cholesterol and triglycerides are lipids.

They are provided in a normal diet, both being present in meat and dairy products. Eggs are a particularly rich source of cholesterol. In addition to dietary sources, cholesterol and triglyceride are synthesised in the body, principally the liver (both cholesterol and triglyceride) and adipose or fat tissue (triglycerides only).

Function of cholesterol and triglycerides

In common with all lipids, cholesterol and triglycerides are essential components of all cell membranes. Their function is, however, not confined to cell structure. In the liver, cholesterol is converted to bile acids and bile salts, which are excreted from the liver, via the gall bladder, to the intestinal tract in the digestive juice, bile. The presence of bile acids and salts in bile is essential for absorption of dietary fats. Cholesterol is the raw material from which steroid hormones are synthesised; examples include cortisol in the adrenal glands, progesterone in the ovaries and

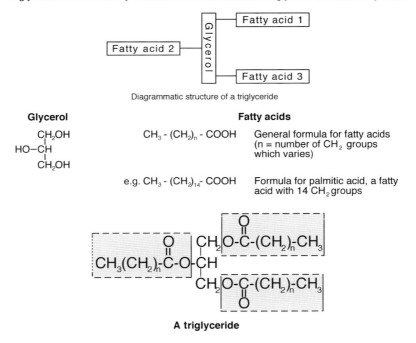

Figure 8.1 Structure of cholesterol and triglycerides.

testosterone in the testis. Vitamin D is synthesised in the skin from a cholesterol-derived compound.

Triglyceride is the principal fat present in adipose (fat) tissue and as such its main function is energy storage; triglycerides provide an alternative energy source to glucose during fasting and starvation when glucose is in short supply. During these periods of relative glucose depletion, triglyceride present in adipose cells is broken down to its constituent parts by an enzyme called lipase; the process is called lipolysis. The free fatty acids that result from lipolysis are transported in blood to cells around the body, where they are oxidised (burnt), providing chemical energy. Meanwhile the other product of lipolysis, glycerol, is converted to glucose in the liver.

Blood transport of cholesterol and triglyceride

Like all lipids, cholesterol and triglyceride are insoluble in water. This poses a difficulty for their transport in blood plasma, which is essentially a water-based solution of chemicals. To overcome the problem, lipids, including cholesterol and triglycerides, are packaged in a water-soluble protein shell called an apoprotein. The total package, lipids plus apoprotein is called a lipoprotein. There are four main types of lipoproteins in blood, each with differing proportions of cholesterol, triglyceride and apoprotein (Figure 8.2). They are defined by their relative density and particle size and are known as:

- chylomicrons (lowest density, largest particle)
- very low density lipoproteins (VLDLs)
- low density lipoproteins (LDLs)
- high density lipoproteins (HDLs).

Around 70% of the cholesterol in blood is present in LDL and most of the remainder is present in HDL. By contrast, most of the triglyceride in blood is contained within VLDL. As will become clear, the distinction between LDL-cholesterol and HDL-cholesterol is clinically important.

Laboratory measurement of plasma/serum cholesterol and triglyceride

Patient preparation

The concentration of cholesterol and triglyceride in blood is affected by diet, smoking, alcohol intake, intercurrent illness and even changes in posture. It is important that where possible blood is sampled under standard conditions to minimise some of these effects.

The patient's normal diet should be followed in the two to three weeks before testing.

There is a transient and quantitatively unpredictable rise in blood triglyceride level immediately after a meal, making interpretation difficult. For this reason, blood for triglyceride estimation must be sampled only after an overnight fast of 12–14 hours. Fasting is not essential if cholesterol only is to be measured.

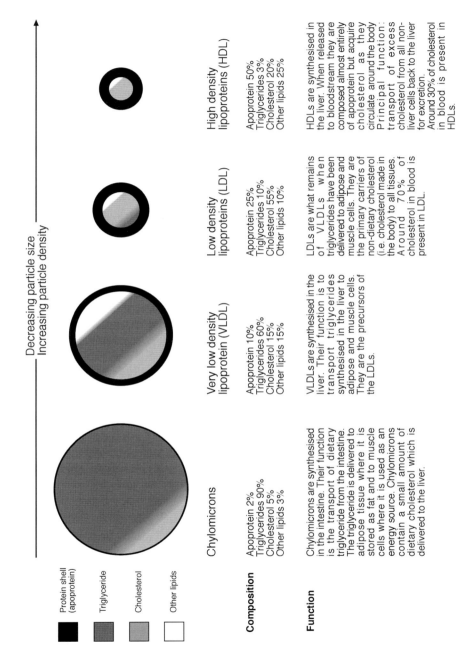

Decreasing particle size
Increasing particle density

Protein shell (apoprotein)

Triglyceride

Cholesterol

Other lipids

Chylomicrons

Very low density lipoprotein (VLDL)

Low density lipoproteins (LDL)

High density lipoproteins (HDL)

Composition

Apoprotein 2%
Triglycerides 90%
Cholesterol 5%
Other lipids 3%

Apoprotein 10%
Triglycerides 60%
Cholesterol 15%
Other lipids 15%

Apoprotein 25%
Triglycerides 10%
Cholesterol 55%
Other lipids 10%

Apoprotein 50%
Triglycerides 3%
Cholesterol 20%
Other lipids 25%

Function

Chylomicrons are synthesised in the intestine. Their function is the transport of dietary triglyceride from the intestine. The triglyceride is delivered to adipose tissue where it is stored as fat and to muscle cells where it is used as an energy source. Chylomicrons contain a small amount of dietary cholesterol which is delivered to the liver.

VLDLs are synthesised in the liver. Their function is to transport triglycerides synthesised in the liver to adipose and muscle cells. They are the precursors of the LDLs.

LDLs are what remains of VLDLs when triglycerides have been delivered to adipose and muscle cells. They are the primary carriers of non-dietary cholesterol (i.e. cholesterol made in the body) to all tissues. Around 70% of cholesterol in blood is present in LDL.

HDLs are synthesised in the liver. When released to bloodstream they are composed almost entirely of apoprotein but acquire cholesterol as they circulate around the body. Principal function: transport of excess cholesterol from all non-liver cells back to the liver for excretion. Around 30% of cholesterol in blood is present in HDLs.

Figure 8.2 Structure, composition and function of lipoproteins.

The test should be deferred for three months if the patient has suffered major illness (e.g. myocardial infarction) or major surgery unless blood can be sampled within 12 hours of such an event. The test should be deferred for two to three weeks after minor illness.

The patients should be well rested and seated for 5–10 minutes before blood collection.

Use of a tourniquet for more than a minute or so before blood collection can cause erroneous results. If possible, avoid the use of tourniquet for this test.

Interpretation of results is not possible if blood is sampled during lipid infusion (e.g. intralipid).

Sample requirement

Around 5 ml of venous blood is required. The test may be performed on either plasma or serum. If local policy is to use serum, then blood must be collected into a plain chemistry tube (i.e. without anticoagulant). If local policy is to use plasma, then blood must be collected into a tube containing an anticoagulant (EDTA or heparin), which prevents blood from clotting.

In the laboratory

Three measurements are made in the laboratory:

- serum or plasma concentration of total cholesterol (i.e. cholesterol contained in LDL, HDL and VLDL)
- serum or plasma concentration of HDL-cholesterol (i.e. only the cholesterol contained in HDL)
- serum or plasma concentration of triglycerides (i.e. triglyceride contained in VLDL, LDL and HDL).

The concentration of serum or plasma LDL-cholesterol is technically difficult to measure and in most laboratories is calculated using the results of analysis in the following equation:

LDL-cholesterol = total cholesterol − HDL-cholesterol − (Triglyceride/2.2)

Interpretation of results

Reference range

Fasting triglycerides   0.45–1.80 mmol/l

Unlike most other blood tests, the concept of a normal or reference range is not considered appropriate for cholesterol testing. This is because a large proportion of apparently healthy individuals from which a reference range would be constructed have a cholesterol level that is associated with an increased risk of cardiovascular disease. In other words, it is 'normal' to have an unhealthy amount of cholesterol in blood. Rather than a *reference* range, the concept of *target* values is used to interpret cholesterol results. Target values will be discussed a little later, but for now it would be helpful to record some data about serum cholesterol concentration in the UK population.

- The mean serum/plasma total cholesterol for UK adults (> 16 yrs) is 5.5 mmol/l for men and 5.6 mmol/l for women.[1]
- The National Service Framework target for CHD prevention is a serum/plasma total cholesterol < 5.0 mmol/l.[2]
- Around 66% of UK adults have total cholesterol > 5.0 mmol/l.[1]

Terms used in interpretation

Hyperlipidaemia	raised concentration of lipids in blood, i.e. total cholesterol > 5.0 mmol/l and/or triglyceride > 1.80 mmol/l
Hypercholesterolaemia	raised concentration of total cholesterol, i.e > 5.0 mmol/l
Hypertriglyceridaemia	raised blood concentration of triglyceride, i.e. > 1.80 mmol/l

Consequences of raised cholesterol or triglyceride

Cardiovascular disease

As the concentration of serum/plasma total cholesterol rises, so too does the risk of those cardiovascular diseases that result from the restricted blood flow through arteries diseased by atherosclerosis and associated thrombotic (blood clotting) consequences. Atherosclerosis may affect any artery, but the most commonly affected are the coronary arteries. The result is coronary heart disease, the most common cardiovascular disease.

Coronary heart disease

Coronary heart disease (CHD) (alternative name ischaemic heart disease) is caused by atherosclerosis in the coronary arteries that supply oxygenated blood to heart muscle (the myocardium). The focal thickening and hardening of the normally elastic walls of coronary arteries that characterises atherosclerosis progressively reduces the internal diameter of the artery, restricting blood flow and therefore oxygen delivery to the cells of which the myocardium is composed. The portion of myocardium affected becomes relatively deficient of oxygen (ischaemic). The first clinical manifestation of this relative oxygen deficit is usually angina pectoris or stable angina, intermittent attacks of chest pain or discomfort precipitated by increased heart rate due to exercise or some other stress. The pain subsides as rest and return of resting heart rate reduces the increased oxygen demand of myocardium.

Atherosclerosis predisposes to the inappropriate activation of the clotting cascade and formation of a blood clot (thrombus) within blood vessels at the site of atherosclerosis. This further occludes or totally occludes blood flow through the artery, effectively starving myocardial cells of the nutrients and oxygen required for survival. The clinical consequence of this is either unstable angina that is chest pain at rest or myocardial infarction (heart attack). The two conditions are referred to as acute coronary syndromes. A diagnosis of unstable angina implies high risk of future myocardial infarction. Myocardial infarction implies tissue necrosis (cell death), i.e. permanent damage to heart muscle as a result of ischaemia. The damage to the heart may result in sudden death if it causes lethal abnormal rhythms (ventricular fibrillation).

Stable angina, unstable angina, myocardial infarction and sudden death represent the most common manifestations of coronary heart disease in order of severity. They do not necessarily present in this ordered sequence and myocardial infarction or sudden death may be the first indication of coronary disease.

Other cardiovascular disease

Other less commonly affected sites affected by atherosclerosis include:

- peripheral arteries that supply oxygenated blood to the limbs
- cerebral arteries, which supply oxygenated blood to the brain
- abdominal aorta, lower half of the main blood vessel (aorta) that delivers oxygenated blood to the body.

Peripheral arterial disease usually affects the legs. Reduced oxygen delivery (consequent on reduced blood flow) to the leg causes calf muscle pain on exercise, which is relieved by rest (intermittent claudication). The most severe presentation occurs if a thrombus forms at the site of atherosclerosis, totally occluding blood flow through the affected artery. Without urgent treatment to restore blood flow, resulting acute ischaemia can lead to necrosis, gangrene and the need for amputation.

Reduced blood flow through cerebral arteries partially occluded by atherosclerosis is a common cause of transient ischaemic attacks. (mini-strokes). Occlusion of cerebral arteries by a thrombus formed at the site of atherosclerosis is the most common cause of cerebrovascular accident (stroke), which can result in permanent disability or death.

Atherosclerosis in the abdominal aorta contributes to the weakening of the wall of this large vessel that results in dangerous dilation (aneurysm). This can be asymptomatic or cause abdominal pain. Without surgical repair to the vessel, progressive dilation can lead to catastrophic rupture of the aneurysm, massive haemorrhage and sudden death.

Blood lipids and cardiovascular disease

Atherosclerosis, the underlying pathology of coronary heart disease and other cardiovascular disease outlined above, is a complex and as yet not fully understood phenomenon, which begins many years before symptoms develop. It is clear, however, that there are well-defined risk factors (Table 8.1) that predispose people to atherosclerosis and subsequent cardiovascular disease. Some, like cholesterol and triglyceride are modifiable, and some are not.

All risk factors must be taken into account to make the most reliable assessment of an individual's overall risk of CHD.

To understand how the lipids in blood, particularly cholesterol, contribute to CHD and other cardiovascular disease it is necessary to examine in a little more detail what is known about the process of atheroma formation, which leads to atherosclerosis and thrombosis.

Atheroma formation begins with damage to the endothelium that lines the internal surface of arteries, allowing entry of cholesterol-rich LDL particles present in blood. The damage attracts protective cells called macrophages, which take up the LDL particles; LDL accumulates in these cells. At this early stage, the only

Table 8.1 Major risk factors for coronary heart disease.

Increasing age
Family history of CHD
Diabetes
   Diabetics have 2 to 4 times the risk of CHD compared with non-diabetics who in all
   other respects have a similar risk status
Cigarette smoking*
Hypertension*
Obesity*
   Defined as body mass index BMI (i.e. weight in kgs/height in metres) > 25
   Obesity associated with hypertension, raised total and LDL cholesterol and reduced
   HDL-cholesterol
Unhealthy diet*
   High fat diet (i.e. fat more than 30% of total calorific intake) ⎫
   High intake of saturated rather then unsaturated fat   ⎬ causes increase in serum
   High intake of cholesterol   ⎭ total and LDL cholesterol
   Diet devoid of fruit and vegetables which provide protective antioxidant vitamins
   High salt diet (predisposes to hypertension)
Excess alcohol*
   Although 1 or 2 drinks per day protects against heart disease, as alcohol intake rises
   above 21 units per week so too does risk of CHD. Excess alcohol causes hypertension
Lack of exercise*
   Exercise reduces body weight and increases serum HDL-cholesterol
Abnormal concentration of blood lipids*
   Raised serum total cholesterol
   Raised serum LDL-cholesterol
   Reduced serum HDL-cholesterol
   High ratio serum total cholesterol: serum HDL-cholesterol

Modifiable risk factors

evidence of atheroma is a barely visible raised yellowish patch on the internal surface of the artery, known as a fatty streak. Development of the fatty streak to the more ominous and complex fatty plaque that protrudes into the lumen of the artery is thought to involve an inflammatory reaction initiated by the death of the cells engorged with LDL-cholesterol. The normal smooth muscle cells of which arterial walls are composed migrate into the plaque, proliferate and synthesise fibrous proteins like collagen, which renders the growing plaque hard. The atherosclerotic plaque has a lipid-rich centre surrounded by a dynamic fibrous cap composed of collagen protein and pro-inflammatory cells. The strength and stability of the cap is of great pathological significance because this determines if thrombosis occurs. A thin and fragile cap may rupture, exposing the platelets in blood flowing through the vessel to substances beneath the cap that promote platelet aggregation and activation at the site of the ruptured plaque. This in turn initiates the clotting cascade with formation of a blood clot (thrombus), which may completely occlude blood flow.

In general, stable angina is associated with a stable plaque, whereas acute coronary syndromes (unstable angina and myocardial infarction) are associated with an unstable plaque, plaque rupture and consequent thrombosis.

The growth of atherosclerotic plaques to the point where they can occlude blood flow sufficiently to cause symptoms of cardiovascular disease is very slow, occurring over a period of many years. There is now evidence that by addressing risk factors such as hyperlipidaemia it is possible to halt or even reverse plaque progression.[3]

Research directed at better understanding of the complexities of atherosclerosis continues, but some aspects are clear.

- Accumulation of cholesterol, specifically LDL-cholesterol is an important requirement for atheroma formation.
- The LDL-cholesterol found in atherosclerotic plaques is derived from the blood.
- The higher the concentration of cholesterol in blood, the greater is the risk of CHD and other cardiovascular disease.
- It is specifically LDL-cholesterol that is damaging; the higher the LDL, the greater is the risk of CHD.
- By contrast, HDL is protective against CHD because it clears the blood of cholesterol. The lower the HDL-cholesterol, the greater is the risk of CHD. A high level of HDL-cholesterol is associated with reduced risk of CHD.
- Reducing the concentration of total cholesterol in a patient with raised levels is effective in reducing the overall risk of CHD.
- The link between blood triglyceride and CHD is currently less clear. There is evidence that particularly among those who have an increased LDL-cholesterol or a reduced HDL-cholesterol, a raised blood triglyceride increases yet further the risk of CHD.
- There is little evidence, however, to suggest that reducing raised triglyceride levels decreases the risk of CHD.

It must be emphasised that blood lipid testing determines *risk* only; results cannot be used to diagnose or definitively predict CHD for a particular individual. Some have a raised LDL-cholesterol and do not suffer CHD; and there is no safe level of cholesterol or triglyceride below which one can be guaranteed not to suffer CHD. The best we can say is that the higher the level of LDL-cholesterol, the greater is the risk of CHD; that risk is increased if triglycerides are also raised, and reduced by a high HDL-cholesterol level.

Other effects of raised blood lipids

There are few signs or symptoms to suggest that an individual may have an increased level of cholesterol or triglyceride and the onset of anginal pain or myocardial infarction may be the first indication. Lipid deposits (xanthomata) visible as nodules may form in subcutaneous tissue among those with very high levels. Lipid may also accumulate in the cornea. Severe hypertriglyceridaemia is associated with abdominal pain and is a rare cause of acute pancreatitis.

Causes of raised cholesterol and/or triglycerides

Many genetic defects in lipid metabolism have been identified which result in either a raised cholesterol, a raised triglyceride or both, so it is possible to inherit a predisposition to raised blood lipids. This in part explains the observation that coronary heart disease runs in families. One of these inherited conditions is extremely common, several are less common and most are extremely rare. All are grouped together in the term *primary hyperlipidaemias*. A raised cholesterol or triglyceride may arise as a complication of another disease process; this is called *secondary hyperlipidaemia*. Treatment of the underlying disease often corrects secondary hyperlipidaemia.

Primary hyperlipidaemia

The most common cause of primary hyperlipidaemia is known as 'polygenic' hypercholesterolaemia. As its name implies many genes interact to cause raised cholesterol. The condition results in mild to moderate increase in LDL-cholesterol, the actual level depending to a great extent on diet. Triglyceride levels are usually normal. Much higher levels of LDL-cholesterol, often greater than 9.0 mmol/l, characterise a less common inherited condition known as familial hypercholesterolaemia which affects around 1 in 500 in the UK. This single gene defect is associated with high risk of myocardial infarction in early middle age.

Although rare, it is possible to inherit a predisposition to raised triglyceride levels. Familial hypertriglyceridaemia is the most common genetic cause of raised triglyceride. Levels are usually very high (> 10 mmol/l). Cholesterol levels are usually normal. Risk of CHD is not greatly increased for this group of patients.

Secondary hyperlipidaemias

The most common cause of secondary hyperlipidaemia is diabetes mellitus. Untreated diabetic patients tend to have a mild increase in LDL-cholesterol and moderate to severe increase in triglyceride. This is, at least in part, the reason why diabetic patients are at high risk of coronary heart disease. Other causes of secondary hyperlipidaemia include hypothyroidism, nephrotic syndrome, cholestatic liver disease and alcohol abuse.

National guidelines (recommendations) for prevention of cardiovascular disease[4]

The Joint British Societies guidelines[4] identify the following groups of people who require careful monitoring of blood cholesterol and cholesterol-lowering drug intervention to reduce blood cholesterol because they are all at equally high risk of future cardiovascular disease:

- those with a history of atherosclerotic cardiovascular disease (e.g. angina, myocardial infarction, stroke, etc.)
- those with diabetes (types 1 and 2)
- those with elevated blood pressure (> 160 mm Hg systolic or > 100 mm Hg diastolic)
- those with hypercholesterolaemia (defined as total cholesterol to HDL-cholesterol ratio > 6)
- those without cardiovascular but whose quantified risk of CVD during the next 10 years is > 20%.

(It is recommended that all adults over the age of 40 who have no *history of cardiovascular disease be assessed in primary care every five years using the new Joint British Societies risk charts to quantify their 10-year risk of cardiovascular disease. This risk assessment is based on consideration of the following five major risk factors: age, sex, smoking habit, systolic blood pressure and ratio of total to HDL-cholesterol.*)

The optimal total cholesterol target for all those in these high risk groups is < 4 mmol/l, and that for LDL-cholesterol < 2.0 mmol/l. The previous recommended targets contained in the National Service Framework for CHD prevention (total cholesterol < 5.0 mmol/l and LDL-cholesterol < 3.0) have thus been revised downwards in the light of accumulating evidence that reducing total and LDL-cholesterol yet further has benefit in terms of reducing both morbidity and mortality due to cardiovascular disease.

Case history 7

Michael Oliver, a 41-year-old accountant in good health attended a 'well man' clinic at his GP's surgery. A family health history and lifestyle questionnaire revealed a family history of heart disease; his 61-year-old father was currently recovering from a heart attack and his grandfather had died of 'heart disease' at the age of 71. His father's recent illness had prompted Michael to quit smoking but he took little exercise. As part of the health screen Michael was weighed, his blood pressure was taken and blood was sampled for blood glucose and lipid screen. Body weight and blood pressure were normal. Clinical examination was unremarkable. The laboratory reported the following blood results:

Blood glucose	5.6 mmol/l
Plasma total cholesterol	5.9 mmol/l
Plasma LDL-cholesterol	4.3 mmol/l
Plasma HDL-cholesterol	0.97 mmol/l
Plasma triglyceride	1.0 mmol/l

In view of his father's illness, Michael was most concerned about his own risk of heart disease. Consider the advice that might be given.

Discussion of case history

To advise Michael it is necessary to consider all risk factors for coronary heart disease. The recommended method for making this risk assessment is the new Joint British Societies risk assessment charts, which take account of age, sex, systolic blood pressure, smoking habit and ratio of total cholesterol to HDL-cholesterol. In Michael's case, the cholesterol ratio (5.9/0.97) is 6.1, which places him in a high-risk group irrespective of the results of global risk assessment. This indicates that Michael would benefit from reducing his total and LDL-cholesterol. The recommended targets are total cholesterol < 4.0 mmol/l and LDL-cholesterol of < 2.0 mmol/l. This might be achievable by lifestyle changes (e.g. dietary changes, increased exercise) but if this fails, a cholesterol-lowering drug, most commonly a statin, might be advised. However, before embarking on this course it is important to confirm the hyperlipidaemia on two further occasions, because of the biological variability of serum cholesterol. Due consideration should also be given to the possibility that raised cholesterol is due to some underlying disease.

References

1. Peterson S, Peto V et al. (2005) Coronary heart disease statistics. London: British Heart Foundation.
2. Department of Health (2000) National Service Framework for Coronary Heart Disease: Modern standards and service models. Product no 16602, DoH.
3. Okazaki S, Yokoyama T et al. (2004) Early statin treatment in patients with acute coronary syndrome: demonstration of the beneficial effect on atherosclerotic lesions by serial volumetric intravascular ultrasound analysis during half a year after coronary event: the ESTABLISH study. Circulation 110: 1061–68.
4. Joint British Societies (2005) Joint British Societies guidelines on prevention of cardiovascular disease in clinical practice. Heart 91(suppl v): v1–v52.

Further reading

Nelson M & Tonkin A (2004) Secondary prevention of CHD. Aust Fam Physician 34: 433–40.
Lindsay G & Gaw A (eds) (2003) Coronary Heart Disease Prevention: A handbook for the healthcare team (2nd edn). Edinburgh: Churchill Livingstone. ISBN 0443071179.

Chapter 9

CARDIAC MARKERS

Chest pain is a common reason for adults to seek medical help, either in primary care or at the hospital emergency department. This chapter is concerned with how laboratory testing contributes to the differential diagnosis of patients presenting with chest pain. The tests to be considered are measurement of the concentration in serum or plasma of troponins (cTnT and cTnI); myoglobin; and creatine kinase (CK(MB)). Although functionally and structurally unrelated, all are present in cardiac muscle cells and released to blood during cardiac muscle injury; they are known as cardiac markers. The principal use of the tests is to help identify those patients whose chest pain is due to myocardial infarction, the acute and life-threatening manifestation of coronary heart disease commonly known as a 'heart attack'.

Every year in the UK around 250 000 people suffer myocardial infarction.[1] The damage to the heart may be sufficient to cause immediate lethal arrhythmia, cardiac arrest and sudden death; around 20% die before medical help arrives. For the remaining victims, early diagnosis and treatment can be life saving and minimises permanent damage to the heart. Some emergency care and coronary care units have dedicated analysers for measurement of these cardiac markers, allowing rapid point of care testing. In these circumstances, nursing staff may have delegated responsibility for the analytical process.

Normal physiology

Troponin

There are three main muscle types in the human body: smooth muscle, present in the wall of those hollow organs whose function depends on muscle wall contraction (gastrointestinal tract, uterus, blood vessels etc); skeletal muscle; and cardiac muscle (the myocardium) which makes up the bulk of the heart wall.

Troponin (Tn) is a constituent of cardiac and skeletal muscle cells where it functions as a structural component of the contractile assembly (myofibrils) that enables muscles to contract. It is composed of three polypeptide sub-units: troponin C (TnC), troponin I (TnI) and troponin T(TnT). The whole troponin complex is located on the actin filament of the myofibril. The interaction between actin and myosin filaments that facilitates muscle contraction is initiated by calcium ions binding to troponin C. Troponin I binding of actin inhibits contraction. By these two opposing effects, one initiating contraction of myofibrils, the other inhibiting the process, troponin plays a major role in regulating contraction of both skeletal and cardiac muscle.

There are tissue specific isoforms of troponins C, I and T. This means that it is possible to distinguish cardiac muscle troponin (cTn) from skeletal muscle troponin. Normally all the troponin in the body is contained within skeletal and cardiac muscle cells; it is virtually undetectable in blood. However, if muscle cells are damaged, their contents, including troponin, are released to the bloodstream and plasma concentration rises. If only cardiac muscle is damaged, only troponin composed of the cardiac isoforms of troponin sub-units C, I and T (i.e. cTnC, cTnI, and cTnT) will appear in blood. There are two troponin tests currently used for assessment of patients with chest pain. Some laboratories measure serum or plasma concentration of cTnT; others measure serum or plasma concentration of cTnI. Of many potential candidates, the troponins cTnT and cTnI have emerged as the cardiac markers of choice because of their superior specificity and sensitivity for cardiac damage.[2]

Creatine kinase (MB) CK(MB)

Creatine kinase (alternative name, creatine phosphokinase, CPK) is an enzyme which catalyses the transfer of phosphate from creatine phosphate to adenosine diphosphate. The products of the reaction are creatine and the energy rich compound, adenosine triphosphate.

Creatine phosphate + Adenosine diphosphate →
Creatine + Adenosine triphosphate

CK is present in many types of tissue cells, but three sorts of tissue contain most of the body's CK. They are: cardiac muscle (myocardium), skeletal muscle and the brain.

Creatine kinase is composed of two protein sub-units, M and B, allowing three functionally identical, but structurally different isoenzymes: CK(MM), CK(BB) and CK(MB). CK isoenzymes are tissue specific. Most of the CK(BB) is found in the brain; most of the CK(MM) is in skeletal muscle and most of the CK(MB) is in cardiac muscle cells. Thus CK(MB) is a fraction of total CK which is confined to the cells of which heart muscle are composed. Normally blood plasma contains very little CK(MB) but following damage to heart muscle, blood plasma concentration rises. CK(MB) is considered the best alternative cardiac marker, if troponin is not available.[2]

Myoglobin

Myoglobin is a protein, present only in cardiac and skeletal muscle cells, that is structurally and functionally related to haemoglobin, the oxygen-carrying protein present in red cells (erythrocytes). Like haemoglobin, myoglobin reversibly binds oxygen, but whereas haemoglobin has four oxygen binding sites myoglobin has just one. The principal function of myoglobin is storage of oxygen in muscle cells for release under conditions of relative oxygen deficiency. There is normally negligible or undetectable amount of myoglobin in blood but damage to muscle cells (either skeletal or cardiac muscle) results in release to blood and rising plasma levels. Myoglobin is less suitable as a cardiac marker than either troponin or CK(MB) because it is present in skeletal muscle and therefore less specific for cardiac damage. However, it does allow earlier diagnosis than either of the above tests. It is less widely available than either of the other tests.

Laboratory measurement of troponins (cTnT cTnI), myoglobin and CK(MB)

Patient preparation

No particular patient preparation is necessary.

Timing of blood collection

Most hospitals have a protocol for timing of blood sampling for cardiac markers among patients presenting with chest pain. Commonly blood is sampled on admission and again 9–12 hours later. Further testing at 24 hours may be necessary. Interpretation of test results depends crucially on knowing when the blood was sampled in relation to the time of onset of symptoms of chest pain. For these reasons, it is important to record on the accompanying request card both the time blood is sampled and the time of onset of symptoms (if known) or time of admission.

Amount and type of sample

Around 5 ml of blood is sufficient for cardiac markers. The assays are performed on either plasma or serum, although there is some evidence to suggest that plasma samples are less suitable for cTnT than serum samples.[3] If local policy is to use plasma, then blood must be collected into a tube containing the anticoagulant lithium heparin. If local policy is to use serum, then blood must be collected into a plain glass tube, without any additive. Haemolysed samples (see pages 59–60 for explanation) are unsuitable for troponin testing – repeat blood sampling is necessary if haemolysis is present.

Interpretation of results

Reference ranges

It would be inappropriate to provide definitive reference ranges for these four tests because of varying and currently evolving laboratory methodology. Interpretation of patient results should always be made using reference ranges (or diagnostic cut off values) provided by the laboratory that performed the test(s). Suffice to say there is normally very little (often undetectable quantities) of any of these cardiac markers in blood.

To give some indication of the numbers and units of measurement involved, below is a range of upper limit of reference range (ULRR) or cut off values for diagnosis of myocardial infarction for each of the four cardiac markers that have appeared in the medical literature over the past decade:

Serum/plasma cTnT	0.03–0.5 ng/ml
Serum/plasma cTnI	0.1–3.1 ng/ml
Serum/plasma myoglobin	70–110 ng/ml
Serum/plasma CK(MB)	4.0–9.0 ng/ml.

(Confusingly, some laboratories use µg/l as the unit of concentration rather than ng/ml as above. They are in fact the same, i.e. 10 ng/ml = 10 µg/l)

Causes of raised serum or plasma concentration of cTnT, cTnI, myoglobin and CK(MB)

Cardiac muscle cell death (myocardial necrosis) is the only cause for an increase in serum or plasma concentration of cTnT and cTnI. It is also the principal but not the sole cause for an increase in plasma or serum concentration of both CK(MB) and myoglobin. The most common cause of myocardial necrosis is myocardial infarction.

Myocardial infarction and coronary heart disease

All cells require a continuous supply of oxygen rich blood for survival. Ischaemia is the term used to describe deficient blood supply to an area of tissue and infarction is the term for the death of tissue that results if ischaemia is sufficiently severe or prolonged. Myocardial infarction is the death of an area of heart muscle tissue due to ischaemia. Almost invariably in cases of myocardial infarction, ischaemia is the result of coronary heart disease.

The atherosclerotic plaque is the pathological lesion that defines coronary heart disease. This is a focal accumulation of lipid and cellular material beneath a fibrous cap on the internal surface of a coronary artery. During a long subclinical period of many years, the plaque may grow to the point where it reduces blood flow sufficiently to cause symptoms of reduced oxygen delivery to an area of heart muscle. The main symptom is ischaemic chest pain, which is often experienced as discomfort rather than as a sharp or stabbing pain. Tightness, pressure, constriction and strangling are common descriptors of ischaemic chest pain. It is usually diffusely located across the chest and may radiate to neck, throat, jaw, shoulders or arm.

The least severe and most common manifestation of coronary heart disease is the ischaemic chest pain associated with stable angina. A patient with stable angina experiences chest pain or discomfort only during periods of increased oxygen demand, for example during exertion or other stress (e.g. emotional stress) that causes heart rate to increase. Symptoms disappear as the heart's demand for oxygen is reduced by rest. The reduced oxygen delivery to heart muscle cells that causes ischaemic pain in those with stable angina is not sufficient to cause cell death. There is therefore no increase in the serum or plasma concentration of any of the four cardiac markers among patients whose chest pain is the result of stable angina.

The first manifestation of coronary heart disease may not be stable angina but the more serious acute coronary syndrome (ACS). This is not a single entity but a spectrum of disease of increasing severity that includes myocardial infarction. The pathological feature that defines ACS is plaque instability. For reasons that remain poorly understood, the fibrous cap which protects the underlying lipid and cellular contents of an atherosclerotic plaque from the blood flowing through an affected artery, may be thin, fragile and prone to disruption (rupture). It is the patients whose plaques have these vulnerable characteristics that are most at risk of the life-threatening consequences of coronary heart disease. Plaque rupture exposes the platelets in blood to the pro-coagulant environment of the plaque contents. A single thrombus may form at the site of the exposed plaque, partially or totally occluding blood flow. Alternatively debris from the plaque, along with fragments of thrombi, may embolise to smaller vessels where they may occlude blood flow at a site remote from the plaque. It is in the context of these variable effects of plaque disruption that ACS is evident.

The mildest clinical presentation of ACS is unstable angina. This is the same ischaemic chest pain or discomfort as that experienced by patients suffering stable angina. However, in the case of unstable angina, symptoms are experienced at rest or on minimal exertion, and are generally of longer duration and greater intensity. A definitive feature of unstable angina and one that distinguishes it from the more serious presentation of ACS, myocardial infarction, is the absence of myocardial necrosis. As with stable angina, the ischaemia associated with unstable angina is not sufficient to cause cell death, so cardiac markers remain within normal limits. However, unstable angina is clinical evidence of an unstable plaque and therefore high risk of myocardial infarction in the immediate future or later. Around 15% of patients with unstable angina suffer myocardial infarction during the seven days following diagnosis.

Myocardial infarction and cardiac markers

If the ischaemia induced by thrombus or other occlusion of an artery is severe and prolonged, the myocardial cells that are supplied by the vessel simply die. This is myocardial infarction. The volume of myocardium affected varies greatly from < 1 to > 25 g depending on the site of occlusion, and this is reflected in the variable electrocardiographic (ECG) changes and mortality associated with myocardial infarction.[4] In all cases there is an increase in the plasma concentration of cardiac markers; indeed an increase in the plasma concentration of troponin (either cTnT, or cTnI) or CK(MB) is an essential criterion for diagnosis of myocardial infarction (Table 9.1). The magnitude of the increase reflects the amount of tissue destroyed and therefore severity of the infarct.

Crushing ischaemic chest pain or discomfort at rest, usually lasting not less than 20 minutes, marks the onset of severe myocardial infarction in the majority of

Table 9.1 Definition of myocardial infarction[1].

The following criteria satisfy the diagnosis of acute, evolving or recent MI:
  Typical rise and gradual fall (troponin) or more rapid rise and fall (CK-MB) of biochemical markers of myocardial necrosis with at least one of the following:

- ischaemic symptoms (see text)
- development of Q waves on ECG
- ECG evidence of ischaemia (ST segment elevation or depression)
- coronary artery intervention (e.g. coronary angioplasty)

cases. Additional symptoms include breathlessness, lightheadedness, sweating, nausea, and vomiting. Extensive tissue ischaemia is reflected in the early characteristic electrocardiograph (ECG) change (ST elevation) that gives this severe presentation its name: ST elevation myocardial infarction (STEMI). Myocardial necrosis is not immediate and begins only after a finite period ($\approx$10–15 minutes) of ischaemia. Necrosis of all the tissue at risk occurs gradually over the following 4 to 6 hours or longer, providing a window of therapeutic opportunity to limit the damage with thrombolytic/reperfusion therapy.

The rise in plasma concentration of cardiac markers following myocardial infarction is a transitory phenomenon, related to the time of infarction. No change occurs during the first hour after onset of symptoms.

Myoglobin is the first of the four cardiac markers to be released to blood and a rise in plasma myoglobin concentration is detectable within 1–2 hours after the onset of symptoms. (Figure 9.1). Peak concentration is reached at 6–7 hours, followed by a gradual return to normal between 12–24 hours onset of symptoms.

The rise in cTnI, cTnT and CK(MB) is a little delayed compared with myoglobin and typically begins between 4–8 hours after onset of symptoms, although may be earlier in particular cases. Peak levels occur at about 12–24 hours after onset of symptoms.

CK(MB) concentration returns to normal within 2–3 days but both cTnI and cTnT remain raised for much longer, up to 2 weeks in some cases.

Myocardial infarction can usually be excluded as the cause of chest pain if plasma or serum concentration of either CK(MB), cTnT, or cTnI remains within normal limits during the 12 hours following onset of symptoms. There may still be clinical doubt, in which case repeat testing at 24 hours is indicated. If this confirms previous normal results, myocardial infarction is definitively excluded. However, this does not exclude the possibility that chest pain is of cardiac origin, because cardiac markers always remain within normal limits in patients with stable and unstable angina.

Other causes of myocardial necrosis

Although the ischaemia associated with myocardial infarction is the most common cause of myocardial necrosis, it is not the only cause, so cardiac markers may be raised in conditions other than myocardial infarction.[5]

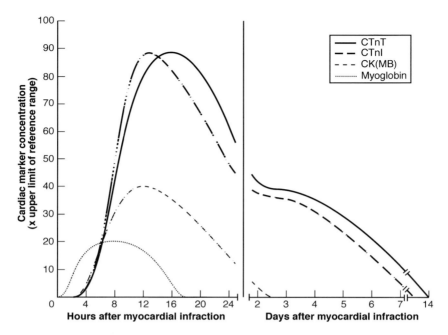

Figure 9.1 Typical time-related change in cardiac marker concentration following myocardial infarction.

These conditions include myocarditis (inflammatory infection of heart muscle), pericarditis (inflammation of the membrane that covers the heart), pulmonary embolism, renal failure, trauma to the heart (e.g. during cardiac surgery) and sepsis. In general, these conditions are associated with only slight increase in cardiac markers.

Skeletal muscle disease

Myoglobin is present in skeletal muscle and serum myoglobin concentration is raised in conditions associated with muscle cell destruction e.g. rhabdomyolysis, severe trauma, etc.

Case history 8

Henry Jarvis, a 58-year-old retired teacher with a history of myocardial infarction three years previously, developed chest pains while working in the garden. Within an hour, he arrived by ambulance at his local hospital emergency department. Clinical history and examination suggested a provisional diagnosis of myocardial infarction but ECG trace was normal, save evidence of previous infarct. He was admitted to coronary care. Blood was collected for measurement of cardiac markers according to local protocol, on admission (sample 1); at 9 hours post admission (sample 2); and again at 24 hours post admission (sample 3).

Sample 1	serum cTnI	0.4 µg/l
	serum CK(MB)	3.9 µg/l
Sample 2	serum cTnI	3.1 µg/l
	serum CK(MB)	3.8 µg/l
Sample 3	serum cTnI	2.4 µg/l
	serum CK(MB)	4.1 µg/l

Laboratory upper limit of the reference range

| troponin | 0.5 µg/l |
| CK(MB) | 5.0 µg/l |

Questions

(1) Would you expect the results of sample 1 to show elevated cTnI and CK(MB) if Mr Jarvis had suffered a myocardial infarction?

(2) What do the serum cTnI results indicate?

(3) What do the serum CK(MB) results indicate?

(4) Did Mr Jarvis suffer myocardial infarction? Explain.

Discussion of case history

(1) Not necessarily. There is a delay between the onset of chest pain and a rise in the concentration of cardiac markers. The increase in cTnI and CK(MB) starts on average between 4 and 6 hours after onset of pain and Mr Jarvis's blood was sampled just an hour after onset of symptoms. Normal cardiac markers on admission cannot be used to exclude a diagnosis of myocardial infarction.

(2) The serum cTnI results at 9 hours and 24 hours were marginally raised. The combination of raised cTnI and typical clinical symptoms of ischaemic disease allow a diagnosis of myocardial infarction. The magnitude of the increase in cTnI was small, indicating only minimal tissue loss. The results indicate minimal or micro-infarction.

(3) The serum CK(MB) remains normal throughout the period of 24 hours following the onset of chest pain. These results are sufficient evidence to exclude a diagnosis of myocardial infarction.

(4) Yes. Based on the cTnI results Mr Jarvis did suffer a minimal or micro-myocardial infarction. These results demonstrate the superior sensitivity of cTnI for detecting myocardial necrosis. In this case, the amount of tissue destroyed during infarction was not sufficient to cause an increase in CK(MB). The ischaemia that caused the minimal loss of tissue was not sufficiently extensive to cause any of the ECG changes normally associated with evolving myocardial infarction.

References

1. Melville M, Brown N *et al.* (1999) Outcome and use of health services four years after admission for acute myocardial infarction: case record and follow up study. *Br Med J* **319**: 230–31.

2. The Joint European Society of Cardiology/American College of Cardiology Committee (2000) Myocardial Infarction Redefined – A Consensus Document of the Joint European Society of Cardiology/American College of Cardiology Committee for the Redefinition of Myocardial Infarction. *J Am Coll Cardiol* **36**: 959–69.

3. Dominici R, Infusino I & Valente C (2004) Plasma or serum samples: measurements of cardiac troponin T and of other analytes compared. *Clin Chem Lab Med* **42**: 945–51.
4. Fox K (2004) Management of acute coronary syndrome: an update. *Heart* **90**: 698–706.
5. Roongsritong C, Warraich I & Bradley C (2004) Common causes of troponin elevations in the absence of acute myocardial infarction. *Chest* **125**: 1877–84.

Further reading

Babuin L & Jaffe A (2005) Troponin: the biomarker of choice for detection of cardiac injury. *CMAJ* **173**: 1191–1202.
French J & White H (2004) Implications of the new definition of myocardial infarction. *Heart* **90**: 99–106.

Chapter 10
THYROID FUNCTION TESTS

This chapter is concerned with endocrinology, that branch of medical science concerned with organs or parts of organs responsible for production and secretion of hormones. These hormones or 'biochemical messengers' are transported in blood to distant target organs where they exert their various and specific effects. The thyroid gland is an endocrine organ responsible for production and secretion of thyroid hormones, thyroxine (T4) and triiodothyronine (T3). Of all endocrine disorders, those involving the thyroid are the most common; thyroid disease affects around 5% of the adult population,[1] so thyroid hormones are the most frequently measured hormones in clinical laboratories. In this chapter, we consider how the laboratory contributes to diagnosis and monitoring of the thyroid disorders.

Normal anatomy and physiology

Thyroid gland

The thyroid gland (Figure 10.1), weighing around 20 g, is butterfly-shaped and situated in the neck. The two lobes of the thyroid sit on either side of the trachea, just below the larynx and are connected by a bridge of tissue, the thyroid isthmus. Thyroid enlargement (goitre), a feature of many thyroid disorders, may be visible as a swelling of the neck or at least palpable on physical examination.

The gland is composed of two types of hormone-producing cell, the bulk of the cells are so-called follicle cells that produce the two thyroid hormones, thyroxine (T4) and triiodothyronine (T3). Interspersed between these cells are the parafollicular cells or C-cells which produce calcitonin, a hormone not considered here, that is involved in calcium metabolism.

Function of thyroid hormones T3 and T4

Thyroid hormones are delivered via the bloodstream to every part of the body and with few exceptions have an effect on the cells of all tissue types. Although T3 is the more potent of the two hormones, both increase the speed of many cellular metabolic reactions. For example, mobilisation and breakdown of body fat

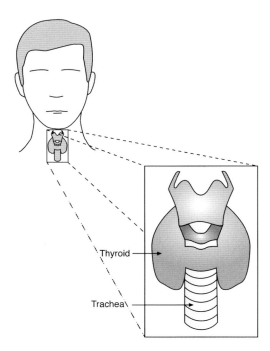

Figure 10.1 The thyroid gland.

is increased in the presence of thyroid hormone as is the speed of many reactions involved in the metabolism of carbohydrates and proteins. This overall stimulatory effect on the body's metabolism determines that thyroid hormones are essential for normal growth and development, including sexual maturation. Specific effects of thyroid hormones are evident in relation to the heart and central nervous system. Cardiac output is influenced by the concentration of thyroid hormones in blood. Mental development from birth is dependent on adequate amounts of thyroid hormone: a deficiency at this time can lead not only to impaired growth but also to severe and irreversible mental retardation.

Thyroid hormone production

Around 95% of the body's iodine is concentrated in the thyroid. This element is present in a normal diet and absorbed to blood from the small intestine in the form of iodide. By an energy consuming process, iodide is removed from blood and 'trapped' in thyroid follicular cells, where it is required for production of the two thyroid hormones, thyroxine (T4) and triiodothyronine (T3). In the thyroid follicular cells, iodide is oxidised and hormone synthesis begins with addition of this oxidised iodide to the amino acid tyrosine, a process called iodination (Figure 10.2). Both the oxidising process and iodination are facilitated by the action of a key enzyme, thyroid peroxidase (TPO).

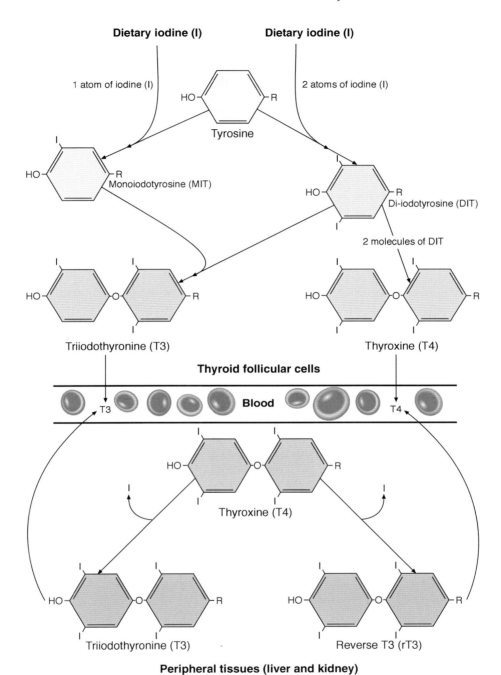

Figure 10.2 Formation of thyroid hormones T4, T3 and reverse(r)T3.
Note: R = CH₂·CHNH₂·COOH.

Iodination results in monoiodotyrosine and diiodotyrosine. Two molecules of diiodotyrosine combine to form thyroxine (T4) and one molecule of monoiodotyrosine combines with one molecule of diiodotyrosine to form triiodothyronine (T3). Both T4 and T3 are released into the bloodstream from follicular cells, although 80% of circulating T3 is formed not in the thyroid but by enzymatic deiodination (removal of one molecule of iodine) of T4 in peripheral tissue, notably the liver and kidney. Two forms of T3 are formed in this way: physiologically active T3 and physiologically inactive reverse T3 (rT3). More than 99% of both T4 and T3 that circulates in blood is bound to specific proteins, predominantly thyroxine binding globulin (TBG). In this protein bound form, the hormones are inactive but serve as a reservoir or store of thyroid hormones. Less than 0.05% of total T3 and T4 in blood is present in a free (i.e. unbound to protein) and therefore physiologically active form.

Control of thyroid hormone production

The maintenance of thyroid hormone blood concentration within normal limits is essential for good health so that production and secretion from the thyroid gland is finely controlled. This control depends on the pituitary gland, a pea-sized organ located at the base of the brain (Figure 10.3). Among several hormones that this tiny gland produces is thyroid-stimulating hormone (TSH), also called thyrotropin. As its name implies, TSH stimulates production and secretion of thyroid hormones from the thyroid gland. The secretion of TSH is in turn controlled by thyrotropin-releasing hormone (TRH) secreted by the hypothalamus in the brain. Release of both TSH and TRH is controlled by the plasma concentration of circulating free thyroid hormone (T4 and T3). As thyroid hormone concentration falls, TRH and TSH secretion increases, stimulating the thyroid to secrete more thyroid hormone. Conversely, as thyroid hormone concentration rises, TRH and TSH secretion decreases and consequently thyroid hormone production and secretion decreases. This continuous process of negative feedback maintains the amount of thyroid hormone in blood within normal limits.

Normal concentration of thyroid hormones (T3 and T4) in blood is dependent on:

- an adequate amount of dietary iodine for manufacture of thyroid hormones
- a normally functioning thyroid gland
- adequate production of TSH and therefore normally functioning pituitary gland
- adequate production of TRH and therefore normally functioning hypothalamus.

Laboratory assessment of thyroid function

Patient preparation

No particular patient preparation is necessary.

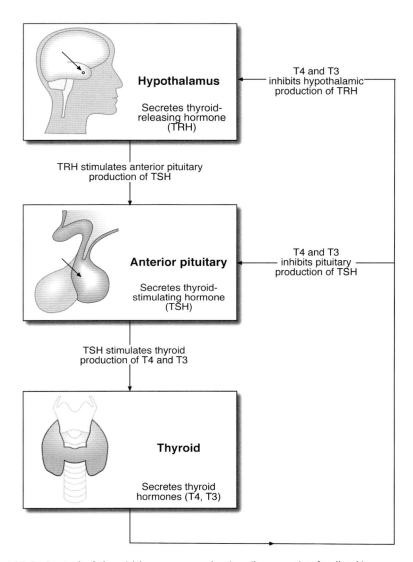

Figure 10.3 Control of thyroid hormone production (by negative feedback).

Sample requirements

Around 5 ml of venous blood is required. The tests may be performed on blood plasma or blood serum; if local policy is to use plasma, then blood must be collected into a tube containing an anticoagulant (usually heparin) but if local policy is to use serum, blood must be collected into a plain tube (i.e. without any additive).

Request card information

Since drugs and pre-existing non-thyroid disease can affect interpretation, it is important to record drug and brief clinical history. In addition to its role in the diagnosis of thyroid disorders, the test may also be used to monitor the effectiveness of therapy among those already diagnosed; it is important that the reason for requesting the test and dosage of any prescribed thyroxine replacement or antithyroid drugs is recorded.

In the laboratory

Two tests are used in the first line investigation of patients suspected of suffering thyroid disease.

Thyroid-stimulating hormone (TSH). The TSH test measures concentration in blood serum or plasma of the pituitary hormone TSH.

Free thyroxine (FT4). The FT4 test measures the concentration in blood plasma or serum of free thyroxine (the biologically active fraction of total thyroxine that is not bound to protein).

A third test may be useful in particular circumstances:

Free triiodothyronine (FT3). The FT3 test measures the concentration in blood serum or plasma of free triiodothyronine (the biologically active fraction of total triiodothyronine that is not bound to protein).

Before development of the highly sensitive laboratory methods required to detect the minute (picomole) concentration of free thyroid hormones (FT4 and FT3) present in blood, the only way of assessing thyroid function was to measure the concentration of total (free plus bound) T4 and T3. Although technically less demanding, measurement of total T4 and T3 (TT4, TT3) concentration is a less satisfactory means of assessing thyroid function, not least because results are affected by the plasma concentration of thyroid-binding globulin (TBG), which varies in both healthy and disease states. The concentration of TBG has no effect on free hormone concentration, allowing clearer interpretation of results. Most laboratories now only offer the FT4 and FT3 tests but some may still be using the older TT4 and TT3 tests. For completeness, these older tests will be included in the list of reference ranges below, but for the rest of the chapter attention will be focused on the now preferred tests, FT4 and FT3.

Interpretation of test results

Approximate reference ranges

TSH	0.3–4.5 mU/l
FT4	9–26 pmol/l
FT3	3.0–9.0 pmol/l
TT4	60–150 nmol/l
TT3	1.1–2.6 nmol/l

Terms used in interpretation

Euthyroid (ism)	normal thyroid activity
Hyperthyroid (ism)	overactive thyroid gland
Hypothyroid (ism)	underactive thyroid gland
Goitre	enlargement of the thyroid gland – depending on the cause, goitre may be a feature of euthyroidism, hyperthyroidism or hypothyroidism
Thyrotoxicosis	the clinical syndrome that results from hyperthyroidism, often used as a synonym for hyperthyroidism
Myxoedema	a clinical syndrome that results from severe hypothyroidism

Causes of abnormal thyroid function test results

Overactivity of the thyroid gland and associated increased production of thyroid hormones are called hyperthyroidism. In most instances, this is due to disease of the thyroid gland itself, in which case the condition is known as primary hyperthyroidism. Very rarely, hyperthyroidism occurs because a normally functioning thyroid gland is being overstimulated by inappropriately increased secretion of TSH from a diseased pituitary gland; this is known as secondary or central hyperthyroidism.

Similarly, underactivity of the thyroid gland and concomitant reduced production of thyroid hormones, called hypothyroidism, is most commonly due to disease of the thyroid gland (primary hypothyroidism) but can rarely result from decreased production of TSH by the pituitary gland (secondary or central hypothyroidism).

Primary hyperthyroidism

Graves' disease is the most common cause of primary hyperthyroidism, accounting for around 80% of cases. This is an autoimmune disease of unknown cause that affects around 1–2% of the adult population and is significantly more common among women.[2] Newly-diagnosed patients often report a family history of the condition, so it is possible to inherit a predisposition to Graves' disease. The thyroid gland of those suffering Graves' disease is diffusely enlarged (smooth or diffuse goitre) and non-tender. The cause of the increased hormone production is abnormal thyroid-stimulating antibodies, produced by the patient's immune system, which act in the same way as TSH and stimulate the thyroid to produce thyroid hormones. Unlike TSH, however, the production and action of these antibodies is not under negative feedback control, and continues despite rising thyroid hormone levels.

Three other less common conditions, toxic adenoma, toxic multinodular goitre and subacute thyroiditis, account for most of the remaining 20% of primary hyperthyroidism cases. Toxic adenoma is characterised by a single abnormal 'nodule' in the thyroid gland that secretes excessive thyroid hormone autonomously, whereas in toxic multinodular goitre the problem is many hypersecreting nodules. Leakage of thyroid hormone from follicular cells damaged by inflammation is the

Table 10.1 Major signs and symptoms of hyperthyroidism.

Thyroid hormone excess causes a general speeding of body metabolism, resulting in the following signs and symptoms:

- Weight loss
- Increased appetite
- Intolerance of heat
- Increased sweating; warm moist skin
- Increased heart rate (tachycardia)
- Palpitations
- Diarrhoea
- Nervousness
- Anxiety
- Inability to concentrate
- Fine hand tremor
  'Staring' prominent eyes (exopthalmus)
- Disturbance of menstrual cycle

cause of the hyperthyroidism in those with subacute thyroiditis, a self-limiting, usually painful and debilitating condition that follows viral infection. The hyper-thyroid phase is typically followed by a hypothyroid phase before recovery, which may take many months.

Amiodarone is the most significant of a number of drugs that can cause hyper-thyroidism. Whatever the cause, primary hyperthyroidism is characterised by increased concentration of thyroid hormone in blood and it is this feature which accounts for the many signs and symptoms (Table 10.1) that reflect the signific-ance of thyroid hormones for all organ systems.

Since increased thyroid hormone production suppresses pituitary secretion of TSH (Figure 10.3), a reduction in serum or plasma TSH is an important diagnostic feature of primary hyperthyroidism. Measurement of TSH is the single most import-ant biochemical test for investigation of those suspected of suffering primary hyperthyroidism because a diagnosis can usually be excluded if TSH is within the normal range.

The blood results that would be expected in primary hyperthyroidism, no matter what the cause, are:

- serum/plasma TSH concentration always reduced (often undetectable in severe cases)
- serum/plasma FT4 and FT3 concentrations increased
- occasionally FT4 is normal and only FT3 is increased (this is called T3 thyrotoxicosis).

Secondary (central) hyperthyroidism

Very rarely, excessive thyroid hormone production is the result not of a problem within the thyroid but rather a result of uncontrolled secretion of TSH due to disease (overactivity) of the pituitary gland. For example, pituitary tumours secrete abnormally high amounts of TSH. In these rare cases, the thyroid is responding normally to abnormal stimulation. Typical blood results in secondary hyperthyroidism are:

- serum/plasma TSH concentration raised
- serum FT4 and FT3 concentration raised.

Subclinical (mild) primary hyperthyroidism

Sometimes patient testing reveals reduced plasma concentration of TSH (indicating primary hyperparathyroidism) in association with a normal, usually high normal plasma concentration of FT4 and FT3 (indicating euthyroidism). This pattern indicates that production of thyroid hormones is sufficiently increased to partially suppress TSH production, but there remains sufficient TSH to maintain thyroid hormone concentration within the reference range, albeit often at the high end of that range. It is not usually associated with symptoms because thyroid hormone concentration is not increased, so it is called subclinical hyperthyroidism. However, it is not normal and represents a stage between normality and overt hyperthyroidism. Patients with subclinical hyperthyroidism are at greater than normal risk of developing overt hyperthyroidism, usually Graves' disease in the long term and should be offered thyroid testing every 6–12 months. In addition, there is evidence that subclinical hyperthyroidism is a risk factor for atrial fibrillation in the elderly[3] and osteoporosis in postmenopausal women.[4] Blood results to be expected in subclinical hyperthyroidism:

- serum/plasma TSH raised
- serum/plasma FT4 and FT3 normal.

Primary hypothyroidism

Primary hypothyroidism affects around 2–3% of the adult population. The condition is, like primary hyperthyroidism, much more common among women; an estimated 1 in 10 women over the age of 45 are thought to have some degree of hypothyroidism.[5] Most cases of hypothyroidism are the result of slowly progressive autoimmune mediated destruction of thyroid tissue. There are two main forms: atrophic autoimmune thyroiditis and goitrous autoimmune thyroiditis (alternative name Hashimoto's thyroiditis). In the first, the thyroid is shrunken in size (atrophic) and function and in the second the thyroid is enlarged (goitrous) – but still 'shrunken' in function. In both cases, destructive autoantibodies are detectable in the patient's serum and the same infiltration of the thyroid by inflammatory cells is evident; they are probably different stages of the same disease, with atrophy of the gland being the final stage.

Destruction of thyroid tissue by thyroid surgery or administration of radioactive iodine is frequently used to treat hyperthyroidism so that treatment of primary hyperthyroidism is associated with an increased risk of hypothyroidism later in life. Taken together, treatments for hyperthyroidism constitute the second

Table 10.2 Major signs and symptoms of primary hypothyroidism.

Deficiency of thyroid hormone causes a general slowing of body metabolism, resulting in the following signs and symptoms:

- Weight gain
- Puffy face particularly below the eyes
- Decreased appetite
- Intolerance of cold
- Dry skin, dry 'lifeless' hair
- Decreased heart rate (bradycardia)
- Constipation
- Lethargy
- Depression
- Slowing of mental agility
- Hoarse, 'gruff' voice

most common cause of primary hypothyroidism. Autoimmune destruction and treatment of hyperthyroidism account for more than 90% of all cases of primary hyperthyroidism.

Some drugs, notably lithium (Chapter 14) can cause hypothyroidism.

Around 1 in 3500–4000 babies are born with a deficiency of thyroid hormone (congenital hypothyroidism) usually due to either absence or abnormal development of the thyroid gland. If not treated with replacement hormone within the first few weeks of life, congenital hypothyroidism leads to severely impaired growth and permanent mental retardation (cretinism). All newborn babies are routinely screened for the condition soon after birth by measurement of the concentration of TSH in blood recovered from a heel prick. This is part of the Guthrie test familiar to neonatal nurses and midwives.

In some parts of the world, a diet deficient of iodine and consequent reduced thyroid hormone production is a major cause of hypothyroidism.

Whatever the cause, primary hypothyroidism is associated with reduced thyroid hormone production and it is this hormone deficiency that accounts for symptoms in adults (Table 10.2). The normal response of the pituitary to reduced thyroid hormone production is increased production of TSH. An increased concentration of TSH in blood is the most important diagnostic feature of primary hypothyroidism.

The blood results that would be expected in primary hypothyroidism whatever the cause are:

serum/plasma TSH concentration always increased (usually > 10 mU/l)
serum/plasma FT4 concentration reduced.

Secondary (central) hypothyroidism

There are several very rare forms of hypothyroidism that are the result not of thyroid disease but of an inability to adequately stimulate a normal thyroid gland because of a deficiency of TSH. These are all the result of damage to, or disease of, the pituitary gland. Damage to the hypothalamus has the same effect. The blood results that would be expected in secondary hypothyroidism, whatever the cause are:

- serum/plasma TSH concentration reduced
- serum/plasma FT4 concentration reduced.

Subclinical (mild) hypothyroidism

Relatively frequently, patient testing reveals raised serum TSH (indicating primary hypothyroidism) in association with serum FT4 within the reference range (indicating euthyroidism). This pattern indicates that although the thyroid gland is producing enough thyroid hormone to maintain concentration within the reference range, it is not producing sufficient to suppress TSH production so that it also remains within the reference range. So despite normal concentration of thyroid hormones, thyroid hormone production is reduced. Since thyroid hormone concentration is normal, there are usually no symptoms, so the condition is called subclinical hypothyroidism. This represents a stage between normality and overt hypothyroidism. Patients with subclinical, sometimes called mild hypothyroidism are at long-term risk of developing overt hypothyroidism, especially if TSH is found to be particularly high (> 10 mu/l), and should be offered annual thyroid testing.

The effect of non-thyroid illness on TSH, FT4 and FT3

The laboratory diagnosis of hyper- and hypothyroidism, whether mild or overt, is rarely a problem in otherwise well patients, but interpretation of thyroid function test results is often more difficult in patients who are suffering acute illness. The term euthyroid sick syndrome is applied to those patients whose thyroid function tests (TSH, FT4, FT3) are transiently abnormal due to acute illness. By definition, the thyroid of these patients is working normally – the cause of the abnormal thyroid blood tests is the acute illness. Euthyroid sick syndrome may reflect a protective adaptive response to acute illness or perhaps a pathological result of acute illness. Either way, the practical clinical problem is that there is often no way of knowing if abnormal blood tests results are due to euthyroid sick syndrome or thyroid disease.

The range of acute illnesses that might be associated with euthyroid sick syndrome is long and includes: acute infectious disease (especially sepsis), myocardial infarction, malignancy, severe trauma, e.g. surgery, indeed any acute illness may be affected in this way. Those being cared for in intensive care are a patient group with particularly high prevalence of euthyroid sick syndrome.

Abnormal results of all three tests may be found in those with severe acute illness; the most consistent finding is reduced FT3. FT4 may be normal, reduced or raised. TSH is usually normal but this too may be reduced or raised, depending on the phase of the illness (acute or recovery).

The confounding effect of acute illness makes detection of mild subclinical thyroid disease particularly difficult. Repeat testing after resolution of the acute illness may be the only way of making or excluding such a diagnosis.

Table 10.3 Summary of typical changes to thyroid function test results in thyroid and non-thyroid disease.

Thyroid disease	FT4	T3	TSH
Primary hyperthyroidism (thyrotoxicosis) Common causes: Graves' disease Rarer causes: Plummer's disease (single toxic nodule) Toxic multinodular goitre Sub-acute thyroiditis	Increased occasionally normal	Increased	Marked decrease may be undetectable
Primary hypothyroidism Common causes: Hashimoto's disease Treatment of hyperthyroidism Rarer causes: Congenital disease Iodine deficiency (common in some parts of the world)	Decreased (may be low end of normal range in early or mild disease)	Decreased occasionally normal	Marked increase
Non-thyroid disease			
Secondary hyperthyroidism (Rare) Cause: overactivity of pituitary or hypothalamus	Increased	Increased	Increased
Secondary hypothyroidism (Rare) Cause: underactivity of pituitary or hypothalamus	Decreased	Decreased	Decreased
Euthyroid sick syndrome May be a feature of any acute, severe illness e.g. cancer, severe liver disease, renal failure, major trauma or surgery, extensive burns, severe infection, starvation	Normal (though may be decreased in particularly severe illness)	Decreased	Normal (may be transiently decreased during recovery)

Note: Use of many drugs affects one or more thyroid function tests. These include: oral contraception, corticosteroids, propanalol, carbamazepine, phenytoin, lithium and amiodarone.

A summary of the abnormal changes in thyroid function tests for both thyroid and non-thyroid disease is contained in Table 10.3.

Monitoring treatment of thyroid disease

The blood tests described above for the identification of patients suffering thyroid disorders are also useful in monitoring the effectiveness of therapy among those already diagnosed.

Treatment of hyperthyroidism

There are three possible treatment regimes for those with hyperthyroidism. Most patients are treated with anti-thyroid drugs. In the UK carbimazole, a drug that inhibits the key enzyme TPO required for normal thyroid hormone production, is most often prescribed. Typically, a daily dose of carbimazole for 12 to 18 months effects a cure for around a half of patients. For those in whom drug therapy is either contraindicated or unsuccessful, an alternative is radioactive iodine treatment. Like all ingested iodine, radioactive iodine is concentrated in the thyroid gland. Here the radioactivity destroys thyroid tissue. Surgical removal of thyroid tissue (partial thyroidectomy) offers a third treatment option.

The object of therapy is to reduce thyroid hormone levels to normal (biochemical euthyroidism) and thereby remove symptoms, that is, achieve a state of clinical euthyroidism. All therapies carry a high risk of 'overtreatment', rendering patients hypothyroid so that monitoring of blood hormone levels during and after treatment is an essential part of the care of patients being treated for hyperthyroidism. The dose of anti-thyroid drug is adjusted in the first instance in the light of serum FT4 results; the serum TSH often remains suppressed for a month or two after treatment begins but will eventually return to normal. Since there is a long-term risk of hypothyroidism developing or recurrence of hyperthyroidism in those treated for hyperthyroidism, continued blood testing of thyroid function (FT4 and TSH) at least every 12 months is necessary for all patients.

Treatment of primary hypothyroidism

The only treatment for primary hypothyroidism is thyroid hormone replacement therapy, usually in the form of thyroxine tablets to be taken daily, for life. The object is to increase thyroid hormone levels (T4 and T3) to normal; this will reduce the abnormal high level of TSH secretion to normal and remove symptoms. The dosage required to achieve this state of biochemical and clinical euthyroidism varies and can only be assessed by gradually increasing the dose at four- to six-week intervals in the light of serum TSH results, the primary target being to achieve a serum TSH that is within the reference range. Too low a dose and symptoms of hypothyroidism persist; to high a dose and T4 and T3 levels rise above normal, TSH levels drop below normal and the patient develops symptoms of hyperthyroidism. Once a maintenance dose has been achieved which results in both biochemical and clinical euthyroidism, the dose usually remains the same for life and blood levels (TSH and FT4) need only be checked annually.

Case history 9

Mrs Hollingsworth, a 35-year-old PE teacher, has visited her current GP only for antenatal visits during two uneventful pregnancies in her 20s and for annual 'well woman' checks over the previous five years. She now goes to see her GP because for a period of several months she has been feeling 'constantly tired and washed out' despite increasingly less activity at work and sleeping more than usual. She tells the doctor that she thinks she might be anaemic because of several 'heavy periods' over the past few months. The doctor feels that this normally lively woman appears unusually depressed. On questioning she admits feeling depressed but attributes this to tiredness and hopes that some 'iron tablets' will put things right. She also reports being frustrated at recent increase in body weight despite eating less than normal; she feels she has lost her appetite for food. The weight gain is confirmed by comparing her current weight with measurements made at previous well woman clinics. Although there are no clinical signs of anaemia, the doctor agrees to take blood to test for anaemia but also takes a further sample for thyroid function tests.

The full blood count results are entirely normal, excluding anaemia as a cause for the tiredness.

The thyroid function test results are:

FT4   8.0 pmol/l
TSH   26 mIU/l

Questions

(1) What symptoms suggested that thyroid function tests were appropriate?
(2) Are the thyroid function results normal?
(3) What do the results suggest?

Discussion of case history

(1) As the GP suspected from clinical examination, Mrs Hollingsworth was not anaemic. Tiredness, depression, excessive menstrual blood flow (menorrhagia) and weight gain without increased food intake can all result from a deficiency of thyroid hormone i.e. hypothyroidism. The condition is particularly common in middle-aged women. The extent and severity of symptoms among patients with hypothyroidism vary greatly so that the absence of more clinical features of hypothyroidism does not exclude the diagnosis.

(2) No. FT4 is reduced and TSH is increased.

(3) The results suggest a diagnosis of primary hypothyroidism (Table 10.3). Mrs Hollingsworth's thyroid is producing insufficient thyroid hormone despite increased secretion of TSH by the pituitary gland and would benefit from thyroid replacement therapy if repeat testing confirms these abnormal results.

References

1. Clark J (1993) Thyroid disease. *The Practitioner* **237**: 264–68.
2. Vanderpump M, Tunbridge W *et al.* (1995) The incidence of thyroid disease in the community: a twenty-year follow-up of the Wickham survey. *Clin Endocrinol* **43**: 55–68.
3. Swain C, Geller A *et al.* (1994) Low serum thyrotropin concentrations as risk factor for atrial fibrillation in older persons. *New Eng J Med* **331**: 1249–52.
4. Schneider D, Barrett-Connor E & Morton D (1994) Thyroid hormone use and bone mineral density in elderly women. Effects of oestrogen. *JAMA* **271**: 1245–49.
5. Clark J (1995) Current management of thyroid disease. *Prescriber* **May 5**: 31–38.

Further reading

Tews M, Shah S & Gossain V (2005) Hypothyroidism: mimicker of common complaints. *Emerg Med Clin North Am* **23**: 649–67.

Reid J & Wheeler S (2005) Hyperthyroidism: diagnosis and treatment. *Am Fam Physician* **72**: 623–30.

Topliss D & Eastman C (2004) Diagnosis and management of hyperthyroidism and hypothyroidism. *Med J Aust* **180**: 186–93.

Umpierrez G (2002) Euthyroid sick syndrome. *South Med J* **95**: 506–13.

Guidelines Development Group (2006) UK Guidelines for the use of thyroid function tests. Available at: *www.acb.org.uk/docs/TFTguidelinefinal.pdf*

Chapter 11

LIVER FUNCTION TESTS: ALANINE TRANSFERASE (ALT), GAMMA GLUTAMYL TRANSPETIDASE (GGT), ALKALINE PHOSPHATASE (AP), BILIRUBIN AND ALBUMIN

This chapter is concerned with the measurement of five substances present in blood plasma. Although structurally and functionally distinct, they are treated together here because they are routinely measured together in a profile commonly known as liver function tests (LFTs). The principal use of the profile is identification of patients who are suffering liver or biliary tract disease. Depending on the exact nature of liver disease, one or more of these tests may be normal but it is unlikely that all would be normal in any patient suffering significant liver or biliary tract disease. Thus, the combination of five liver function tests has more power to detect liver or biliary tract disease than each individual test. None of the five tests is specific for liver disease, so that there are other diseases, not involving the liver or biliary tract, in which one or more of these tests might be abnormal.

Normal anatomy and physiology

The liver

The liver, one of the largest of the body's organs, weighing around 2 kg, is located in the right upper quadrant of the abdomen, protected for the most part by the lower rib cage. (Figure 11.1a) The narrower left lobe extends from the ribcage over the stomach. It is red-brown in colour due to its copious blood supply: the organ receives around 30% of total cardiac output every minute from two sources, the portal vein and hepatic artery. The products of ingested food are transported to the liver directly from the gastrointestinal tract in blood via the portal vein and oxygenated blood is supplied via the hepatic artery. Blood leaves the liver by way of the hepatic vein, draining into the inferior vena cava for return to the heart (Figure 11.1b).

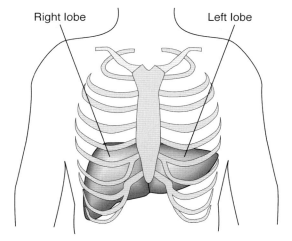

Figure 11.1a Location of the liver.

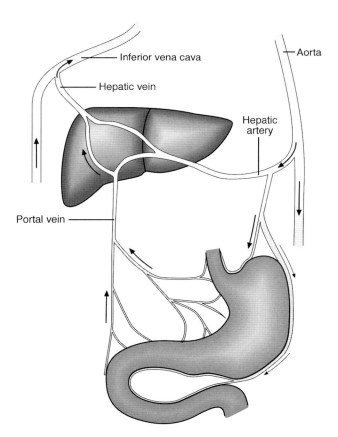

Figure 11.1b Hepatic circulation.

The complexities of liver function can be broadly summarised under three inter-connected headings:

- metabolic function
- synthetic function
- excretory function.

Hepatocytes, the cells of which the bulk of the liver is composed, play a central role in the metabolism of ingested carbohydrates, proteins and fats. This is why these products of digestion are transported first to the liver, via the portal vein. Glucose derived from ingested carbohydrates can be stored until required, in hepatocytes, as glycogen. Between meals when glucose is in short supply, these glycogen stores are mobilised. During starvation, when even glycogen stores are depleted, hepatocytes are able to convert amino acids derived from ingested and body proteins to glucose. By these effects on carbohydrate metabolism, the liver plays a central role in regulating blood glucose concentration.

Dietary derived amino acids are synthesised into proteins in the liver; these include many of the proteins, like albumin, that are present in blood plasma. The vital process of blood clotting depends on the liver synthesis of the specific plasma proteins (clotting factors) of the clotting cascade. Urea, a waste product of amino acid metabolism, is synthesised in the liver before transport in blood to the kidneys, where it is excreted in urine. The liver plays a major role in the metabolism of ingested fats (lipids) by synthesising the lipoproteins necessary for transport of these fats including cholesterol and triglycerides around the body, in blood. Synthesis of bile acids from cholesterol provides a further example of the way liver affects lipid metabolism and leads nicely to the excretory role of the liver.

Production of bile: the biliary tract

The liver is the source of bile, an alkaline watery yellow-green fluid that contains the bile acids produced from cholesterol. These bile acids have to be conveyed in bile to the intestine where they are required for absorption of dietary lipids. Bile also provides the route for excretion of drugs and other waste products of metabolism that are not excreted from the body by the kidneys in urine. The production of bile thus fulfils the excretory role of the liver.

Bile is produced within and secreted from hepatocytes to microscopic tube-like structures called bile canaliculi that coalesce within the liver to form larger bile ducts. These in turn join to form the larger hepatic bile ducts that conduct bile from the liver. Left and right hepatic bile ducts join outside the liver forming the common hepatic bile duct, and this is connected via the common bile duct to the duodenum of the intestinal tract. The pancreatic duct that conveys pancreatic digestive juice from the pancreas joins the common bile duct a few centimetres from the duodenum, so that bile and pancreatic juice enter the intestinal tract through the same opening in the duodenum.

Bile production by the liver is continuous, amounting to around 500 ml/day. Between meals, when its digestive property is not required the passage of bile (and pancreatic juice) to the duodenum is blocked by closure of a sphincter (sphincter of Oddi) sited at the junction of common bile duct and duodenum. When this sphincter is closed, bile is stored in the gall bladder, which is connected to the common bile duct via the cystic duct. When food is ingested, the sphincter opens and bile passes from the gall bladder via the cystic duct and common bile duct, to the lumen of duodenum. The biliary tract is the totality of structure that conveys bile from hepatocytes to the intestine and includes bile ducts within the liver, hepatic bile ducts, gall bladder, common bile duct and sphincter of Oddi.

Although bile acid represents a major constituent of bile, it is by no means the only one; bile is a chemically complex fluid containing many waste products of metabolism destined for excretion in faeces. Among them is bilirubin, a waste product of haemoglobin metabolism.

Bilirubin

Many patients suffering liver disease have a yellow discoloration of the skin and mucous membranes, first evident in the sclerae (whites) of the eye. This clinical sign, known as jaundice (derived from the French word for yellow, *jaune*) which is not confined to those suffering liver disease, is due to an abnormally high concentration in the blood of the potentially toxic yellow pigment, bilirubin.

Most of the 250–300 mg bilirubin normally produced each day is derived from the breakdown (catabolism) of haemoglobin, the oxygen carrying protein contained in red blood cells (Figure 11.2). At the end of their normal 120-day life span, red blood cells are removed from general circulation by the spleen and other parts of the reticuloendothelial (RE) system. Within the RE system, haemoglobin released from dead red cells is split into its constituent parts, haem and globin. The haem portion is converted to bilirubin, which is then tightly bound to albumin and transported in blood to the liver for excretion in bile. Before entry to liver cells, bilirubin is released from albumin. Bilirubin is water insoluble and must be made water soluble for excretion in bile. This is achieved within the hepatocytes by conjugation (joining) of bilirubin to a substance called glucuronic acid. The resulting so-called conjugated bilirubin is secreted from the hepatocyte to bile canaliculi and onwards in bile, out of the liver to the duodenum. The action of bacteria normally present within the gut deconjugates bilirubin (that is releases bilirubin from glucuronic acid) and converts bilirubin to the brown pigment stercobilinogen and then stercobilin. Almost all of these final products of bilirubin metabolism are excreted from the body in faeces; they are responsible for the brown colour of faeces. A little stercobilinogen is reabsorbed to blood during passage through the gut. Most of this is recycled by the liver and re-excreted into the gut, but some is excreted in urine as urobilinogen.

Albumin

Blood plasma contains a mixture of many proteins, each with its own function. These include proteins required to fight infection (immunoglobulins or antibodies), enzymes, blood clotting factors, specific transport proteins and many more.

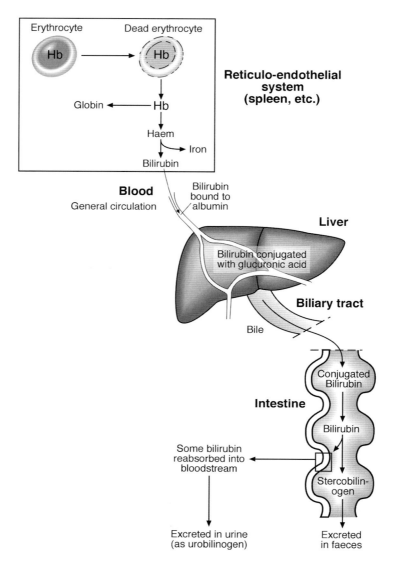

Figure 11.2 Bilirubin production and excretion.

Albumin is the single most abundant protein in plasma comprising as it does around 40–60% of total plasma protein; it is the most frequently measured plasma protein in clinical laboratories.

Like many other proteins present in plasma, albumin is synthesised from amino acids in the liver. It has two main functions. The first of these is as a transport protein. Many water-insoluble substances can only be transported in blood plasma when bound to specific proteins. Albumin is one of these proteins and is, as we have already seen, required for transport of bilirubin. Around half the calcium present in blood plasma is bound to albumin, as are free fatty acids and many drugs.

The other important function of albumin is maintenance of blood plasma volume. As the single most abundant protein in plasma, albumin is a major contributor to colloid osmotic pressure or plasma oncotic pressure. This pressure opposes the tendency of fluid to escape from capillary blood vessels into the surrounding interstitial space due to blood pressure within vessels. Oedema (which may be visible as swelling) is the term used to describe an abnormal accumulation of fluid in the interstitial space and this occurs if albumin concentration of plasma and therefore plasma oncotic pressure fall below normal.

Solution of albumin may be administered therapeutically via an intravenous line to patients who have suffered major trauma, burns or clinical shock, to restore plasma volume.

Gamma glutamyl transpeptidase (GGT), alanine transferase (ALT) and alkaline phosphatase (AP)

GGT, ALT and AP are all enzymes. They are present in the cells of the liver and biliary tract where they function as catalysts of specific metabolic reactions. The enzymes have no function in blood plasma and the small amount that is normally present (compared with that in cells) is due to normal cell turnover. As cells die they release their contents to blood plasma. The cell injury associated with liver or biliary tract disease results in increased amounts of these intracellular enzymes being released to blood plasma.

If the source of these enzymes were only liver or biliary tract tissue, then raised levels would always indicate liver or biliary tract disease. In fact, although GGT, ALT and AP are frequently referred to as 'liver enzymes', they are also present in other tissues, and damage or disease of these non-liver, non-biliary tract tissues may also be associated with a rise in serum concentration of either GGT, ALT or AP. The most significant non-liver non-biliary tract source of GGT is the pancreas. ALT is present predominantly in the hepatocytes of the liver but also, albeit at far lower concentration, in kidney tissue, heart muscle (myocardium) and skeletal muscle. AP is present not only in the liver cells of the bile canaliculi, but also in bone cells, intestinal tissue cells and placental tissue cells.

Laboratory measurement of liver function tests (LFTs)

Patient preparation

No particular patient preparation is necessary.

Timing of sample

Blood for LFTs may be sampled at any time. It is, however, important that there is not undue delay (more than a few hours) in transporting specimens to the laboratory for separation of serum (or plasma) from cells.

Sample requirement

Around 5 ml of venous blood is required for LFTs. Blood should be collected into a plain tube without additives if local policy is to use serum for analysis; and into a tube containing the anticoagulant lithium heparin if local policy is to use plasma. A falsely raised albumin level occurs if a tourniquet is left in position for a more than a minute or two before sampling blood. If possible, the use of a tourniquet should be avoided. Bilirubin is slowly destroyed by both artificial light and sunlight, leading to falsely low results. To reduce this effect, samples should be protected as far as possible from exposure to light both before and during transport to the laboratory.

Neonatal measurement of bilirubin only

For reasons to be discussed later, newborn babies (particularly premature babies) frequently need monitoring of serum bilirubin concentration. In these cases, only bilirubin need be measured, reducing the sample requirement to around 0.5 ml or less. Capillary blood obtained by a heel stab (Chapter 2) is usually used in these circumstances. Particular care is required to avoid haemolysis during blood collection, as such samples are unsuitable for bilirubin estimation. A special dark plastic container (to protect bilirubin from exposure to light) is often used for collection of blood samples for neonatal bilirubin measurement.

Interpretation of results

Approximate reference ranges

Serum/plasma bilirubin	< 17 µmol/l
Serum/plasma albumin	35–50 g/l

Methods used to measure serum/plasma ALT, GGT and AP enzymes levels vary between laboratories; each method has its own reference range. It would be misleading, therefore, to quote even approximate reference ranges for these enzyme tests. Always use local laboratory range when interpreting results. The amount of AP in serum/plasma is age-dependent, being much higher in childhood and adolescence than during adulthood. Each laboratory publishes AP reference ranges for each of these age ranges. It is important that the age of the patient is taken into account when interpreting AP results. The presence of AP in placental tissue determines that AP is higher during pregnancy.

Causes of raised bilirubin

Jaundice
The concentration of bilirubin in serum reflects the balance between the amount produced by the normal process of red cell destruction and that removed from

the blood by the liver and excreted in bile. An abnormally raised serum bilirubin occurs in three broad pathological situations.

- Diseases in which the rate of bilirubin production exceeds the normal rate of liver processing and excretion. Bilirubin consequently accumulates in blood. These are the haemolytic anaemias, which are characterised by increased red cell destruction and therefore increased catabolism of haemoglobin and consequent increased bilirubin production. Liver and biliary tract are functioning normally, so that haemolytic anaemias serve to remind that jaundice can occur in patients without liver disease.
- Diseases in which rate of bilirubin production is normal but the rate at which the liver can process a normal bilirubin load is compromised by disease. These are diseases solely of the liver.
- Diseases in which the rate of production of bilirubin is normal, the rate at which liver cells process bilirubin is normal but the rate of excretion is reduced due to disease of the biliary tract (either within the liver or at some other point in the biliary tract between the liver and the duodenum). The disorders in this group are characterised by cholestasis, which means reduction in bile flow.

Generally speaking, haemolytic anaemias are associated with only a slight increase in bilirubin; concentration rarely rises above 70 μmol/l. An important exception is haemolytic disease of the newborn (see later). Since the liver is functionally normal, all other LFTs are normal.

Higher serum bilirubin concentration is seen in liver disease in which there is injury to liver cells. For example, acute inflammation of the liver (acute hepatitis), usually the result of viral infection (Table 11.1) or alcohol abuse (alcoholic hepatitis) causes peak concentrations (up to 300 μmol/l) at around the 10th day after symptoms develop. During the 4–8 week recovery period, bilirubin gradually returns to normal. In some cases, inflammation does not resolve and becomes chronic and progressively destructive. The term chronic active hepatitis is used to describe such cases, and bilirubin, though not as high as during acute hepatitis, may remain raised. Cirrhosis, that is irreversible liver damage, most often the result of prolonged alcohol abuse or unresolved viral hepatitis (there are many rarer causes), may be associated with a near normal serum bilirubin concentration in the early stages but rises as the disease progresses over many years to liver failure. Secondary spread (metastases) of primary cancers to the liver is often associated with raised bilirubin; jaundice is a poor prognostic sign in patients with such secondary cancer spread.

Obstruction of bile flow and consequent failure to excrete conjugated bilirubin is the cause of the raised serum bilirubin that can complicate gallstone disease if gallstones become lodged in the cystic duct or common bile duct. A similar mechanism accounts for the very high bilirubin that can occur in cancers of the biliary tract and cancer of the head of pancreas. In these cases, it is the malignant growth that obstructs bile flow.

Table 11.1 Viral causes of hepatitis and therefore abnormal liver function tests.

	Hepatitis A Virus (HAV)	Hepatitis B Virus (HBV)	Hepatitis C Virus (HCV)	Hepatitis D Virus (HDV)	Hepatitis E Virus (HEV)	Hepatitis G Virus (HGV)
Relative significance as a cause of hepatitis in the UK	Most common cause of viral hepatitis; accounts for 40% of all cases	Common cause of viral hepatitis; accounts for 35% of all cases	Less common cause of viral hepatitis; accounts for 15% of all cases	Can only occur in association with HBV infection. Never the sole cause of hepatitis	Rare. Cases are almost always the result of travel to areas where the virus is endemic, e.g. Far East, India	Newly discovered virus thought to be a rare cause of hepatitis
Mode of transmission Risk factors	Faecal-oral route. Close personal contact Eating uncooked contaminated food or water	Inoculation with infected blood. Can be sexually transmitted. Those at risk include injecting drug abusers, health care workers	As for HBV. Evidence of sexual transmission less clear cut. Blood transfusion before 1993 is a risk factor for chronic infection	As for HBV	Faecal-oral route, eating contaminated food and water in areas of the world where virus is endemic	Transmitted like HBV HCV and HDV via infected blood. Blood transfusion an additional risk factor, as blood is not tested
Symptoms of acute infection	Infection does not always result in symptoms particularly during childhood. When they do occur symptoms begin with a 'flu like illness with fever and generalised aches and pains. This is followed a few days later by nausea, vomiting, abdominal pain and fatigue which may be extreme. Generally speaking Hep A results in less severe symptoms. For the great majority of patients symptoms gradually resolve over a period of six to eight weeks. Rarely, acute viral hepatitis can result in liver failure					
Long-term consequences of infection: progression to chronic liver disease (chronic active hepatitis, cirrhosis) or liver cancer	No long-term consequences	Around 5–10% of infected patients progress to chronic liver disease. Some of these susequently develop primary liver cancer	Common. Around 70% of HCV infected patients progress to chronic liver, with high risk of cirrhosis and liver cancer	Risk of chronic liver disease among those infected with HBV is greater if they are also infected with HDV	No long-term consequences	Unclear at the present time

Other viral causes of hepatitis
- *Epstein-Barr virus, the cause of glandular fever (infectious mononucleosis)*
- *Cytomegalovirus and herpes simplex virus only in immunocompromised patients.*

Some inherited defects of bilirubin metabolism result in raised bilirubin but all are rare, except Gilbert's syndrome. This is an entirely benign condition affecting around 5% of the population and usually discovered quite by chance during routine blood testing. The only abnormality is a slight increase in serum bilirubin, which rarely rises above 70 μmol/l.

Neonatal jaundice

All babies have a raised bilirubin at birth and concentration rises sufficiently during the first week of life to cause jaundice in around 50% of full-term healthy neonates. In the vast majority of cases, this is due to so called 'physiological' jaundice. Two factors contribute to 'physiological' jaundice. Firstly, the days after birth are associated with increased red cell destruction and therefore increased bilirubin production. In addition, liver metabolism is not fully mature at this time so that newborn babies are unable to conjugate bilirubin at a sufficient rate for excretion to balance production. Physiological jaundice is transitory, with serum bilirubin peaking no higher than 200 μmol/l on the third or fourth day of life before falling to a level at which jaundice is no longer evident over the next few days. Jaundice persisting beyond 10 days after birth or jaundice associated with bilirubin levels in excess of 250 μmol/l cannot be regarded as physiologic and 'normal'. The most common reason for persistence of jaundice is breast milk feeding. Around 2.5% of breastfed babies develop jaundice that can persist for up to 16 weeks. Less benign causes include haemolytic disease of the newborn (HDN), which is discussed in Chapter 20, hypothyroidism, neonatal hepatitis, biliary atresia and some rare inherited defects of bilirubin metabolism.

Causes of abnormal serum albumin concentration

Since albumin is synthesised in the liver, it might be expected that liver disease is always associated with abnormally low levels. This however is not the case. Albumin is reduced only in chronic liver disease (e.g. cirrhosis) and liver failure but usually remains normal if damage is acute and self-limiting. (e.g. acute hepatitis). Albumin may also be reduced in conditions other than liver disease. Inadequate supply of dietary amino acids required for albumin synthesis is the cause of the low albumin associated with severe malnutrition and malabsorption. Abnormal loss of albumin from the body may also result in low levels. For example, the abnormal loss of albumin in urine accounts for the low serum albumin in diseases of the kidney (particularly marked in nephrotic syndrome). Albumin is frequently low in patients who have suffered extensive burns due to the loss of albumin through skin.

The level of hydration, although not affecting the total amount of albumin in the body, does affect the concentration of albumin. In dehydrated patients, serum albumin concentration is raised and in overhydrated patients, serum albumin concentration is reduced.

Causes of abnormal enzyme results

Alanine transferase (ALT)

Highest ALT results (in extreme cases up to 50 or even 100 times the upper limit of normal) are seen in any disease associated with acute and massive liver cell necrosis. In acute viral hepatitis for example, liver cell death causes ALT to rise to a peak during the first few days following development of first symptoms, usually before jaundice develops. As the disease resolves over the following 6–8 weeks, ALT gradually falls back to normal. A similar picture follows the liver cell death that results from acute circulatory failure (clinical shock) and that which results from ingestion of liver toxins (e.g. overdose of paracetamol in which ALT levels may be in excess of 100 times the upper limit of normal). A persistently moderately raised ALT (up to 10 times the upper limit of normal) suggests the development of chronic liver disease. Chronic hepatitis, cirrhosis and malignant disease of the liver are frequently associated with such moderate rises. ALT is usually normal or only slightly increased in diseases associated with reduced bile flow.

An isolated mild increase in ALT (up to five times the upper limit of normal) with all other liver function tests normal is a very common finding. Causes of this pattern include chronic hepatitis C infection and drug-induced hepatic damage but the most common cause is non-alcoholic fatty liver disease (NAFLD) an increasingly recognised liver disease strongly associated with obesity and type 2 diabetes, that can, in a minority of cases, progress over many years to liver failure.

Gamma glutamyl transpeptidase (GGT)

Gamma glutamyl transpeptidase (GGT) is usually raised (up to five times the upper limit of normal) in all types of liver and biliary tract disease (acute and chronic hepatitis, cirrhosis, obstructive jaundice, etc.) The test can help to identify those with disease of the liver or biliary tract disease but is not very useful in establishing the exact nature of that disease. Measurement of GGT has, however, been found to be particularly useful in the management of patients who are at risk of liver disease due to alcoholism. Unlike the other two liver enzymes, GGT production is induced by alcohol, so that if patients are drinking alcohol, GGT is raised, even if there is no liver damage. Levels return to normal on cessation of drinking. If GGT of an alcoholic patient remains persistently high, it is likely that the patient continues to drink alcohol or that some damage to the liver has occurred (alcoholic hepatitis or cirrhosis).

Some drugs, including the anticonvulsants phenytoin, phenobarbitone, tricyclic antidepressants and paracetamol, also induce GGT production. For patients taking these and other drugs, a slight increase in GGT can be expected and does not necessarily imply any liver damage. Disease of the pancreas (e.g. acute pancreatitis) usually results in an increased GGT and a slight increase in GGT is sometimes noted in diabetic patients.

Alkaline phosphatase (AP)

Alkaline phosphatase levels may be raised in liver, biliary tract and some diseases of the bone. As far as liver and biliary tract disease is concerned, highest levels are seen in diseases that obstruct the flow of bile, after it has left the liver (e.g. gallstones in the common bile duct, carcinoma of the head of the pancreas). AP is also usually raised in cirrhosis and liver cancers (including liver metastases). Levels are generally only slightly raised in acute hepatitis and may be normal.

Alkaline phosphatase is present in high concentration in the osteoblastic cells of bone. The function of these cells is formation and constant remodelling of bone. Any condition associated with increased osteoblastic activity results in increased levels of alkaline phosphatase in blood. The increase in osteoblastic activity associated with growth spurts in childhood, as new bone is formed, accounts for the increased levels of plasma alkaline phosphatase throughout childhood. Some diseases of the bone are associated with abnormally increased osteoblastic activity. Among these is Paget's disease, a painful and bone-deforming condition usually diagnosed in middle age, and osteomalacia (called rickets in children) caused usually by Vitamin D deficiency. Paget's disease is characterised by particularly high levels of plasma alkaline phosphatase. A raised AP is often seen during the healing process, following bone fracture, as new bone is formed. Finally, AP is raised in patients who have tumours of the bone (either primary or secondary). Primary tumours often metastasise first to the bone. An isolated raised alkaline phosphatase in a cancer patient is a poor prognostic sign as it may indicate tumour spread beyond the primary site.

Drugs and liver function tests

Liver damage can be caused by a wide spectrum of drugs, including some antibiotics (especially those used in the treatment of tuberculosis), paracetamol, aspirin, some antidepressants, cytotoxic drugs, etc. It has been estimated that 10% of cases of jaundice among hospital patients are the result of drug therapy. A full drug history is essential for interpretation of liver function test results in particular cases. The main causes of abnormal bilirubin, albumin, ALT, GGT and AP are summarised in Tables 11.2a and 11.2b.

Specific clinical effects of abnormal liver function tests

Bilirubin

A raised bilirubin is the cause of jaundice, although this clinical sign is not evident if concentration is below around 50 µmol/l. At serum bilirubin concentration in excess of 100 µmol/l, jaundice is clearly evident to the untrained observer. Jaundice during the neonatal period is due to a rise in unconjugated bilirubin. If unconjugated bilirubin concentration rises above 350 mmol/l, there is risk of a devastating complication of neonatal jaundice called kernicterus. This is the deposition of bilirubin in the basal ganglia of the brain with neuronal death. The permanent brain damage caused by kernicterus can result in severe physical disability due to athetoid cerebral palsy and loss of hearing. Severely jaundiced neonates at risk of kernicterus are treated with ultraviolet (UV) phototherapy. UV light destroys bilirubin so the therapy prevents kernicterus. An exchange transfusion, in which blood of normal bilirubin concentration is transfused in exchange for affected babies'

Table 11.2a Most common causes of abnormal bilirubin and albumin result.

Increased serum/plasma bilirubin	Reduced serum/plasma albumin
Failure of liver cells to conjugate or excrete conjugated bilirubin	Failure to synthesise normal amount of albumin
• acute/chronic hepatitis • cirrhosis • toxic liver cell damage (e.g. paracetamol overdose) • primary biliary cirrhosis • liver metastases (spread of cancer to the liver from some other primary site) • primary liver cancer congestive cardiac failure	• any chronic liver disease, e.g. cirrhosis, chronic hepatitis • malnutrition • diseases associated with malabsorption, e.g. Crohn's disease, coeliac disease Abnormal losses of albumin in urine:
Failure to excrete bilirubin due to obstruction of bile flow after it has left the liver	• nephrotic syndrome • chronic renal failure
• gallstones obstructing the common bile duct • carcinoma head of pancreas	Movement of albumin from plasma to interstitital space (total albumin in the body remains normal)
Increased production of bilirubin due to abnormal rate of red cell destruction	• any severe acute illness or tissue damage (e.g. common finding postoperatively)
• the haemolytic anaemias	Albumin level affected by patient's state of hydration: raised in those who are dehydrated and reduced in those who are overhydrated.
In neonates raised bilirubin may be due to	
• physiological jaundice (very common particularly among premature babies and those being breast fed) haemolytic disease of the newborn (HDN) (less common) • liver disease (rare) • inherited metabolic defect (rare)	

blood, is sometimes indicated for those in whom the rate at which bilirubin is being formed is faster than the rate at which it can be destroyed by UV light.

Albumin

A reduced plasma albumin concentration is one of several contributory causes of oedema, the abnormal accumulation of fluid within the interstitial fluid, sometimes causing visible swelling (e.g. ankle oedema). Of particular relevance to liver disease is the abdominal swelling that complicates the course of cirrhosis in some patients. This swelling is the result of accumulation of so-called ascitic fluid in the peritoneal cavity. This form of oedema, known as ascites, is thought in part to be due to low plasma albumin concentration, a feature of cirrhosis.

ALT, GGT, AP

There are no clinical signs or symptoms that can be directly attributable to raised liver enzymes.

Table 11.2b Most common cause of abnormal liver enzyme levels.

Increased plasma/serum ALT	Increased serum/plasma AP	Increased serum/plasma GGT
Marked increase (up to 100 times the upper limit of normal) in all conditions associated with acute severe liver cell death	Liver and biliary tract disease Highest levels (up to 5 times the upper limit of normal) seen in liver and biliary tract disease which obstructs the flow of bile	Liver and biliary tract disease
• acute viral hepatitis • acute toxic hepatitis (e.g. paracetamol overdose) • acute liver failure due to circulatory failure (i.e. shock)	• gallstones in common bile duct • carcinoma of head of pancreas • primary biliary cirrhosis • primary liver cancer • secondary spread of cancer to the liver	• acute hepatitis (whatever the cause) • infectious mononucleosis • gallstones • carcinoma of head of pancreas • primary liver cancer • secondary liver cancer
Moderate increase (up to 10 times the upper limit of normal) in other liver disease	Moderately raised levels (up to 3 times the upper limit of normal) may be a feature of any acute or chronically active liver disease	Non-liver disease
• cirrhosis • chronic hepatitis • primary liver cancer • secondary cancer spread to the liver • infectious mononucleosis (glandular fever)	• acute viral hepatitis • acute toxic hepatitis • chronic active hepatitis • cirrhosis • infectious mononucleosis	• pancreatitis • diabetes Alcohol and some drugs result in increased production of GGT
Mild increase (up to 5 times the upper limit of normal) may occur in disorders which do not affect the liver	Bone disease Very high levels (may be up to 10 times the upper limit of normal)	• alcohol use • drugs including phenytoin and phenobarbitone
• severe tissue damage, e.g. major trauma or surgery • severe myocardial infarction • muscle disease	• Paget's disease of the bone Also raised • during recovery of bone fracture • secondary spread of cancer to bone • primary bone tumour	

Case history 10

Jamie Conrad, a 22-year-old heroin addict, attended his GP surgery complaining of a two-day history of vomiting, abdominal pain and unusual tiredness. On questioning, he revealed that he had felt unwell and feverish for a day or two a fortnight before, but those symptoms had passed. Apart from that, he judged himself to have been in good health until the current symptoms developed. The GP considered hepatitis might be the cause of his symptoms and sampled blood for LFTs. The laboratory reported the following results:

Bilirubin	28 µmol/l
Albumin	42 g/l
ALT	104 U/l (laboratory normal range < 20 U/l)
AP	56 U/l (laboratory normal range < 150 U/l)
Gamma GT	203 U/l (laboratory normal range < 50 U/l)

Questions

(1) What might have persuaded the GP to investigate Jamie for possible hepatitis?
(2) What laboratory results are abnormal?
(3) Are the results consistent with a diagnosis of hepatitis?

Discussion of case history

(1) Some viruses that cause hepatitis (notably Hep B virus) can be transmitted by inoculation with infected blood. For this reason, injecting drug users like Jamie who may share syringes with those harbouring the virus are at particular risk of hepatitis. The symptoms that Jamie describes are consistent with a diagnosis of early hepatitis.

(2) The bilirubin level is raised, though not sufficiently to cause visible jaundice. There is a significant increase (5 times the upper limit of normal) in serum AST. Gamma GT is also raised (4 times the upper limit of normal).

(3) The results are consistent with early hepatitis. If Jamie does indeed have hepatitis, then it can be expected that increase in bilirubin and AST particularly will become more marked over the next 7–10 days. Peak bilirubin concentration is usually sufficient to cause jaundice.

Further reading

Bjornsson E, Ismael S et al. (2003) Severe jaundice in Sweden in the New Millenium: causes, investigations, treatment and prognosis. Scand J Gastroenterol 38: 86–94.

Boyd S (2004) Treatment of physiological and pathological neonatal jaundice. Nursing Times 100(13): 40–43.

Giannini E, Testa R & Savarino V (2005) Liver enzyme alteration: a guide for clinicians. CMAJ 172: 367–79.

Johnston D (1999) Special considerations in interpreting liver function tests. Am Fam Physician 59: 2223–30.

Limdi J & Hyde G (2003) Evaluation of abnormal liver function tests. Postgrad Med J 79: 307–12.

Machado M & Cortez-Pinto H (2005) Non-alcoholic fatty liver disease and insulin resistance. Eur J Gastroenterol Hepatol 17: 823–26.

Pratt D & Kaplan M (2000) Evaluation of abnormal liver enzyme results in asymptomatic patients. New Eng J Med 342: 1266–71.

Whitehead M, Hainsworth I & Kingham J (2001) The causes of obvious jaundice in South West Wales: perceptions versus reality. Gut 48: 409–13.

Chapter 12
SERUM/PLASMA AMYLASE

The measurement of amylase in blood serum or plasma is used almost exclusively in the investigation of patients with acute abdominal pain, a very common symptom, especially among patients admitted urgently to hospital. Acute abdominal pain is almost invariably a major presenting symptom of common surgical emergencies such as acute appendicitis, intestinal obstruction, perforated peptic ulcer and ruptured aortic aneurysm, so that rapid diagnosis, sometimes with the help of blood and urine tests, is important. A small proportion (around 3%) of patients whose principal symptom is acute abdominal pain will be suffering acute pancreatitis, a potentially life-threatening inflammatory disease of the pancreas. The serum amylase test is particularly useful in identifying these patients; a marked increase in serum amylase in a patient with acute abdominal pain is strongly suggestive of acute pancreatitis.

Normal physiology

The pancreas

The pancreas is a soft, pale yellow-tan coloured organ, around 12 to 15 cm in length and weighing approximately 100 g. Its shape somewhat resembles a tadpole, with a just recognisable 'head', 'body' and 'tail'. The organ lies transversely across the upper abdomen, with the 'head' positioned in the inner curve of the C-shape formed by the first loop of the duodenum, the 'body' lying behind the stomach and the 'tail' extending from behind the stomach towards the spleen (Figure 12.1). The microanatomy of the pancreas reveals two sorts of functionally distinct tissue reflecting the dual (exocrine and endocrine) role of the pancreas. Around 90% of the pancreas comprises so-called acinar (exocrine) tissue, which is responsible for the production of pancreatic juice, a thin watery fluid required for intestinal digestion of dietary foodstuffs.

Pancreatic acinar cells are arranged like a bunch of grapes around a microscopical central tube or duct; acinar tissue comprises millions of these functional units. The ducts from each unit join, forming progressively larger ducts, which eventually drain all the pancreatic juice from the acinar cells into one large central duct

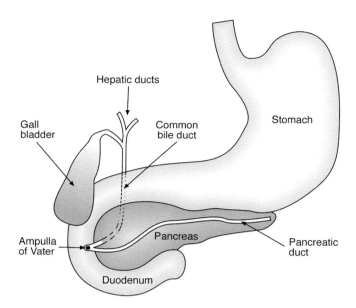

Figure 12.1 Gross anatomy of the pancreas and spatial relationship to nearby organs.

called the duct of Wirsung, running the length of the pancreas. This central duct leaves the head of the pancreas and joins with the bile duct conveying bile from the gall bladder before joining with an opening in the duodenum called the hepatopancreatic ampulla. Here, pancreatic juice (and bile) drains into the duodenum. Some people (around 20%) have a second pancreatic duct which drains pancreatic juice into the duodenum around 1 cm above the hepatopancreatic ampulla.

Dispersed throughout the acinar tissue of the pancreas are highly vascularised islands of quite distinct (endocrine) cells that have no ductal connection with the duodenum. These are the islets of Langerhans, which are responsible for the production of pancreatic hormones. There are three main cell types within the islets: alpha (α), beta (β) and delta (δ), each producing a specific hormone. β cells, by far the most numerous, produce insulin; α cells produce glucagon; and δ cells produce somatostatin. These pancreatic hormones are released directly into the blood flowing through the islets and have their effect on cellular metabolism throughout the body. The function of insulin and glucagon in regulating blood glucose concentration is discussed in Chapter 3.

Pancreatic juice

The exocrine product of pancreatic acinar tissue, pancreatic juice, is a thin watery alkaline fluid (pH around 8) containing a mixture of many digestive enzymes, and electrolytes, most notably sodium, potassium, chloride and bicarbonate ions. With the exception of bicarbonate, electrolytes are present at similar concentration to that found in blood plasma; bicarbonate concentration of pancreatic juice is around four times higher. The relatively high bicarbonate concentration accounts for the alkaline reaction of pancreatic juice.

Pancreatic juice drains into the duodenum at the rate of between 1500 and 3000 ml per day. Its principal function is to continue the process of digestion of food in the small intestine, already begun in the mouth and stomach. The alkaline pH of pancreatic juice ensures that acid chyme (partially digested food) emptying from the stomach into the duodenum is rendered sufficiently alkaline (pH 7–7.5) for optimum pancreatic enzyme activity. The many digestive enzymes contained in pancreatic juice can be broadly divided into three groups according to the substrates in food on which they act: amylase for the digestion of carbohydrates, lipases for the digestion of fats, and proteases for the digestion of proteins. Amylase and lipases are secreted in their active form, whereas proteases are secreted as proenzymes, capable of digesting proteins only after they have been activated within the duodenum. For example, trypsin, a protease present in intestine, is derived from the inactive pancreatic proenzyme trypsinogen. Pancreatic production and secretion of inactive proenzymes rather than their highly reactive product protects the pancreas from enzymic destruction.

The volume and content of pancreatic juice is principally controlled by hormonal pathways. Cholecystokinin-pancreozymin, a gut hormone released in response to gastric emptying of food into the duodenum, stimulates acinar cell production of digestive enzymes. Secretin, another gut hormone, promotes acinar cell production of bicarbonate. Neural pathways also affect pancreatic juice production. The vagal nerve, which is stimulated by the site, smell and thought of food, as well as the presence of food in the mouth, stimulates production of pancreatic juice. Release of pancreatic juice to the duodenum is controlled by the sphincter of Oddi, sited at the hepatopancreatic ampulla. The sphincter opens when food is present in the duodenum. By a synergy of these and other subtle hormonal and neural mechanisms, the body is able to adjust the volume, content and release of pancreatic juice to suit its digestive requirement at the time.

Once pancreatic juice has performed its digestive function, around 99% of the water and electrolyte content of pancreatic juice is reabsorbed into the bloodstream as it passes through the large intestines.

Amylase

Amylase is just one of several digestive enzymes secreted in pancreatic juice. It is also secreted in saliva by three pairs of salivary glands in the mouth. Salivary and pancreatic amylase function only within the gastrointestinal tract where together they are responsible for the breakdown of starch, the principal form of dietary carbohydrate. Starch is essentially many glucose molecules joined together. The product of amylase action on starch is a mixture of three sorts of molecule: the disaccharide maltose (two molecules of glucose joined together); dextrin, a short chain of around eight glucose molecules; and some single molecules of glucose. Any glucose formed by the action of amylase on starch is absorbed to blood by active transport across the cells of the intestinal wall, but maltose and dextrin require further enzymic degradation by the intestinal enzymes maltase and iso-maltase to single glucose molecules, before absorption can occur.

As with all enzymes, amylase will only work to maximum effect within a narrow pH range; for amylase, the optimum pH is 7.1. Digestion of starch begins in the mouth with the action of salivary amylase, during the process of chewing. As soon as food reaches the acidic medium of the stomach (pH 2–3), salivary amylase action ceases. In practice, unless food is masticated in the mouth for a prolonged period, salivary amylase contributes little to overall starch digestion and most starch is broken down in the duodenum and jejunum by pancreatic amylase.

Normally a small amount of amylase circulates in blood plasma. Most of this is of pancreatic origin; some is derived from salivary glands. Amylase has no function in blood plasma and is present there only as a result of normal pancreatic and salivary cell turnover. By comparison with most other enzymes, amylase is a small molecule. Indeed, it is small enough to pass through the glomeruli of the kidneys, so that it is one of very few plasma enzymes normally found in urine.

Laboratory measurement of serum amylase

Patient preparation

No particular patient preparation is necessary.

Sample requirements

Between 2 and 5 ml of venous blood is required.

The test is performed on either blood serum or blood plasma. If local policy is to use serum, then blood must be collected into a plain tube containing no anti-coagulant. If local policy is to use plasma, then blood must be collected into a tube containing an anticoagulant (usually heparin).

Timing of blood sampling and transport

Blood may be collected without reference to time. In many instances the result is required urgently so must be transported to the laboratory without delay. If the request is non-urgent, the sample may be stored at room temperature before routine transport to the laboratory.

Interpretation of results

Approximate reference range

Serum (plasma) amylase   50–200 U/l

(Note: it is particularly important to use local reference range when interpreting enzyme results.)

Terms used in interpretation of results

Hypoamylasaemia   serum amylase below normal
Hyperamylasaemia   serum amylase above normal

An abnormally low serum amylase is a rare finding which has little or no clinical significance. Discussion will be confined to the interpretation of a raised serum amylase.

Causes of raised serum (plasma) amylase

Acute pancreatitis

Acute pancreatitis is a relatively common condition with an annual incidence of 10–20 per million population[1] that predominantly affects the middle aged and elderly. There is evidence that it has become more common over the past 30 years.[2]

There are two main causes: gallstones and alcohol abuse. Together these account for around 80% of cases. A long list of much less common causes include trauma to the pancreas, overactivity of the parathyroid gland (hyperparathyroidism), viral infections (e.g. mumps virus, Epstein–Barr virus, cytomegalovirus), parasitic worm infection and raised blood lipids. Very rarely, acute pancreatitis occurs as a postoperative complication following upper abdominal surgery. Equally rare are those cases caused by prescribed drugs (e.g. thiazide diuretics, angiotensin-converting enzyme (ACE) inhibitors and steroids). Acute pancreatitis is a well documented but rare complication of the invasive diagnostic procedure, endoscopic retrograde cholangiopancreatography (ERCP).

Acute pancreatitis is an acute inflammatory disease that is thought to result from the premature activation of the proteolytic (protein splitting) enzyme. Activation of these enzymes within the pancreas leads to a process of 'autodigestion', in essence self-destruction of the pancreas. Activation of trypsinogen to trypsin has been proposed as an initiating event.[3] It remains unclear precisely how alcohol abuse or gallstone disease triggers the initiating event. Temporary obstruction to the flow of pancreatic juice by gallstones transiently lodged in the hepatopancreatic ampulla is probably significant.

The cardinal symptom is sudden onset of severe upper abdominal pain, which often radiates to the back. Vomiting and pyrexia is common. The course of acute pancreatitis is variable. In the majority of patients, the inflammation is self-limiting, confined to the pancreas and resolves over a period of a few days to a week with no serious long-term consequences. However, this is not the case for the 20–25% of patients who suffer severe acute pancreatitis. This is a life-threatening condition in which the local inflammation leads to systemic inflammatory response syndrome (SIRS) with high risk of sepsis and multiple organ failure. Complications of severe disease include overwhelming infection consequent on massive tissue necrosis, (which may not be confined to pancreas), acute respiratory distress syndrome, jaundice, anaemia, hyperglycaemia, hypocalcaemia, disseminated intravascular coagulation and haemorrhage. Multiple organ failure and death occurs in between 30 and 50% of patients with severe acute pancreatitis.[3]

Damage to acinar cells, the central pathological feature of acute pancreatitis, results in a sudden and massive increase in release of pancreatic enzymes into the bloodstream; among these is amylase. This increase in serum amylase has no clinical consequences of itself, that is, no signs or symptoms of acute pancreatitis can be attributed to an increase in serum amylase. It does, however, provide a marker in the blood of damage to the pancreas. Serum amylase begins to rise 2 to 12 hours after the onset of symptoms and remains elevated for three to five days in most cases. An amylase level of greater than five times the upper limit of normal (i.e. > 1000 U/l) in a patient with acute abdominal pain is widely considered to be almost diagnostic of acute pancreatitis. The probability that acute pain is due to pancreatitis increases as amylase level rises above 1000 U/l. A minority of patients with acute pancreatitis do not show such a marked increase so that a serum amylase of < 1000 U/l cannot be used to exclude the diagnosis.[4] Very rarely, the serum amylase may be normal in a patient with acute pancreatitis. It might be assumed that the higher the serum amylase, the more severe the pancreatitis; this is not the case. In fact, no prognostic information can be derived from measurement of serum amylase at the time of diagnosis.[4] However, failure of amylase to return to normal following an acute attack suggests the presence of a pancreatic pseudocyst (a late complication of acute pancreatitis).

Chronic pancreatitis

Natural repair of the damage caused by inflammation of acute pancreatitis leaves the pancreas of someone who has recovered from acute pancreatitis functioning normally. By contrast, chronic pancreatitis is a chronic inflammation in which damage to the pancreas is slow but irreversibly progressive. The most common cause is long-term alcohol abuse. It may be a feature of haemochromatosis, a disease of iron overload in which excess iron is deposited in the pancreas and other organs. Continuous or at least recurrent abdominal pain is the cardinal symptom of chronic pancreatitis. Long term, the condition results in malabsorption of food and consequent weight loss due to failure of pancreatic enzyme production and diabetes as a result of islet cell damage. Serum amylase may be slightly raised in the early stages but as acinar cell production of digestive enzymes (including amylase) becomes increasingly compromised, serum amylase falls to normal or even to levels below normal. Since amylase may be raised, normal or reduced, the test serves no useful purpose in the diagnosis of chronic pancreatitis.

Cancer of the pancreas

Apart from acute and chronic pancreatitis, cancer of the pancreas is the only other significant disease of the pancreas. Serum amylase is either marginally raised or normal; the test is not useful for the diagnosis of cancer of the pancreas.

Table 12.1 Principal causes of raised serum/plasma amylase.

- Acute pancreatitis
- Chronic pancreatitis
- Renal failure
- Diabetic ketoacidosis
- Intestinal obstruction
- Perforated peptic ulcer
- Acute cholecystitis
- Abdominal trauma
- Mumps
- Macroamylassaemia

Non-pancreatic disease

Serum amylase may be mildly to moderately raised (i.e. rarely greater than 1000 U/l) in some non-pancreatic disorders e.g. perforation of peptic ulcer, intestinal obstruction, and gall bladder disease (acute cholecystitis). All these conditions are usually associated with acute abdominal pain, so a patient with a raised serum amylase in association with acute abdominal pain is not necessarily suffering acute pancreatitis. Abdominal trauma, not necessarily involving the pancreas, may result in an increased amylase; a significant minority of patients who receive abdominal surgery have a transient rise during the postoperative period.

Amylase is cleared from the blood by the kidneys, so that patients in acute or chronic renal failure typically have slight to moderate increases in serum amylase.

A moderate to marked increase is often a feature of diabetic ketoacidosis. Disease of, or damage to the parotid glands where salivary amylase is produced may result in an increase in serum amylase. Examples include infection with the mumps virus, maxillofacial surgery, and parotid gland irradiation.

Finally, raised serum amylase is a feature of a rare and entirely benign condition called macroamylasaemia, in which amylase circulates in serum in the form of macromolecular aggregates of amylase or bound to serum proteins. Because they are so large, these macromolecules cannot pass across the glomerular membrane of the kidneys and are not excreted in urine; instead they accumulate in serum.

Table 12.1 provides a summary of the principal causes of raised serum amylase.

Case history 11

Mrs Campbell, a 40-year-old pharmacist, arrived by ambulance at the emergency department of her local hospital in considerable pain and distress, looking pale and shocked. The pain, which had only become severe four hours earlier, was localised in the mid-epigastric region; she described it as 'shooting through her back'. She was vomiting. Her temperature was 100°C, blood pressure 90/60 mm Hg and respiratory rate 30/min. During initial examination, Mrs Campbell told the admitting doctor that she had been diagnosed as having gallstones and was currently on a weight reduction diet in preparation for cholecystectomy (surgical removal of gall bladder). The doctor suspected Mrs Campbell might be suffering acute pancreatitis. Blood was sampled for U&E, glucose, amylase and full blood count. The laboratory results included:

Serum amylase   1700 U/l
Blood glucose   15.6 mmol/l

Questions

(1) What suggested to the admitting doctor that Mrs Campbell might be suffering acute pancreatitis?
(2) Are the serum amylase and blood glucose normal?
(3) Do the laboratory results support the initial diagnosis?
(4) Why might a patient suffering acute pancreatitis have a raised blood glucose?

Discussion of case history

(1) Sudden onset of severe abdominal pain is the most common finding in patients with acute pancreatitis; in around a half of cases, this pain is referred to the back. Vomiting is also a common symptom. Mrs Campbell was hypotensive, suggesting hypovolaemic shock. Loss of pancreatic secretion into the peritoneal space and haemorrhage due to vessel erosion by pancreatic enzymes, can lead to hypovolaemic shock in acute pancreatitis. Finally, acute pancreatitis is a complication of gall bladder disease.

(2) No. Both serum amylase and blood glucose are markedly raised; amylase is more than 7 times the upper limit of normal.

(3) Yes. An increase in amylase of this degree is almost diagnostic of acute pancreatitis. Amylase may be raised in a number of non-pancreatic conditions that result in abdominal pain, but very rarely to this degree. Transient hyperglycaemia is sometimes a feature of acute pancreatitis, requiring insulin therapy and regular blood glucose monitoring.

(4) Acute pancreatitis may involve damage to the endocrine (islet) cells of the pancreas, where insulin is produced. Insulin is the principal hormone of blood glucose regulation; a deficiency of the hormone results in raised blood glucose concentration. Islet cells damage may be minimal, in which case normal insulin production and secretion continues and hyperglycaemia does not occur.

References

1. Beckingham I & Bornman P (2001) Acute pancreatitis. *Br Med J* **322**: 595–98.
2. Goldacre M & Roberts S (2004) Hospital admission for acute pancreatitis in an English population, 1963–1998: database study of incidence and mortality. *Br Med J* **328**: 1466–69.
3. Bhatia M, Wong F *et al.* (2005) Pathophysiology of acute pancreatitis. *Pancreatology* **5**: 132–44.
4. Lankisch P, Burchard-Recjkert S & Lehnik D (1999) Underestimation of acute pancreatitis: patients with only a small increase in amylase/lipase levels can also have or develop severe acute pancreatitis. *Gut* **44**: 542–44.

Further reading

Despins L, Kivlahan C & Cox K (2005) Acute pancreatitis: diagnosis and treatment of a potentially fatal condition. *Am J Nurs* **105**: 54–57.

Imrie C (1993) Acute pancreatitis. In: Bouchier L, Allan R, Hodgson H, Keighly M (eds) *Gastroenterology: Clinical Science and Practice*. Philadelphia: WB Saunders.

Chapter 13

DRUG OVERDOSE: PARACETAMOL AND SALICYLATE

Clinical laboratory staff are often requested to analyse blood or urine samples for the presence of drugs. Such analyses are valuable in two usually separate clinical contexts: deliberate or accidental drug overdose and therapeutic drug monitoring. Chapter 14 is concerned principally with the latter, while this chapter is concerned with how laboratory measurement of serum or plasma concentration of salicylate and paracetamol contributes to the care of patients who have, or are suspected of having, taken a deliberate or accidental acute overdose of paracetamol (acetaminophen) or aspirin (acetylsalicylic acid).

Despite government initiatives to restrict over the counter sales,[1] paracetamol remains the most common drug to be taken in overdose, accounting for a half of all drug overdose-related attendances at UK hospital emergency departments [2] It is the sole or contributory cause of death for around 500 people every year in England and Wales.[3] Overdose with aspirin is less common but still accounts for 5–7% of drug overdose-related hospital admissions and around 30–40 deaths in the UK each year.[4]

Clinical use of aspirin and paracetamol: safety of therapeutic dose

Both aspirin and paracetamol are analgesics and antipyretics, that is, they reduce pain and body temperature. They are frequently self-prescribed for the relief of temporary symptoms associated with minor viral infections (e.g. influenza, colds, etc.) and for the relief of headaches and minor muscular aches and pains. Aspirin has two further major pharmacological properties: at high dose (> 3 g/day) it has an anti-inflammatory effect and at lower dose (75–300 mg/day) an antithrombotic (anti-blood clotting) effect. These two properties have determined that long-term prescription of aspirin is useful in the treatment of chronic inflammatory conditions like arthritis, and for the prevention of myocardial infarction and strokes among high-risk patients. The use of aspirin for primary prevention of myocardial infarction and strokes in the general population is currently under investigation. There is evidence that long-term aspirin use protects against many common cancers including bowel,[5] lung[6] and breast[7] cancer.

The maximum recommended dose of paracetamol for adults and children over the age of 12 is two 500 mg tablets, with an interval of at least four hours between doses. No more than eight tablets should be taken in 24 hours (i.e. a maximum dose of 4 g/day). As long as this dose is not exceeded, paracetamol has no adverse effect and is a remarkably safe drug, even if used for a prolonged period.

Long-term aspirin use, even at prescribed therapeutic doses, is less safe. In common with other non-steroidal anti-inflammatory drugs (NSAIDs), long-term aspirin use is associated with irritation of the stomach wall lining (gastric mucosa) and the risk of gastrointestinal bleeding and stomach ulcers. Patients with a history of peptic ulcer or an increased tendency to bleed are prescribed aspirin only rarely. Some patients on long-term, high-dose aspirin therapy may experience some of the symptoms of acute overdose, even if they are taking what, for others, is a safe therapeutic dose. There is evidence that aspirin use among children with a viral infection precipitates a serious life threatening condition known as Reye's syndrome. For this reason aspirin is not recommended for use in children. The recommended dose for analgesic and antipyretic effect is one to two 325 mg tablets every four hours; no more than 12 tablets in 24 hours should be taken. For anti-inflammatory effect, that dose has to be increased to around two 500 mg tablets, usually every six hours. Just 75–150 mg/day is sufficient for anti-thrombotic effect.

Paracetamol

Absorption, metabolism and acute toxicity

Paracetamol is quickly absorbed from the gastrointestinal tract to blood over a period of 30 minute to two hours for a therapeutic dose. A small amount (up to 5%) is eliminated unchanged in urine, but the remainder is metabolised in the liver (Figure 13.1). Like most other drugs, paracetamol must be made more water soluble for appreciable elimination in urine. This is achieved in the liver, by synthetic conjugation (joining) of paracetamol with sulphate, glucuronate, glycine and phosphate. The resulting water-soluble conjugates of paracetamol are non-toxic. Around 90% of an ingested paracetamol dose is eliminated safely via urine in this way. The rest of the paracetamol (between 5 and 10% of an ingested dose) is oxidised in the liver, to a highly reactive and toxic free radical, called N-acetyl-p-benzoquinoneimine (NAPQI). NAPQI is responsible for the toxic effects of paracetamol. At normal paracetamol dose the liver is able to inactivate this potentially damaging NAPQI by reaction with a substance called glutathione, which is synthesised in the liver. The product of the reaction between NAPQI and glutathione is non-toxic and is eliminated safely in urine and bile.

If there were no limit to the rate at which the liver could synthesise glutathione, then paracetamol would not be harmful, no matter how much had been taken, but unfortunately this is not the case. If recommended dose is exceeded the production of NAPQI increases, but the ability of the liver to synthesise the inactivating glutathione cannot keep pace, and NAPQI accumulates in liver cells, disrupting cellular mechanisms and eventually causing liver cell death (necrosis).[8] Without

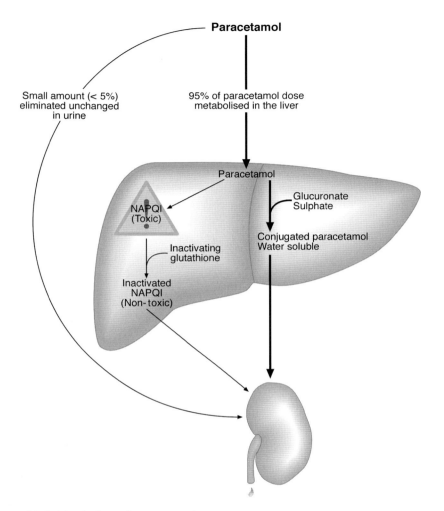

Figure 13.1 Metabolism of paracetamol.
*NAPQI = **N**-**a**cetyl-**p**-benzo**q**uinone**i**mine*

prompt treatment, liver cell necrosis becomes extensive, leading to acute liver failure. At this stage liver transplantation is the only treatment option.

A single dose of paracetamol of between 150–200 mg/kg is sufficient to cause liver cell damage in adults. This means that for an adult weighing an average 70 kg, just 10 g of paracetamol (i.e. 20 tablets) may be significant. Twelve grams (24 tablets) can be fatal, and without treatment 25 g (50 tablets) is inevitably fatal. Certain drugs (notably the anticonvulsants phenytoin, carbamazepine and phenobarbitone) and alcohol result in increased production of the enzymes responsible for NAPQI production. Thus patients who have taken alcohol or these drugs are particularly susceptible to the toxic effects of paracetamol.

Signs and symptoms of acute overdose

The early symptoms of even potentially fatal paracetamol overdose are non-specific and unremarkable. For the first 24 hours, nausea and vomiting are the only symptoms; loss of consciousness is not an early feature. Signs and symptoms of extensive liver cell damage including jaundice, abdominal tenderness, continuing nausea and vomiting begin to develop in the 24 to 36 hours after overdose. Deterioration in liver function over the next few days leads to acute liver failure in the most severe cases. Drowsiness leading to coma is a feature at this late stage.

Principles of overdose treatment

As long as treatment is initiated early enough (i.e. within 12 hours of overdose), a complete recovery can be expected, even after a potentially fatal dose of paracetamol. Because of the speed at which paracetamol is absorbed from the intestine, efforts aimed at reducing absorption of paracetamol, including gastric lavage and administration of charcoal, are only likely to be effective if begun within an hour or two of the overdose. The main treatment is early IV administration of the paracetamol antidote: N-acetylcysteine (NAC). In the body NAC is converted to glutathione, the substance required for inactivation of NAQI, the toxic metabolite of paracetamol. NAC is successful in preventing liver damage if administered within 12 hours of the overdose. Although less effective after 12 hours, some benefit can be gained by administration up to 24 hours, or even 72 hours in some cases, after overdose.

Aspirin

Absorption, metabolism and acute toxicity

Absorption of aspirin from the gastrointestinal tract is dependent on the amount and formulation of the drug. Therapeutic doses of regular (non-enteric coated) aspirin are absorbed rapidly within two hours. Larger quantities (overdose) of regular aspirin however inhibit gastric emptying with a resulting delay of up to six hours in intestinal absorption. Enteric coated formulations of aspirin are designed to be impervious to the acid contact in the stomach and only begin to dissolve after arrival in the alkaline medium of the small intestine; such formulations may take up to 12 hours to be completely absorbed.

After absorption, aspirin is rapidly hydrolysed to salicylic acid (salicylate). This is the substance responsible for the acute toxicity as well as many of the therapeutic effects of aspirin. Before salicylate can be eliminated in urine it must first be conjugated with glycine to form salicyluric acid, or glucuronate to form phenolic glucuronides, but the enzymes for these detoxifying reactions become rapidly saturated at even therapeutic levels. As a consequence, salicylate accumulates in tissues in a dose-dependent manner. Increased serum salicylate concentration stimulates the respiratory centre causing hyperventilation, which results in increased carbon dioxide elimination and respiratory alkalosis (Chapter 6). Salicylate at toxic levels has an effect on cellular metabolism which results in hyperpyrexia, sweating and abnormally high production of metabolic acids. Along with salicylate, itself an acid, these acids accumulate in blood causing a metabolic acidosis. Salicylate causes increased permeability of the vasculature in the lungs, predisposing to the development of pulmonary oedema in salicylate overdose, particularly among smokers and the elderly. Finally, salicylate can adversely affect normal control of blood glucose concentration; overdose of aspirin may result in hypoglycaemia (low blood glucose) or reduced levels of glucose in the brain (neuroglycopaenia), despite normal blood glucose levels. Mild toxicity arises after a single dose of around 150 mg/kg body weight, whereas severe toxicity is associated with a single dose of greater than 500 mg/kg. For an adult of average weight (70 kg) just 20×500 mg tablets or 30×325 mg tablets are sufficient for mild toxicity.

Signs and symptoms of acute toxicity

Salicylate poisoning is much easier to recognise in the early stages than paracetamol poisoning. Mild to moderate poisoning commonly causes nausea, vomiting and tinnitus, with loss of hearing. Patients are usually hyperventilating, hyperpyrexial and sweating. Dehydration secondary to vomiting, sweating and hyperventilation is usually a feature, particularly in severe poisoning. Blood gas analysis reveals disturbance of acid-base (either respiratory alkalosis, metabolic acidosis or a combination of the two). Acidaemia (low blood pH) is a poor prognostic sign because it enhances salicylate entry into tissue cells; entry of salicylate into brain cells causes additional neurological symptoms including confusion, delerium, and extreme agitation. Loss of consciousness may occur, but is rare.

Principles of overdose treatment

There is no antidote for the treatment of aspirin overdose, as there is for paracetamol overdose. Treatment instead is based on three main objectives:

- preventing further absorption of aspirin from the gastrointestinal tract
- increasing urinary elimination of salicylate
- correction of dehydration and deranged blood chemistry (acid-base and electrolyte disturbances, and hypoglycaemia if present).

The delay in intestinal absorption of high-dose aspirin, especially enteric coated formulations, ensures that gastric lavage or repeated administration of activated charcoal are likely to be effective in reducing absorption, for much longer than is the case in paracetamol overdose, although of course, the sooner it is started, the more effective it will be. Urinary elimination of salicylate is increased if urine is made alkaline (pH > 7.5) and urine output increased. This is achieved by administration of large volumes of sodium bicarbonate. Such treatment has the additional advantage of making blood more alkaline and thereby inhibiting the entry of salicylate into cells. Removal of salicylate from blood by haemodialysis or peritoneal dialysis may be considered in the most severe cases. Dextrose may be added to any IV fluid used to correct fluid and electrolyte disturbance since there is evidence that even if blood glucose is normal, the brain is depleted of glucose in moderate to severe salicylate poisoning.

Laboratory measurement of salicylate and paracetamol

Patient preparation

No particular patient preparation is necessary.

Timing of sample

The time of blood sampling and the time of the overdose (if known) must be recorded on the accompanying request card. Because of varying rates of paracetamol absorption, it is impossible to accurately interpret a paracetamol result of a sample taken less than four hours after an overdose. Blood sampling should therefore be delayed until four hours have elapsed since paracetamol was taken. In all cases of salicylate poisoning it is useful to know the peak concentration. This can only be found by repeat sampling (every three hours) until a reduction in concentration is detected.

Sample requirements

Around 5 ml of venous blood is required for paracetamol and salicylate estimation. Analysis can be performed on either serum or plasma. If local policy is to use serum, blood must be collected into a plain (without additives) tube. If local policy is to use plasma, blood must be collected into a tube containing the anticoagulant, lithium heparin.

Transport of samples

The results of paracetamol and salicylate estimation are required for immediate patient management and therefore samples must be considered urgent and transported to the laboratory without delay.

Interpretation of paracetamol result

There seems to be no universal agreement about units of measurement for paracetamol; some laboratories report paracetamol in traditional units (mg/l or μgm/ml); *note that 1 mg/l = 1 µg/ml*. Other laboratories use the SI unit of measurement (µmol/ml or µmol/l); *note 1 µmol/ml = 1000 µmol/l*. A potentially dangerous interpretation is possible if these units are confused.

Interpretation of paracetamol results depends crucially on knowing the approximate time of overdose. Figure 13.2 is a widely used nomogram, which allows assessment of the severity of overdose based on the paracetamol concentration in relation to the time in hours since the overdose. For example, it can be seen from the graph that a paracetamol concentration of 80 mg/l taken four hours after an overdose indicates that liver damage is extremely unlikely. However, the same paracetamol result in a blood sample taken 12 hours after an overdose indicates that

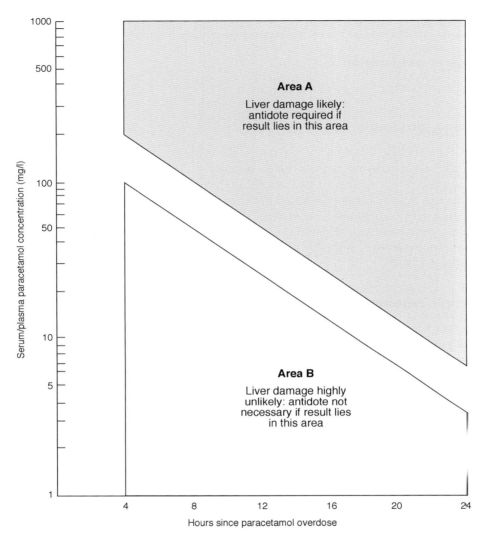

Figure 13.2 Interpretation of paracetamol result following overdose.
Note: If result lies between areas A and B, antidote treatment is normally only considered necessary if patient has also taken alcohol or certain other drugs that increase the toxicity of paracetamol. It is not possible to interpret a result if blood is sampled less than four hours after overdose.

without antidote (N-acetylcysteine) treatment, severe, even fatal liver damage can be expected.

The graph highlights two important features of paracetamol toxicity. Firstly, it is not possible to accurately determine the severity of a paracetamol overdose, based on a serum paracetamol derived from blood sampled less than four hours after an overdose; a repeat sample would be advisable in these circumstances. Secondly, any measurable amounts of paracetamol in serum 24 hours or later after an overdose indicates a poor prognosis, especially as antidote treatment at this late stage is unlikely to be very effective in halting liver cell damage.

Interpretation of salicylate result

Again there is no consensus between laboratories concerning units of measurement. Most laboratories use either mg/l or mg/dl. *Note: a salicylate concentration of 10 mg/dl = 100 mg/l.*

Patients on long-term high-dose aspirin therapy for chronic inflammatory conditions such as rheumatoid arthritis typically have a serum salicylate concentration of 25–35 mg/dl (i.e. 250–350 mg/l). These levels are rarely associated with any symptoms of acute toxicity. Mild to moderate toxicity occurs with peak salicylate concentration in the range 30–80 mg/dl (300–800 mg/l) while peak levels greater than 80 mg/dl (800 mg/ml) are associated with severe toxicity; around 5% of patients admitted to hospital with this level of toxicity do not survive. Serum salicylate levels provide an approximate and useful guide to the severity of a particular overdose but are not as reliable in this regard as serum paracetamol is in cases of paracetamol overdose. The clinical condition of the patient, along with blood gas and electrolyte results, are as important as plasma salicylate results for assessment of prognosis and clinical care planning. However, some general points can be made. Nearly all patients, even those with mild toxicity, will be given gastric lavage and or activated charcoal. The likelihood that a patient will require alkalinisation of urine increases as the serum salicylate increases beyond 50 mg/dl. Finally, haemodialysis is usually reserved for those patients whose serum salicylate is in excess of 80 mg/dl, although it may be considered the treatment of choice for all patients who have significant kidney disease.

A rise in serum salicylate during treatment may indicate continuing salicylate absorption and/or failure to adequately increase urine elimination. A decline in serum salicylate concentration is used to confirm that treatment aimed at increased urinary elimination of salicylate has been effective. Sometimes, however, a reduction in serum concentration merely reflects haemodilution, if high volume fluids have been infused.

Case history 12

Andrew Roberts, a 23-year-old university student, became depressed having failed his final examinations. Following an alcoholic binge he returned to his flat, took 18 paracetamol tablets and fell asleep. On waking early the next morning, some six hours after taking the tablets, he was feeling sick and extremely regretful about taking the tablets. Worried about the possible effects, he rang the local hospital accident and emergency department for advice.

Question

(1) What would your advice be?
(2) Would it have been advisable for Andrew to have received activated charcoal on arrival?
(3) What is the significance of the paracetamol result?

Discussion of case history

(1) Andrew had taken 9 g of paracetamol, well in excess of the maximum recommended single dose, which is 1 g. Assuming an average body weight of 70 kg, 9 g represents a dose of 9000/70 mg/kg (i.e. 129 mg/kg). Liver damage is unlikely if a single dose of < 150 mg/kg has been taken. However, the fact that Andrew also took alcohol must be taken into account, because alcohol increases production of the enzymes necessary for oxidation of paracetamol to the toxic metabolite NAPQI. The toxicity of paracetamol is increased if alcohol has been taken. It would be wise for Andrew to attend casualty urgently so that his serum paracetamol can be checked.

Andrew took the advice given by A&E staff. Within the hour, he arrived at the hospital and was seen immediately by the casualty officer who took blood for serum paracetamol estimation, some eight hours after Andrew had taken the tablets. The laboratory telephoned back the result:

serum paracetamol   42 mg/l

(2) Paracetamol is absorbed from the gastrointestinal tract within a few hours of ingestion. It is highly unlikely that there would have been any paracetamol remaining in Andrew's stomach by the time he arrived in A&E. Both gastric lavage and charcoal administration would have been ineffective at this late stage.

(3) From the nomogram (Figure 13.2) it can be seen that Andrew was not at risk of liver damage and did not require antidote therapy. His physical health was considered not at risk.

References

1. Hawton K, Simkin S et al. (2004) UK legislation on analgesic packs before and after study of long-term effects. Br Med J 329: 1076–80.
2. Greene S, Dargan P & Jones A (2005) Acute poisoning: understanding 90% of cases in a nutshell. Postgrad Med J 81: 204–16.
3. Morgan O, Griffiths C & Majeed A (2005) Impact of paracetamol pack size restrictions on poisoning from paracetamol in England and Wales. J Public Health 27: 19–24.
4. Wood D, Dargan P & Jones A (2005) Measuring plasma salicylate concentrations in all patients with drug overdose or altered consciousness: is it necessary? Emerg Med J 22: 401–403.
5. Chan A, Giovannucci E & Schernhammer E (2004) A prospective study of aspirin use and the risk for colorectal adenoma. Ann Intern Med 140: 157–66.
6. Moyisch K, Menezes R et al. (2002) Regular aspirin use and lung cancer risk. BMC Cancer 2: 31.
7. Rahme E, Ghosn J et al. (2005) Association between frequent use of nonsteroidal anti-inflammatory drugs and breast cancer. BMC Cancer 5: 159.
8. James L, Mayeux P & Hinson J (2003) Acetaminophen-induced hepatotoxicity. Drug Metab Dispos 31: 1499–1506.

Further reading

Dargan P, Wallace C & Jones A (2002) An evidence-based flowchart to guide management of acute salicylate (aspirin) overdose. *Emerg Med J* **19**: 206–209.

Farley A, Hendry C & Napier P (2005) Paracetamol poisoning: physiological aspects and management strategies. *Nurs Stand* **19**(38): 58–64.

Littlejohn C (2004) Management of intentional overdose in A&E departments. *Nurs Times* **100**(33): 38–43.

Wallace C, Dargan P & Jones A (2002) Paracetamol overdose: an evidence based flow chart to guide management. *Emerg Med J* **19**: 202–205.

Chapter 14

THERAPEUTIC DRUG MONITORING: LITHIUM, DIGOXIN AND THEOPHYLLINE

This chapter is concerned with how laboratory measurement of drug concentration in blood helps in determining correct drug dose. Such an approach is either unnecessary or unsuitable for most drug therapies, but for a limited number of drugs, including lithium, digoxin and theophylline, measurement of serum or plasma concentration is the preferred method of optimising dosage and preventing dangerous side effects (toxicity). Measuring drug concentration also provides a means of confirming patient compliance. Other drug therapies, not discussed in this chapter, in which therapeutic drug monitoring is useful, include the anticonvulsant drugs carbamazepine, valproate and phenytoin; some drugs used to treat disturbances of cardiac rhythm (e.g. procainamide, quinidine) and a few antibiotics (e.g. gentamicin, vancomycin).

Lithium

Pharmacological action and clinical use

Although the precise mechanism of action of lithium is poorly understood, the effect of the drug is to stabilise mood; its use is confined to psychiatric patients primarily for the treatment of bipolar disorder.[1] This common psychiatric condition, sometimes called manic-depression or affective disorder affects around 1.5–2% of the population and is characterised by cyclic episodes of depression followed by elation (mania). Normal mood is in the middle of a continuum, which runs from depression at one extreme to mania at the other. Depression is associated with a lack of energy, diminished interest and ability to experience pleasure, along with feelings of despair and pessimism. During the manic phase of bipolar disease, however, symptoms are those of an abnormally expansive mood with increased mental and physical energy. Affected patients are hyperactive and have difficulty sleeping. Inflated self-esteem and false optimism are accompanied by flights of fancy and impulsive behaviour. In its most severe form, mania results in thinking that can race so fast that it becomes fragmented. Speech is fast and may be incoherent. Psychotic symptoms, including hallucination, grandiose delusion and illusion, may be a feature of severe acute mania.

Lithium is an anti-manic drug. Although used to treat acute mania and its less severe form, hypomania among patients presenting with symptoms, the most important use of lithium is to prevent both manic and depressive episodes in patients with bipolar disorder; the result is a marked reduction in mood swings. Patients may need to take lithium for many years in order to remain well. Unfortunately, for unknown reasons, some patients with bipolar disease do not respond to lithium therapy. Lithium may also be used in conjunction with antidepressant drugs to treat severe depression that does not respond to antidepressant drugs alone.

Adverse side effects

All drugs have unwanted side effects and lithium is no exception. Lithium can affect kidney function, causing a condition known as nephrogenic diabetes insipidus, which is characterised by increased urine flow (polyuria) and resulting increased thirst (polydipsia). The thyroid gland of patients on long-term lithium therapy may become underactive, with resulting symptoms of hypothyroidism (Chapter 10). This may contribute to the weight gain that is often associated with lithium use. Patients on long-term lithium therapy should have regular (six-monthly) thyroid function tests and serum creatinine estimation to assess renal function. Special caution should be taken in prescribing lithium during pregnancy, as there is increased risk of congenital malformation of the developing fetus associated with lithium use, particularly during the first three months of pregnancy. Lithium is eliminated from the body almost entirely by the kidneys in urine. For this reason the potential for lithium toxicity is greater in older patients, whose renal function is reduced, and patients with kidney disease. To avoid adverse effects, such patients may need a lower dose of lithium than those with normally functioning kidneys.

Why and when to measure serum lithium

The lithium dose required for treatment or prevention of manic symptoms (called the therapeutic dose) is very close to that which results in toxicity. In common with all three drugs discussed in this chapter, lithium is said to have a low 'therapeutic index' or narrow 'therapeutic window'. Fortunately, there is a well-defined therapeutic range for serum lithium, providing a means of checking that sufficient drug is being administered for maximum therapeutic effect, consistent with minimum risk of toxic side effects. Serum lithium is checked initially after 5–7 days on initial prescription dose. If serum concentration is below the therapeutic range, dose is increased, and if higher than therapeutic range, dose is decreased. Once a safe and effective maintenance dose has been established, serum lithium should be checked every week for four weeks and then every three months.[1] Urgent blood testing is, however, necessary if any signs or symptoms of toxicity arise and in cases of deliberate overdose (parasuicide).

Patients suffering bipolar disease may be reluctant to take their lithium regularly once initial symptoms have subsided; they may falsely believe that they do not require lithium, and stop taking tablets without consultation with their doctor. Measuring serum lithium provides a means of confirming that patients are continuing with their medication.

Digoxin

Principal pharmacological action and clinical use

Digoxin, which is derived from digitalis, a compound extracted from the leaves of the foxglove plant *(digitalis lanata)* is used in the treatment of heart disease. Digoxin inhibits the enzyme (ATPase) required for action of the sodium-potassium pump, present in the membrane of all cells, which maintains the distribution of sodium and potassium between cells and surrounding extracellular fluid (Chapter 3). The net effect of reduced sodium-potassium pump activity (and therefore digoxin administration) is an increase in sodium and calcium concentration within cells and a decrease in concentration of cellular potassium. It is the increase in calcium concentration within the muscle cells of the heart that accounts for the positive inotropic (increased force of cardiac muscle cell contraction) effects of digoxin. Apart from its positive inotropic effects, digoxin also indirectly affects (via vagal stimulation) the pacemaker cells of the sino-atrial (SA) and atrioventricular (AV) nodes in the heart that propagate electrical signals necessary for normal heart rate and rhythm. The only condition for which digoxin is usually prescribed is chronic heart failure (CHF).

CHF is a common condition of the elderly: average age at diagnosis is 76 years. Both incidence and prevalence increase steadily with increasing age, so that 1 in 35 of the 65–74 year age group are affected, rising to a prevalence of 1 in 7 among those over 85 years.[2] The central problem for those with CHF is failure of the pumping action of the heart, so that it is unable to maintain normal cardiac output and supply sufficient blood to adequately meet the oxygen and other nutritional demands of tissues. The two most common causes are coronary heart disease and hypertension.

Breathlessness, brought on by mild exertion and fatigue, are the two most common early symptoms. As a result of the body's compensatory mechanisms for a failing heart, which include water and sodium retention, ankle oedema develops, causing ankle swelling. Accumulation of fluid in lungs (pulmonary oedema) contributes to breathlessness, which eventually occurs even at rest and is made worse by lying flat. More generalised oedema may develop, causing abdominal distension with associated pain and discomfort, and weight gain. CHF is currently incurable, but treatment, including drug therapy, can improve life quality and life expectancy.

For many years digoxin (in combination with diuretics) was the mainstay drug prescribed for all patients with CHF. With the introduction of a more effective drug regime (ACE inhibitors and β-blockers (plus diuretic)), digoxin is used more selectively today. It remains the first line drug of choice for that subset of patients whose CHF is complicated by the cardiac arrhythmia, atrial fibrillation.[3] Around a third of CHF patients have co-existing atrial fibrillation.[4] Digoxin is also recommended for patients whose symptoms are worsening or not improving despite optimal dose of ACE inhibitor, β-blocker and diuretic.[3]

Toxic (unwanted) side effects

Symptoms of digoxin toxicity include nausea, vomiting, diarrhoea and loss of appetite. Abnormal cardiac rhythms, which may result in either slowing of the heart rate (bradycardia) or increased heart rate (tachycardia), are common; in severe overdose, these may be life threatening. Disturbances of normal vision, including blurring of vision and loss of ability to distinguish some colour combinations, may occur. Mental effects include confusion and restlessness; rarely digoxin toxicity can precipitate acute psychoses. The primary effect of digoxin on the sodium–potassium pump determines that digoxin toxicity may be accompanied by raised serum potassium.

Most digoxin is normally eliminated from the body unchanged, by the kidneys, in urine. Patients with diminished kidney function (the elderly and those with renal disease) cannot eliminate digoxin as efficiently as those with normal kidney function and are therefore at greater risk of digoxin toxicity. Abnormally low concentration of serum potassium (hypokalaemia), often the result of diuretic therapy, potentiates digoxin toxicity. A low serum magnesium and raised serum calcium have a similar effect.

Why and when to measure serum digoxin

Routine monitoring of serum digoxin levels for all patients receiving digoxin is not considered necessary. However, the test is useful in certain clinical situations. Like lithium, digoxin has a low therapeutic index. The serum level required for therapeutic effect is close to that which results in toxic symptoms, so digoxin toxicity is relatively common. Unfortunately, many of the signs and symptoms of mild to moderate toxicity are non-specific and may even be due to the underlying disease that digoxin is being used to treat. The only sure way of making or excluding the diagnosis of digoxin toxicity is to measure serum digoxin concentration. A request for blood digoxin level may be made following a poor clinical response to a standard digoxin dose. If the result is below the therapeutic range, an increased dose may be safely prescribed. Finally, the test can be used to assess patient compliance.

Theophylline

Principal pharmacological action and clinical use

Theophylline is a naturally occurring substance related to caffeine, found in the leaves of the tea plant. Although the mechanism of its action is poorly understood, theophylline has three important pharmacological effects: stimulation of cardiac muscle, relaxation of smooth muscle (notably that of the lungs), and stimulation of the central nervous system. The principal clinical use of theophylline, which is derived from its effect on smooth muscle in the lung, is as a bronchodilator in the treatment of asthma and chronic obstructive pulmonary disease (COPD).

Asthma is a common condition of the lungs, affecting up to 5% of children and 2% of adults in the UK, characterised by episodic attacks of airway constriction. Between attacks, patients are usually quite well but during attacks, which may be triggered by any number of factors including respiratory infection, environmental irritants (chemical fumes, smoke etc), exercise and even in some cases laughter, the bronchial airways constrict, become inflamed and produce abnormal amounts of mucus. These result in the common symptoms associated with an asthma attack: cough, wheeze and increased breathlessness. In its most severe manifestation, an asthma attack can cause respiratory failure in which normal gas exchange of oxygen and carbon dioxide is sufficiently compromised to threaten life. Although prompt hospital admission and treatment can be life saving, around 2000 asthma patients die each year.

Theophylline is given orally as part of the ongoing drug treatment of chronic asthma to prevent attacks, and is also administered intravenously in the form of aminophylline (a salt of theophylline) for the emergency treatment of acute asthma attacks. Theophylline acts directly to relax the smooth muscles of the bronchi effectively dilating or 'opening' the airway. The bronchodilator effect of theophylline is more pronounced if the airway is already constricted, as it is in patients with asthma.

Apart from asthma, the bronchodilating properties of theophylline are also used in the treatment of chronic obstructive pulmonary disease. A quite separate property of theophylline, the ability to stimulate the respiratory centres in the central nervous system, is thought to be the reason for its effectiveness in the treatment of apnoea of prematurity. Affected premature babies suddenly stop breathing for 20 seconds or more threatening brain function; there is a risk of permanent brain damage. Both the frequency and duration of these so-called apnoea attacks are reduced with theophylline treatment.

Toxic (unwanted) side effects

Many patients experience minor adverse effects of theophylline therapy, and for this reason the drug is usually only prescribed for the prevention of asthma attacks, after other anti-asthma drugs have failed. Nausea, vomiting and loss of appetite are the most common signs of mild toxicity. Headache, insomnia, nervousness and increased irritability reflect the effect of theophylline on the central nervous system (CNS). While many patients may experience both gastrointestinal and CNS effects when they first take theophylline, a tolerance is usually acquired and symptoms disappear. Theophylline is a gastrointestinal irritant that can reactivate peptic ulcers. In addition to the gastrointestinal and CNS symptoms, marked toxicity may result in palpitations, increased heart rate, and abnormal heart rhythms (usually sinus tachychardia). Cardiac arrest can occur in patients given a single large dose of theophylline (aminophylline) to control an acute asthma attack. Convulsions and loss of consciousness can occur during marked toxicity. Although rare, severe toxicity can be fatal.

Certain diseases (e.g. liver disease, chronic heart failure and any condition associated with persistent fever) cause a decrease in the rate that theophylline can be eliminated from the body and a consequent increase in serum theophylline to a concentration normally associated with toxic symptoms. Asthmatic patients with these additional problems require a lower dose than normal and careful monitoring if they are to avoid the effects of theophylline toxicity. Conversely, smokers eliminate theophylline more efficiently than non-smokers so require a higher dose to achieve the same therapeutic effect. Toxicity may arise after quitting smoking if dose is not reduced. Many drugs, including alcohol and some antibiotics, reduce theophylline elimination, thereby increasing toxicity at a given dosage. A full drug history must be taken into account when prescribing theophylline.

Why and when to measure serum theophylline

Theophylline has a low therapeutic index: the serum concentration required for therapeutic effect is close to that which results in toxic symptoms. Although the serum level for therapeutic effect has been established, the dose required to attain this therapeutic level varies, so all patients should have their serum concentration checked during initiation of therapy. Typically, dose is increased in small increments until serum concentration is within the therapeutic range. Once an effective and safe dosing regime has been established, serum concentration need only be checked at six- or 12-monthly intervals. More frequent monitoring may be considered in the following types of patients whose ability to eliminate theophylline might be diminishing. All these patient types have an increased risk of theophylline toxicity:

- the elderly
- patients with concurrent liver disease (cirrhosis, hepatitis)
- patients with concurrent congestive heart failure
- acutely ill patients (e.g. those receiving intensive care)
- those being prescribed some additional drugs.

All patients presenting with signs of toxicity should have serum concentration checked to decide whether a reduction in dose or even temporary withdrawal of the drug is warranted.

Patients who seem to be failing to respond to theophylline might require a larger dose. If serum concentration is below the therapeutic range an increase in dose may be warranted.

Laboratory measurement of serum lithium, digoxin or theophylline

Patient preparation

No particular patient preparation is necessary.

Sample requirements

Around 5 ml of venous blood is required. This should be collected into a plain glass (without additives) tube.

Timing of sample

The concentration of any drug in blood varies in relation to the time of the last dose, so timing of sample collection is vital for accurate interpretation of routine therapeutic drug monitoring results.

- Blood for lithium should be sampled at 12 hours after the last dose.
- Blood for digoxin should be sampled at 6 hours after the last dose.
- Blood for theophylline should be sampled at 1–2 hours after the last dose.

If a patient is exhibiting signs of toxicity or a deliberate overdose is suspected, an urgent test result may be required. In these circumstances, it is clearly not appropriate to wait before sampling blood, but it is important to record the time that the sample was taken and the time of the last dose or overdose, if known.

Interpretation of results

Serum lithium

Therapeutic range for those with symptoms of acute mania   0.8–1.5 mmol/l
Therapeutic range for maintenance dose to *prevent* symptoms   0.5–1.0 mmol/l

The objective is to maintain serum concentration within the therapeutic range. Patients actually suffering symptoms of acute mania can tolerate slightly higher doses of lithium than those without symptoms; hence the different therapeutic ranges. Once acute symptoms have passed and the patient stabilised, a maintenance dose must be prescribed which results in a serum concentration within the lower therapeutic range.

Symptoms of mild toxicity – vomiting, diarrhoea, nausea and coarse tremor – usually arise as serum concentration rises above 1.5 mmol/l, although a minority of patients may experience lithium toxicity when serum concentration is less than 1.5 mmol/l. More severe symptoms, including confusion, dizziness, tinnitus, irregular heart rate and blurred vision are associated with serum levels above 2.0 mmol/l. Loss of consciousness and fatality can occur in severe overdose (serum lithium > 2.5 mmol/l) if treatment to eliminate lithium is not urgently initiated.

Serum digoxin

Therapeutic range   1.0–2.6 nmol/l

Symptoms of toxicity are usually associated with serum digoxin concentration greater than 3.0 nmol/l. However, some patients (e.g. those with hypokalaemia, hypomagnesia, hypercalcaemia and thyroid disease) have increased sensitivity to the effects of digoxin and symptoms of toxicity might be present at concentration below 3.0 nmol/l, and may even occur at concentration within the therapeutic range. As long as causes of increased sensitivity can be excluded, then serum digoxin level within the therapeutic range indicates that any symptoms suggestive of digoxin toxicity are unlikely to be due to digoxin; another cause must be sought and there is no real justification for reducing dose. Conversely, the finding of a serum digoxin concentration below the therapeutic range in a patient who is not responding clinically as expected to a particular dose, provides good objective evidence that the patient is receiving insufficient digoxin. Under these circumstances, consideration can be given to increasing the dose.

Serum theophylline

Therapeutic range for treatment of asthma   55–110 µmol/l (10–20 mg/l)
Therapeutic range for treatment of apnoea   28–44 µmol/l (8–20 mg/l)

The objective is to maintain serum concentration within the therapeutic range. A serum concentration below the therapeutic range indicates current dose is unlikely to be effective and a serum concentration above the therapeutic range results in unwanted side effects (toxicity). Mild to moderate toxicity is associated with serum concentration in the range 110–165 µmol/l (i.e. 20–30 mg/l). Severe toxicity with seizures and life threatening cardiac arrhythmias do not usually occur until serum concentration is in excess of 165 µmol/l (i.e. 30 mg/l).

Case history 13

Mr Anderson is 75 years old. He was first suspected of having a failing heart 10 years ago, when he noticed that he was becoming breathless on climbing stairs. Over the next year or two, his condition worsened. He became breathless when lying flat, making it difficult to sleep without additional pillows, and he developed ankle oedema. His prescription included digoxin and an oral diuretic. Although he required increasing amounts of diuretics to control oedema, his symptoms were relieved and he became much more physically active, until a month ago when his condition deteriorated. Immediately before hospital admission he was unable to perform any physical activity, preferring to sleep downstairs propped in a chair rather than make the effort of climbing the stairs at night, and his ankles were so swollen with oedema that he was unable to wear shoes. Despite a loss of appetite, his body weight had been rising with progressive accumulation of oedema fluid. On admission, Mr Anderson's serum digoxin was 2.2 nmol/l. and his serum potassium 3.6 mmol/l. Over the next two days, he was given large oral doses of the diuretic frusemide to remove accumulating fluids; by day 3 of admission this had resulted in a 12 kg fall in body weight. Mr Anderson's body weight was now normal, but he felt nauseous, retched frequently, felt very weak and complained of a headache; he became increasingly drowsy. As these are all signs of digoxin toxicity, blood was sampled for serum digoxin; a request for urea and electrolytes request was made at the same time. The laboratory reported the following results:

Serum digoxin   2.1 nmol/l
Serum potassium   2.4 mmol/l
Serum creatinine   110 µmol/l

Questions

(1) Did digoxin results, either at the time of admission or three days later, indicate that Mr Anderson might be receiving too much digoxin?
(2) Are serum potassium results normal? (See Chapter 4).
(3) Why might Mr Anderson be suddenly suffering from digoxin toxicity despite no increase in dose for the past five years?

Discussion of case history

(1) Both digoxin results are within the therapeutic range. The deterioration in Mr Anderson's heart failure before hospital admission cannot be attributed to failure on his part to continue with his digoxin medication. Serum digoxin results do not indicate digoxin toxicity, rather they indicate that he was receiving an appropriate digoxin dose.

(2) The normal range for serum potassium is 3.6–5.0 mmol/l. On admission, Mr Anderson's serum potassium was at the low end of the normal range but after diuretic therapy on day three of admission, his potassium level was markedly reduced.

(3) The water diuresis induced by administration of frusemide which Mr Anderson urgently required, was accompanied by increased losses of potassium in urine. This is a well-documented side effect of some diuretic therapies. Since before this treatment, serum potassium was already at the low end of the normal range, possibly due to low dietary potassium intake because of loss of appetite, this increased loss of potassium in urine sent Mr Anderson's serum potassium plummeting; he became severely hypokalaemic. Reduced serum potassium concentration potentiates the toxicity of digoxin, so that as in Mr Anderson's case, symptoms of toxicity appear despite the fact that serum digoxin is within the therapeutic range.

Treatment of digoxin toxicity in this case is based not on withdrawal of digoxin, which might exacerbate Mr Anderson's underlying heart failure, but on restoring serum potassium to a level within the normal range by administration of potassium supplements.

References

1. Fraser K, Martin M *et al.* (2001) Mood disorders: bipolar conditions. *Pharmaceutical Journal* **266**: 824–32.
2. Davies M, Hobbs F *et al.* (2001) Prevalence of left-ventricular systolic dysfunction and heart failure in the Echocardiographic Heart of England Screening study: a population based study. *Lancet* **358**: 439–44.
3. National Institute for Clinical Excellence (2003) Chronic heart failure. Management of chronic heart failure in adults in primary and secondary care. *Clinical Guideline 5* London: NICE.
4. Cowie M, Wood D *et al.* (1999) Incidence and aetiology of heart failure: a population based study. *Eur Heart J* **20**: 421–28.

Further reading

Digitalis Investigation Group (1997) The effect of digoxin on mortality and morbidity in patients with heart failure. *New Eng J Med* **336**: 525–33.

Frings C (1987) Lithium monitoring. *Clinics in Lab Med* **7**: 545–50.

Grange J (2005) The role of nurses in management of heart failure. *Heart* **91** Suppl 2: ii: 39–42; discussion ii: 43–48.

Jefferson J (1998) Lithium. *Br Med J* **316**: 1330–31.

Rowe D, Watson I *et al.* (1988) The clinical use and measurement of theophylline. *Ann Clin Biochem* **25**: 4–26.

PART 3

Haematology tests

Chapter 15

FULL BLOOD COUNT 1: *RED BLOOD CELL COUNT, HAEMOGLOBIN AND OTHER RED CELL INDICES*

Of all laboratory blood tests, the full blood count (FBC) is the most frequently requested, reflecting the wide range of both common and less common disturbances of health that may be associated with abnormalities in FBC results. It is not one test, but a panel of tests including a count of each of the three cellular or formed elements of blood: red cells (erythrocytes), white cells (leucocytes) and platelets (thrombocytes). In the first of two chapters which focus on the FBC, we consider the red cell count and several other tests included in the FBC which all relate to red cell function. All these tests (listed in Table 15.1) are used primarily to identify those patients who are anaemic; they also help in elucidating the cause of that anaemia. In Chapter 16, we consider the significance of the total and differential white cell count, while the platelet count will be dealt with in Chapter 17, which focuses on tests of blood coagulation.

Normal physiology

Red cell (erythrocyte) production

Red cells are the most abundant of the three formed elements in blood outnumbering leucocytes (white cells) by around 1000 : 1 and platelets by 100 : 1. The process of blood cell production, called haemopoiesis, takes place within the bone marrow. During infancy, the bone marrow of all bones has the capacity to manufacture blood cells, but in adulthood this is limited to the bone marrow within the vertebrae, ribs, sternum, skull and pelvis as well as the ends of the long bones, femur and humeri. All blood cells are derived from bone marrow stem cells, which have the potential to differentiate to cells committed to becoming either mature red cells, white cells or platelets. The most primitive of those cells within bone marrow that are destined to become mature red cells is the pro-normoblast. The pro-normoblast develops by cell division and differentiation through recognisable stages to normoblast, reticulocyte and finally the mature red cell or erythrocyte

Table 15.1 Tests relating to red cells included in routine full blood count (FBC).

Test	What is measured	Units of measurement
Red blood cell (RBC) count	The number of red cells in blood	Number of thousand million cells i.e. 10^9 in every litre of blood (10^9/l)
Haemoglobin (Hb)	Concentration of the protein haemoglobin in blood	Grams in every 100 ml of blood (g/dl)
Red cell indices:		
Packed cell volume (PCV)	The percentage of total blood volume occupied by red cells	Percentage (%)
Mean cell volume (MCV)	The average (mean) volume of red cells	Femtolitre (fl) (1 femtolitre = $^{-15}1 \times 10$ l)
Mean cell haemoglobin concentration (MCHC)	The average (mean) concentration of haemoglobin in red cells	Grams in every 100 ml of red cells (g/dl)
Red cell distribution width (RDW)	The variation in red cell volume	Percentage (%)

Blood film – for this test blood is spread in a thin film on a glass microscope slide, then stained and examined under the microscope. A blood film report includes the details of any abnormalities in appearance or size of red cells. A blood film is only usually examined if results of above test indicate an abnormality.

(Figure 15.1). This development from stem cell to mature red cell referred to as erythropoiesis is characterised by:

- gradual reduction in cell size
- loss of nucleus and therefore ability to divide
- loss of internal cell organelles.

The final stage of maturation, reticulocyte to erythrocyte, occurs both within the bone marrow and in peripheral blood; normally around 1–2% of the circulating red cell population is reticulocytes. No red cell more primitive than the reticulocyte is normally present in blood.

Red cells have a life span of around 120 days. Constant replacement is necessary; on average around 2.3 million red cells are produced every second by the bone marrow throughout life. This is regulated by erythropoietin, a hormone synthesised in the cells of the kidney (Figure 15.2). In response to a falling blood oxygen level, the kidney releases erythropoietin into the blood stream for transport to the bone marrow. Here erythropoietin stimulates red cell production. As red cell numbers increase, the oxygen content of blood rises and kidney production of erythropoietin is stepped down.

Structure and function of red cells

The structure of the mature red cell is well suited to its primary function: transport of oxygen from the lungs to the tissues and transport of carbon dioxide from

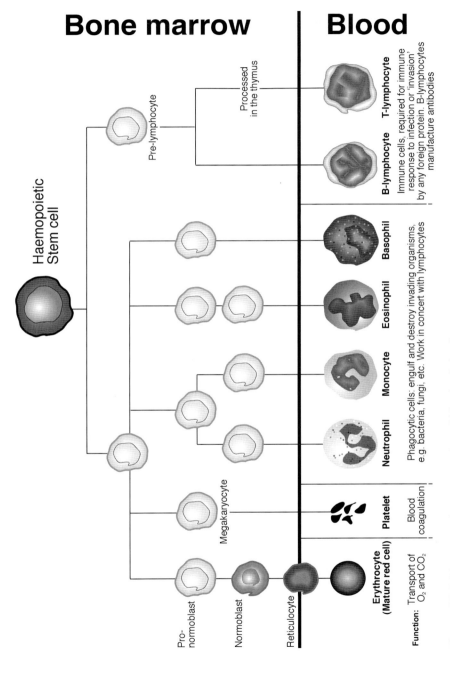

Figure 15.1 Diagrammatic representation of blood cell development.

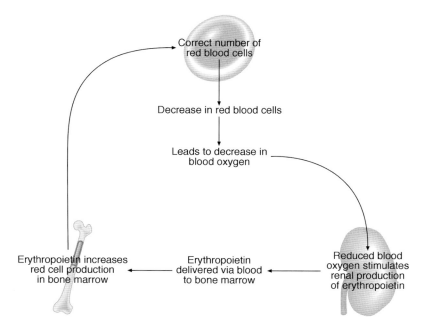

Figure 15.2 Regulation of red cell production.

tissues to the lungs. Central to this function is haemoglobin, the protein contained within the red cell. Haemoglobin production occurs within the red cell during its development in the bone marrow and is complete before full maturation. Each mature red cell (or reticulocyte) leaves the bone marrow with its full complement of 250–300 million molecules of haemoglobin.

Commonly described as a biconcave disc, the mature red cell can be imagined as a flattened sphere with its sides pushed in. This singular shape allows the largest surface area for a given volume, providing maximum possible area for oxygen and carbon dioxide gas exchange.

The diameter of the red cell is around 8 μm, twice the diameter of the smallest blood vessels through which it must pass. The membrane is able to deform itself, altering the overall shape of the red blood cell, so that it can 'squeeze' through the microvasculature within tissues, where gas exchange occurs. Without a nucleus and other internal organelles, the mature erythrocyte may be regarded as little more than a deformable membranous bag, stuffed full of haemoglobin.

Haemoglobin structure and function

Haemoglobin is the oxygen carrying protein pigment present in red cells, which gives blood its colour.

The haemoglobin molecule (Figure 15.3) comprises four folded chains of amino acids. These together form the protein or *globin* portion of the molecule. Each of

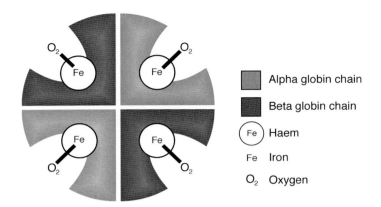

Figure 15.3 Representation of molecular structure of oxygenated adult haemoglobin.

the four globin subunits has a much smaller *haem* group attached, and at the centre of each haem group is an atom of iron in the ferrous state (Fe^{2+}). Whilst the structure of the haem group is always the same, the exact sequence of amino acids in the globin subunits varies slightly, giving rise to four possible globin chains; alpha (α), beta (β), gamma (γ) and delta (δ). Around 97% of adult haemoglobin is haemoglobin A (HbA) comprising 2 α and 2 β globin subunits. The remaining 3% is HbA2 (2 α and 2 δ globins). In the developing fetus and for the first few months of life, fetal haemoglobin (HbF) is the only haemoglobin produced; HbF is composed of 2 α and 2 γ globin subunits. The structure of haemoglobin is of more than passing academic interest. There is a large group of inherited disorders of haemoglobin synthesis and structure. These are collectively known as the haemoglobinopathies. Most are rare, but two – thalassaemia and sickle cell disease – are relatively common and therefore warrant special attention (see boxes 1 and 2).

Haemoglobin transport of oxygen
The oxygen combining property of haemoglobin depends on the single atom of iron present at the centre of each of the four haem groups. An oxygen molecule forms a weak, reversible ionic link with each of these iron atoms in turn; the product of this reaction is oxyhaemoglobin. When all four haem groups are occupied with oxygen the haemoglobin molecule is said to be saturated. The affinity of haemoglobin for oxygen, that is the extent to which it is saturated, depends on the oxygen content of the blood. This is described graphically in the oxygen dissociation curve (Figure 7.2). It is clear from this graph that haemoglobin becomes increasingly saturated with oxygen as the partial pressure of blood oxygen (PO_2) increases. The physiological implications of this relationship are central to the oxygen carriage and delivery function of haemoglobin. In the lungs, oxygen in inspired air diffuses from alveoli to the blood, so PO_2 of blood here is high (around 95 mm Hg). This relatively high PO_2 is associated with high haemoglobin affinity for oxygen and the haemoglobin quickly (within a few seconds) becomes almost

Box 1 Haemoglobinopathies: thalassaemia.

The thalassaemias

These are a group of genetic (inherited) disorders characterised by deficient synthesis of α- or β-globin chains, with resulting low haemoglobin and anaemia. These genetic defects (more than 150 have been identified) are found most frequently in parts of Africa, Mediterranean countries, the Middle East, Indian sub continent and South East Asia. All immigrants from these areas are at risk. There are four genes which code for α-globin production; if the defect lies in these genes, the condition is known as α-thalassaemia, but if the defect lies in the single gene which codes for β-globin production, it is known as β-thalassaemia. The effect of these genetic defects varies greatly depending on the precise nature of the defect and wether the defect is inherited from both parents or just one.

β-thalassaemia-minor (β-thalassaemia trait)   This is the condition when a defective β-globin gene is inherited from just one parent. Since a normal gene is inherited from the other parent, β-globin is only slightly affected and patients can produce near normal amounts of HbA (2α and 2β chains). Synthesis of HbA2 (2α and 2δ chains) is increased (this is used to make the diagnosis), so that patients usually have normal total Hb. They are generally not anaemic and and are usually fit and healthy. Affected women are, however, at high risk of anaemia during pregancy and intercurrent illness.

β-thalassaemia major   This is the much more severe homozygous form of thalassaemia, which occurs when β-thalassaemia trait is inherited from both parents. Production of β-globin is severely affected. This is no problem during fetal development and the early months of life when Hb F (2α and 2γ chains) is the only haemoglobin synthesised. But from around 3 to 6 months when haemoglobin production swtiches from fetal hamoglobin (HbF) to adult haemoglobin (HbA) the deficiency of β-globin chains becomes apparent, with gradual development of severe anaemia. Excessive red cell destruction leads to enlaged liver and spleen. Without regular blood transfusion, (every 4–6 weeks) affected children fail to develop and die in childhood or early adolescence. Iron overload, consequent on repeated blood transfusions, is a major problem, which can be ameliorated by iron sequestering drugs. Bone marrow transplantation is a treatment option.

α-thalassaemia   The genetic defect is actual deletion of α genes. The severity depends on how many of the four genes which code for α chain production are deleted. In the most severe case – known as hydrops fetalis – all four genes are deleted with complete absence of α chain synthesis. Since α chains are required for HbF, HbA and HbA2 the haemoglobin deficency is too severe for fetal survival; death occurs *in utero*. Other forms of α-thalassaemia in which one, two or three genes are deleted result in varying degrees of anaemia.

All forms of thalassaemia, whether severe enough to cause anaemia or not, are associated with changes to red cells which are evident on FBC analysis as reduced MCV and MCH. That is, red cells are microcytic and hypochromic.

Box 2 Haemoglobinopathies: sickle cell anaemia.

Sickle cell anaemia

Sickle cell anaemia is caused by inheritance of a very specific genetic defect in the gene which codes for β globin synthesis. Like all proteins, β globin is composed of amino acids joined in a very precise sequence. The sixth amino acid in normal β globin is valine. The genetic defect of sickle cell anaemia results in synthesis of β globin with the amino acid, glutamic acid instead of valine at position 6. This single amino acid subsitution results in production of abnormal haemoglobin, HbS composed of 2 normal α chains and 2 abnormal β chains. If the defective gene is inherited from just one parent carrier, half of the haemoglobin synthesised is normal HbA and the remainder is HbS. This heterozygous state is known as sickle cell trait. If the defective gene is inherited from both parents, no normal hameoglobin (HbA) is synthesised. Almost all the haemoglobin is abnormal HbS. This is sickle cell disease.

HbS polymerises at low oxygen tensions causing structural changes to the red cell membrane, which becomes rigid. The red cells deform into the familiar sickle shape that gives the condition its name. These deformed red cells are fragile and haemolyse easily, with development of haemolytic anaemia.

The sickle gene is most frequently found in African people and those of African descent (e.g. West Indians). It is also prevalant in some Mediterranean countries, the Middle East and parts of India.

Sickle cell trait   Only around 30–45% of haemoglobin in those with sickle cell trait is HbS. Most of the rest is normal adult haemoglobin HbA. The condition is benign. Those affected are not generally anaemic.

Tissue anoxia, which may occur in severe illnesses (e.g. clinical shock and systeminc infection) may result in a sickling crisis sufficient to cause anaemia. Particular care is required to maintain adequate tissue oxygenation during anaesthesia.

Sickle cell disease   The expression of sickle cell disease varies greatly; a minority are virtually unaffected and live a normal healthy life-span, whilst some die in early childhood. Symptoms may begin after the first six months of life when production of HhF is switched to adult haemoglobin production.

A chronic haemolytic anaemia is the hallmark of the disease. For most, the disease is characterised by periods of good health punctuated by extremely painful sickle cell crises. These crises may be precipitated by a variety of environmental factors including infection, violent exercise, emotional disturbance, anoxia, dehydration, etc. A sickle cell crisis is associated with increased haemolysis and sequestration of sickled cells in the microvasculature of various organs (spleen, bone, lungs, brain) and this accounts for many of the complications of sickle cell disease. Blocked vessels prevent normal blood flow and tissue, starved of oxygen and nutrients, dies. When the microvasculature of the brain is affected patients may suffer a stroke as a result of cerebral infarction. Occlusion of vessels in the eye causes visual impairment. Infarcts in growing bone tissue early in childhood may leave single fingers or toes permanently shorter than the rest. Sickle cell disease is associated with increased risk of infection, due partly to splenic damage. Pneumococcal septicaemia was once a significant cause of death before prophylactic antibiotics were introduced into routine care. Other treatments include regular blood transfusion to replace HbS with normal HbA.

100% saturated. Conversely in the tissues, the blood PO_2 is relatively low (only around 40 mm Hg), reducing affinity of haemoglobin for oxygen. As a result, oxygen is released from haemoglobin and diffuses out of the red cells to tissue cells where it is required for cell metabolism.

Role of red cells and haemoglobin in the transport of CO_2

While the transport of oxygen from lungs to tissues is almost entirely due to haemoglobin in red cells, the transport of carbon dioxide in the reverse direction is slightly more complex. Carbon dioxide, unlike oxygen is soluble in blood plasma, so some carbon dioxide is transported simply dissolved in blood plasma. The remainder is transported in red cells.

In the tissues, carbon dioxide diffuses out of tissue cells into the passing bloodstream; some remains, as discussed above, dissolved in blood plasma, and the rest diffuses into red cells. Within the red cell, some carbon dioxide combines with deoxygenated haemoglobin to form carbamino-Hb and some combines with water in the red cell cytoplasm to form carbonic acid. This reaction is catalysed by the enzyme carbonic anhydrase. Carbonic acid dissociates to hydrogen ions (which are buffered by haemoglobin) and bicarbonate ion, which diffuse out of the red cell into surrounding plasma. In the lungs these red cell reactions are reversed and the CO_2 diffuses out of red cells and pass along with CO_2 dissolved in plasma from the blood to alveoli for excretion in expired air.

The oxygen and carbon dioxide transporting function of haemoglobin is also dealt with in a discussion of respiratory physiology contained in Chapter 7; readers might find it useful to refer to the relevant sections in that chapter.

Normal red cell destruction

After around 120 days circulating in peripheral blood, red cells are no longer viable and are removed from blood by the reticulo-endothelial (RE) system, as blood passes though the bone marrow, spleen and liver. In these RE sites, the red cell membrane is degraded, releasing haemoglobin, which is split into its constituent parts: haem and globin (Figure 10.2). The iron present in haem is recycled for production of new red cells and globin chains are broken down to amino acids, which enter the amino acid pool. What remains of haem after removal of iron is converted to the yellow pigment bilirubin. This is transported in blood to the liver for further metabolism and eventual excretion, mostly via bile in faeces; a little is excreted as the bilirubin metabolites, urobilin and urobilinogen, in urine.

Laboratory measurement of FBC

Patient preparation

No particular patient preparation is necessary.

Timing of sample

There are no special timing requirements, so blood is best sampled at a time that coincides with routine transport to the laboratory. Blood for FBC should not be stored longer than 12 hours before transport to the laboratory. FBC is one of those tests that can be performed urgently and out of normal laboratory hours, if necessary. In such circumstances, it is essential to telephone the laboratory and transport the blood immediately it has been sampled.

Type of sample

Venous blood is preferable, ideally collected without the use of a tourniquet (if used, a tourniquet should not be left for more than a minute or two before blood is sampled). Capillary blood collection is appropriate if venous blood collection poses difficulty (e.g. in babies and those with 'difficult' veins).

Blood collection bottle

Blood for FBC must be collected into a special tube (usually lavender or pink-coloured top) which contains the anticoagulant, K^+EDTA. This prevents the blood from clotting and preserves the structure of blood cells.

Sample volume

The sample bottles for FBC have a 'line to fill' marked on the label. This is usually 2.5 ml or 0.5 ml in the case of paediatric sized bottles for capillary blood sampling. This volume will result in the correct ratio of blood to anticoagulant. It is important for accurate results that neither too much nor too little blood is added to these tubes and that anticoagulant and blood are mixed by gentle inversion, as soon as the blood is sampled. Inadequate mixing can result in formation of tiny blood clots, and inaccurate results.

Interpretation of Hb, RBC and red cell indices results

Approximate reference ranges

red blood cell (RBC)	adult males	$4.5–6.5 \times 10^{12}$/l
	adult females	$3.9–5.6 \times 10^{12}$/l
	at birth	$3.5–6.7 \times 10^{12}$/l
	childhood	$4.1–5.3 \times 10^{12}$/l
haemoglobin (Hb)	adult males	13.5–17.5 g/dl
	adult females	11.5–15.5 g/dl
	at birth	14.0–24.0 g/dl
	childhood	11.0–14.0 g/dl

packed cell volume (PCV) or haematocrit (Ht)

	males	40–52%
	females	36–48%
mean cell volume (MCV)	adults	80–95 fl
	at birth	100–135 fl
	childhood	71–88 fl

mean cell haemoglobin concentration (MCHC) 20–35 g/dl

red (cell) distribution width (RDW)   10–15%

Critical values

haemoglobin	< 7.0 g/dl or > 20.0 g/dl
PCV (haematocrit)	< 20% or > 60%

Terms used to describe red cells

Normocytosis	average size of red cell is normal
Microcytosis	average size of red cells is smaller than normal
Macrocytosis	average size of red cells is larger than normal
Anisocytosis	red cells vary in size
Poikilocytosis	red cells vary in shape
Normochromasia	red cells stain normally indicating they contain normal amount of haemoglobin
Hypochromasia	red cells appear weakly stained indicating they contain less haemoglobin than normal

Conditions associated with reduction in RBC, Hb, PCV(Ht)

Anaemia

Anaemia (literally, without blood) is the collection of signs and symptoms that result from reduced oxygen delivery to tissues, due to a decrease in the total number of red blood cells and/or reduction in haemoglobin concentration of blood. There are many possible causes, so anaemia is not a disease entity itself, rather a sign or symptom of some underlying disease, which must be identified if treatment of anaemia is to be successful. Diagnosis of anaemia is established if Hb concentration is below the lower limit of the reference range, i.e. less than 13.5 g/dl for adult males and less than 11.5 g/dl in adult females. In children who normally have slightly lower levels of haemoglobin, a diagnosis of anaemia is made if Hb is less than 11.0 g/dl. The lower the Hb, the more severe is the anaemia, and anaemia is excluded by the finding of Hb concentration within the reference range.

Reduced red cell count and PCV are also a feature of anaemia, although the magnitude of the reduction of red cell count depends not only on the severity of the anaemia, but also its cause. The main pathological effect of anaemia is reduced delivery of oxygen to the tissues but the extent to which this causes symptoms, depends on several factors including:

- *severity of the anaemia:* many patients with mild anaemia, i.e. Hb greater than 10 g/dl have no symptoms but severe anaemia, Hb < 6 g/dl is almost always associated with symptoms
- *speed of onset:* rapid onset of anaemia is more likely to result in symptoms than that which has developed slowly.

Signs and symptoms of anaemia

There are some generalised signs and symptoms of anaemia, no matter what the cause. Most are the result of reduced oxygenation of tissues (tissue hypoxia). Some reflect the body's attempt to compensate for the reduced oxygen in tissues. The main symptoms include:

- pallor
- tiredness and lethargy
- shortness of breath, particularly on exertion
- dizziness, fainting
- headaches
- increased heart rate (tachycardia), palpitations.

The absence of symptoms does not preclude anaemia; many mildly anaemic individuals remain asymptomatic, particularly if anaemia has developed slowly. The elderly represent a group in which quite severe anaemia may not be symptomatic

Causes of anaemia

While Hb, RBC and PCV measurement all help in identifying those patients who are anaemic and in assessing the severity of anaemia, they provide no information about cause. Anaemia may be caused by:

- acute blood loss (haemorrhage) e.g. trauma or surgery
- deficiency of iron (required for haemoglobin production), the most common cause of anaemia
- chronic inflammation, infection and malignancy – collectively called the anaemia of chronic disease (ACD), this is the second most common cause of anaemia and the most common cause in the elderly who are most likely to be suffering the underlying chronic diseases
- deficiency of vitamins B_{12} and/or folate (required for production of red cells) – pernicious anaemia accounts for most cases of anaemia in this group
- inadequate production of erythropoietin (required for regulation of red cell production) – this is cause of the anaemia that occurs in chronic renal failure
- increased rate of red cell destruction – these are the haemolytic anaemias, examples include sickle cell anaemia, transfusion reactions, haemolytic disease of the newborn

- bone marrow stem cell failure (aplastic anaemia), usually the result of cyto-toxic drug or radiation therapy for treatment of cancer
- malignant disease of bone marrow (e.g. the leukaemias, myeloma).

The red cell indices, MCV, MCHC, MCH and RDW, along with microscopic examination of red cells, help in identifying the cause of anaemia. Initially when investigating the cause of anaemia, MCV is the most useful because all anaemias can be classified according to the average size of red cell (MCV) to one of three groups:

Microcytic anaemia (low MCV)
Normocytic anaemia (normal MCV)
Macrocytic anaemia (raised MCV)

The microcytic anaemias are those that result from iron deficiency and thalassaemia. Some patients whose anaemia is due to chronic disease have a microcytic anaemia, but this is not typical.

Most patients with anaemia of chronic disease have a normocytic anaemia. Other causes of anaemia in this normocytic group include acute blood loss (haemorrhage); the haemolytic anaemias; anaemia caused by decreased erythropoietin production (chronic renal failure), anaemia caused by damage to bone marrow stem cells (aplastic anaemia), and anaemia which results from malignant disease of the bone marrow, (i.e. the leukaemias, etc).

Macrocytic anaemias are confined to those that result from vitamin B_{12} or folate deficiency.

RDW is helpful in further distinguishing the cause within these three groups; for example iron deficiency and thalassaemia are both associated with microcytic anaemia. However, iron deficiency is associated with a raised RDW, whereas RDW is normal in those with thalassaemia. Similarly, RDW is able to distinguish different causes of normocytic anaemia. For example, anaemia of chronic disease is associated with normal RDW whereas haemolytic anaemias are associated with raised RDW. Simply by examining MCV and RDW results of anaemic patients, it is possible to narrow down the likely cause of anaemia.

The examination of a stained blood smear under the microscope may also be useful because the shape and staining characteristics of red cells from an anaemic patient may give important clues as to cause. For example, the red cells of patients with sickle cell anaemia have a characteristic sickle shape, which gives the condition its name. Relatively small red cells that stain weakly (due to abnormally low concentration of haemoglobin) indicate possible iron deficiency while large cells, typically oval in shape, indicate anaemia is probably due to Vitamin B_{12} or folate deficiency. Many more anaemias are associated with characteristic changes in red cell shape.

Causes of increased red cell count, haemoglobin and PCV

Polycythaemia

Polycythaemia (literally many blood cells) is the opposite of anaemia. *Increased* red cell count and haemoglobin concentration is the hallmark of polycythaemia. Since PCV is dependent on the number of red cells, this too is raised in polycythaemia. Polycythaemia may arise as a response to any physiological or pathological condition in which blood contains less oxygen than normal. In response to a low blood oxygen level, the kidney increases erythropoietin production, resulting in increased red cell production. This so-called secondary polycythaemia is a feature of:

- living at high altitude (where inspired air has relatively less oxygen)
- cigarette smoking (carbon monoxide present in inhaled cigarette smoke binds to haemoglobin, displacing oxygen)
- chronic lung disease (oxygen transfer from lungs to blood is compromised)
- cyanotic heart disease (blood is less well oxygenated than normal due to congenital structural defects in the heart).

Primary polycythaemia or *polycythaemia vera* is a quite separate malignant disease of the bone marrow in which bone marrow stem cell proliferation results in marked overproduction of red cells (white cell and platelet numbers are also often increased). This huge increase in red cell numbers increases the viscosity (fluidity) of blood and several of the signs and symptoms (headache, increased blood pressure) are related to this increased blood viscosity.

Effect of hydration on RBC, Hb and PCV(Ht)

Measured red cell count, haemoglobin and PCV are all affected by the state of hydration of the patient. Dehydration is associated with increased RBC, Hb and PCV simply because plasma volume is reduced. The absolute number of red cells and amount of haemoglobin in blood, however, remains unchanged. Conversely, a patient who has received too much fluids and is overhydrated will have a reduced red cell count, Hb and PCV. This effect of hydration has to be taken into account when interpreting results from patients who are either dehydrated or overhydrated. An increased plasma volume is a normal physiological effect of pregnancy so pregnancy is associated with a decrease in Hb, PCV and RBC, even though absolute numbers of red cells and haemoglobin are normal. Thus a pregnant woman with a slight reduction in Hb is not necessarily anaemic.

Other causes of a raised MCV

It is worth noting that MCV may be raised in patients who are not anaemic, i.e. have a normal Hb. The principal causes of an isolated increase in MCV are alcohol abuse and cirrhosis of the liver. An isolated raised MCV in a patient suspected of alcohol abuse is considered objective evidence of continued alcohol use.

Case history 14

Jane Baker, a 32-year-old solicitor, attends her GP surgery complaining of feeling 'washed out'. Although normally an active woman, who enjoys horse riding at weekends and regular visits with her children to the local swimming pool, Jane now reports becoming increasingly tired over the past month or two. She feels unable to do much more than a normal day's work. During examination of Jane's eyes, her GP noted a degree of pallor in conjunctival membrane, suggesting anaemia might be the cause her tiredness. No other abnormal signs were detected. He sampled blood for a full blood count (FBC). The laboratory report, which he received two days later, contained the following results.

Hb	9.2 g/dl
RBC	3.8×10^{12}/litre
PCV	28%
MCV	73 fl
MCHC	20 g/dl
RDW	16%

Questions

(1) What is the laboratory evidence of Jane's anaemia; is it severe?
(2) Using the red cell indices, classify the anaemia to either:
    (a) microcytic anaemia
    (b) normocytic anaemia
    (c) macrocytic anaemia
(3) Suggest possible causes of the anaemia.
(4) What further test(s) is/are indicated?

Discussion of case history

(1) The haemoglobin concentration (Hb) is used to confirm or exclude anaemia. Jane's Hb is well below the reference range for adult females. This is sufficient evidence to make a diagnosis of anaemia. An Hb of 9.2 g/dl indicates that Jane is moderately anaemic; anaemia is usually considered severe only if Hb is less than 6.0 g/dl. Although not required to make a diagnosis, both PCV and RBC results are low, reflecting anaemia.

(2) The MCV (mean cell volume) is a measure of the average size of red cells. Jane's MCV is reduced, which means that her red cells are, on average, smaller than normal; her anaemia is microcytic in nature.

(3) Almost all cases of microcytic anaemia are due to one of:

● iron deficiency
● thalassaemia (an inherited disorder of haemoglobin synthesis found particularly in those of Mediterranean descent)
● particularly severe anaemia of chronic disease (infection, inflammation, malignancy).

Of these, iron deficiency is by far the most common, and thalassaemia the least common. Since Jane has no medical history of chronic disease, iron deficiency is the most likely cause of her anaemia. The RDW result provides supportive evidence for such a diagnosis since it is usually raised in iron deficiency and normal in both thalassaemia and anaemia of chronic disease.

(4) A serum iron and serum ferritin test (Chapter 18) will confirm the diagnosis of iron deficiency anaemia. As will be made clear in Chapter 18, there are many causes of iron deficiency. If iron deficiency is confirmed, Jane may require further investigation to establish the cause of the deficiency in her case.

Further reading

Hoffbrand A, Pettit J & Moss P (2001) Blood cell formation. In: *Essential Haematology* (4th edn) Oxford: Blackwell Science Publications.

Hoffbrand A & Provan D (1997) ABC of clinical haematology: macrocytic anaemia. *Br Med J* **314**: 430–33.

Frewin R, Henson A & Provan D (1997) ABC of clinical haematology: iron deficiency anaemia. *Br Med J* **314**: 360–63.

Weatherall DJ (1997) ABC of clinical haematology: the hereditary anaemias. *Br Med J* **314**: 492–96.

Chapter 16

FULL BLOOD COUNT 2:
WHITE CELL COUNT AND DIFFERENTIAL

In this second of two chapters devoted to the full blood count, the most commonly requested blood test, the clinical value of the white blood cell count is considered. Unlike the mature red cell population, which is homogenous in nature, the white cell (leukocyte) population is heterogeneous, composed as it is of five morphologically and functionally distinct populations. These are: neutrophils, eosinophils, basophils, monocytes and lymphocytes. The total white cell count (WBC) is the sum of all of these white cell types, while the differential white cell count or 'diff' is a count of each of the five types. An increase in white cell numbers is a very common feature of disease, which can be attributed to one of several pathological processes, including the big three: infection, inflammation, and malignancy. A reduced white cell count, which is much less common, implies a reduction in immunity and therefore high risk of infectious disease.

Normal physiology

In common with all other formed elements in blood, white cells (leukocytes) are derived from the pluripotent stem cell present in bone marrow (Figure 15.1). Mature white cells have a limited life span so constant bone marrow production is necessary throughout life. An increase in bone marrow production of white cells is part of the body's normal (inflammatory) response to any insult to the body (i.e. any tissue injury, whatever the cause). The purpose of the inflammatory response is to contain and control injury, to eliminate potential pathogens (bacteria, viruses, fungi, protozoa, parasitic worms) and initiate healing and tissue repair. As key players in the inflammatory response, white cells must leave the blood and enter the tissues. Although as we shall see, each type of white cell has a different and well-defined job to do in the overall process of inflammation, they operate in concert, communicating via a range of chemical messengers called cytokines.

Neutrophils
Comprising between 40 and 70% of the total white cell population, the neutrophil is the most abundant of all white cells in blood. The mature neutrophil has a multi-lobed purple staining nucleus and dark blue staining granules in the cytoplasm.

It has a diameter of about 15 μm, around twice that of a red cell. The function of these cells is to enter the tissues and kill invading bacteria. On release from the bone marrow, mature neutrophils spend only around eight hours in the blood stream and the rest of their 4–5 day maximum life span in the tissues. Chemicals called chemotactic factors released from bacteria and other cells (including basophils, macrophages and lymphocytes, see below) attract neutrophils to the site of tissue infection or inflammation. In the tissues, neutrophils surround and engulf bacteria, by a process called phagocytes. Once inside the neutrophil, bacteria are killed by enzymes and highly reactive free radical chemicals produced within the darkly staining granules of the neutrophil cytoplasm. Pus, the yellow-ish fluid that oozes from an infection site, is a visible reminder of neutrophil function. It is largely composed of dead and dying neutrophils, bacterial debris and other cellular detritus produced during the fight against infection.

Eosinophils

Although much fewer in number, comprising only between 0.2 and 5% of total white cell population, eosinophils have similarities, both in appearance and function, to neutrophils. The nucleus of the eosinophil is like the neutrophil, lobed in appearance, although whereas the neutrophil nucleus is multi-lobed, the eosinophil nucleus has just two lobes. The granules of the eosinophil cytoplasm stain orange-red in contrast to the dark blue of the neutrophil, due to the presence of chemicals peculiar to the eosinophil. Like neutrophils, eosinophils are capable of phagocytosis, although it seems unlikely that they have a role in the killing of bacteria. Instead, it is thought that they target foreign material too large for normal phagocytosis. For example, they bind parasitic worms and inflict damage by releasing enzymes and then phagocytose the products. Their main function is protection against infection by organisms larger than bacteria and viruses.

Eosinophils are present at the site of inflammation caused by allergic reactions, such as the airways of allergic asthma and hay fever sufferers. Release of chemicals from eosinophils contributes to the pathogenesis of allergic inflammatory disease.

Basophils

These are so few in number that they are only rarely seen during microscopical examination of blood. They have a multi-lobed nucleus that is hidden by dense dark blue staining granules. Basophils migrate into tissues where they mature to mast cells. When activated, mast cells release many chemical mediators of the inflammatory response, which include a chemotactic factor that attracts neutrophils, histamine (a chemical that dilates blood vessels, increasing the blood flow to damaged areas) and heparin, an anticoagulant required to begin the process of repair to damaged blood vessels.

Monocytes

The monocyte is the largest blood cell and has a lobulated nucleus, with a usually clear (non-granulated) voluminous cytoplasm. After a short period of 20–40 hours circulating in the blood, these phagocytic cells migrate to the tissues where they mature to cells called macrophages. Macrophages phagocytose and kill foreign organisms in the same way that neutrophils do but have a second important role in processing and presenting foreign proteins or antigens (derived from bacteria, etc.) to T-lymphocytes for initiation of a cell mediated immune response (see below).

Lymphocytes

Between 20 and 40% of the circulating white cell population are lymphocytes; these are the second most abundant type of white cell in blood. Like all other blood cells they are derived from the bone marrow, but a proportion undergo further processing within the thymus; these are thymus dependent lymphocytes or T-lymphocytes, which comprise around 70% of all circulating lymphocytes. Most of the remaining 30% are B-lymphocytes. There is an additional small population of non-B, non T-lymphocytes called natural killer (NK) lymphocytes. The routine lymphocyte count is the sum of these three types.

Like neutrophils, lymphocytes are required for immunity (protection) from infection. B-lymphocytes differentiate to plasma cells, which produce antibodies. These are proteins that bind specifically with complementary proteins called antigens. Micro-organisms (bacteria, viruses etc.) all have specific surface proteins which act as antigens. Antibody binding of these surface antigens prevents bacteria and viruses from invading tissue cells. Furthermore, antibody-coated bacteria are much more easily phagocytosed (destroyed) by neutrophils and macrophages. Antibodies can also bind to, and thereby neutralise bacterial toxins.

Although antibodies are effective in the process that leads to destruction of microbes outside cells, they cannot enter cells and therefore have no effect on the microbes harbouring within cells. The body's defence against these depends on T-lymphocytes.

T-lymphocytes can 'recognise' and destroy tissue cells that are infected, thereby preventing further spread. Since all viruses must infect cells in order to replicate, and many bacteria parasitise body cells, this so-called cell mediated immunity invoked by the T-lymphocyte is a vital component of the body's defence against infection. T-lymphocytes also have the capacity to recognise and kill cancerous cells, so are part of the body's defence against cancer.

An important feature of lymphocyte mediated immunity, whether it be B-lymphocyte (i.e. antibody) mediated or T-lymphocyte (i.e. cell) mediated is that, unlike all other white blood cells, both classes of lymphocytes have the capacity to 'remember' an invading organism, so that the response to a subsequent encounter is greater and more rapid. This so-called 'acquired' immunity explains why we seldom suffer more than once from a particular infection. First exposure provides immunity from subsequent infections with the same organism.

Laboratory measurement of full blood count

See pages 206–207.

Interpretation of WBC and diff results

Approximate reference ranges

Total white blood cell (leukocyte) count

	Adult males	$3.7–9.5 \times 10^9/l$
	Adult females	$3.9–11.1 \times 10^9/l$
Neutrophils	(40–75% of total white cells)	$2.5–7.5 \times 10^9/l$
Lymphocytes	(20–40% of total white cells)	$1.5–4.0 \times 10^9/l$
Monocytes	(2–10% of total white cells)	$0.2–0.8 \times 10^9/l$
Eosinophils	(1–5% of total white cells)	$0.04–0.44 \times 10^9/l$
Basophils	(< 1% of total white cells)	$0.01–0.10 \times 10^9/l$

At birth the total white cell count is very high ($5.0–26.0 \times 10^9/l$). This falls sharply to around $8.0–18.0 \times 10^9/l$ during the first two months of life and to normal adult levels by 12–15 years of age.

Critical values

Total white cell count (WCC) $< 2.0 \times 10^9/l$ or $> 30.0 \times 10^9/l$

Terms used in interpreting results

Polymorphonuclear cells (polymorphs)   Literally 'many shaped nucleus' cells, refers to all white blood cells with a lobed nucleus i.e. neutrophils, eosinophils, and basophils. Lymphocytes and monocytes are non-polymorphs because they have a more regular shaped nucleus.

Granulocytes   All white cells with visibly staining granules in the cytoplasm (i.e. neutrophils, eosinophils and basophils.) Lymphocytes and monocytes are non-granulocytes.

Agranulocytosis   Complete or near absence of granulocytes in blood.

Phagocytes and non-phagocytes   Phagocytes are cells that are able to phagocytose foreign material (bacteria, etc.). Neutrophils, eosinophils, basophils and monocytes are all phagocytes. Lymphocytes do not have this ability; they are non-phagocytes

Leucocytosis   increase in total white cell count

Neutrophilia, eosinophilia, basophilia   selective increase in neutrophil, eosinophil and basophil count respectively

Lymphocytosis   increase in lymphocyte count

Leucopaenia   reduced total white cell count

Neutropaenia   reduced neutrophil count

Lymphopaenia   reduced lymphocyte count.

Pancytopaenia   reduction in all blood cells (red cells, white cells and platelets)

Terms used to describe white cells when viewed under the microscope

'Increase in band forms'   band cells are slightly immature neutrophils recognisable by the non-segmented shape of the nucleus. Normally only 3% of total neutrophils in peripheral blood are of this sort. An increase implies the bone marrow is increasing white cell production in response to infection or inflammation.

'Shift to left'   an alternative term to 'increase in band cells' denoting increase in immature neutrophils in peripheral blood.

Blast cells   very primitive white cells never normally seen in peripheral blood. Their presence almost always indicates a haematological malignancy (e.g. acute leukaemia).

Causes of an increase in total white cell numbers

General considerations

An increase in white cell numbers (leukocytosis) occurs most commonly as a result of infection, inflammation or indeed any significant tissue damage. Since the role of white cells is to defend the body against infection, it is entirely appropriate that numbers should increase under these circumstances. This so-called benign or reactive leukocytosis must be distinguished from the much less common and entirely inappropriate leukocytosis that may be a feature of haematological malignancies, including the leukaemias.

The leukaemias are a group of malignant diseases of the bone marrow, characterised by the unregulated proliferation of one sort (a clone) of immature blood cell at the expense of normal blood cell production. Nearly all cases can be classified to one of four groups depending on whether the clinical course of the disease is rapid (acute) or slow (chronic); and whether the immature cells are derived from the myeloid bone marrow cells or lymphoid bone marrow cells. (Myeloid bone cells normally mature either to red cells, platelets, neutrophils, eosinophils, basophils or monocytes; while lymphoid bone cells normally mature to lymphocytes.) The four main types of leukaemia are: acute myeloid leukaemia (AML), chronic myeloid leukaemia (CML), acute lymphoblastic leukaemia (ALL) and chronic lymphoid leukaemia (CLL). Some of the distinguishing features of the four sorts of leukaemia are outlined in Table 16.1. Since in all cases normal blood cell development is impaired, anaemia (due to deficiency of normal red cells), impaired blood coagulation with increased tendency to bleed (due to low platelet count) and high risk of infection (due to reduced numbers of normal white cells) can be a feature of all leukaemias.

Whether it is benign (reactive) or malignant, leukocytosis is usually the result of a predominant, although not necessarily entirely selective increase in one of the five types of white cell. The differential count thus provides clues as to the cause of an increased total white cell count. A more detailed account of the cause

Table 16.1 Some features of the four main types of leukaemia.

Acute myeloid leukaemia (AML)	Acute lymphocytic leukaemia (ALL)	Chronic myeloid leukaemia (CML)	Chronic lymphocytic leukaemia (CLL)
Most common form of acute leukaemia. Rare in childhood. Incidence increases with increasing age.	Majority (80%) of cases occur in children with peak incidence at age 3–4 years.	Accounts for around 15–20% of all cases of leukaemia. Occurs predominantly in those aged between 40–60 years but may occur at any age.	Most common form of leukaemia. Accounts for around 30% of all cases. Occurs almost exclusively in those aged more than 50 years.
French-American-British (FAB) classification based on appearance of abnormal blood cells allows identification of eight types (M0–M7).	French-American-British (FAB) classification based on appearance of abnormal blood cells allows identification of three types (L1–L3).	No FAB classification of type.	No FAB classification of type.
Rapidly fatal without treatment.	Rapidly fatal without treatment	Disease typically progresses slowly over a period of several years. Later a rapidly progressive (acute) phase may occur.	Disease typically progresses slowly over a period of several years.
May or may not be acutely ill at the time of diagnosis. Symptoms include tiredness and lethargy due to anaemia. Fever and infection due to low numbers of mature functioning white cells. Bruising and increased tendency to bleed (low platelets).	Typically acutely ill at the time of diagnosis. Symptoms include tiredness and lethargy due to anaemia. Fever and infection due to low numbers of mature functioning white cells. Bruising and increased tendency to bleed (low platelets). Infiltration of central nervous system is common, resulting in headaches and vomiting.	Not usually acutely ill at the time of diagnosis. Symptoms incude tiredness and breathlessness on exertion due to slowly progressive anaemia. Bruising due to low platelets. History of weight loss. Night sweats.	Around 25% of patients are symptom free at the time of diagnosis when the disease is identified by chance blood testing. This symptom free period may last for several years. In symptomatic patients symptoms similar to CML.
Initial treatment is with chemotherapy (combination of three cytotoxic drugs). Bone marrow transplantation considered for young patients if chemotherapy fails. Although 80–90% of young patients achieve remission only 30% are cured. Older patients fare less well.	Initial treatment is with chemotherapy (a combination of three or four cytotoxic drugs). Radiation therapy for CNS disease treatment or prevention. Bone marrow transplantation considered if chemotherapy fails. Chemotherapy effects a cure in the majority of children but only around 30% of adults.	Bone marrow transplantation first line treatment of choice for younger patients (less than 40 yrs) otherwise: Drug chemotherapy • bisulphan • alpha interferon • imatinib (Glivee) Only BMT can effect a cure.	No treatment necessary until the onset of symptoms. Control of symptoms but no cure possible with chemotherapy. Survival variable 1–20 years. Median 3–4 years.

of increased white cell numbers follows focusing on each type of white cell in turn.

Causes of increased neutrophil count (neutrophilia)
Neutrophilia is the most common derangement of white cell numbers. Reactive neutrophilia is a feature of:

- most acute bacterial infections, particularly high (up to $50 \times 10^9/l$) in pyogenic (pus-forming) infections, e.g. those caused by *Staphylococcus* and *Streptococcus* bacterial species
- non-infective acute inflammation (e.g. rheumatoid arthritis, inflammatory bowel disease, etc.)
- tissue damage (surgery, trauma, burns, myocardial infarction)
- solid tumours, e.g. lung cancer (an appropriate response to the tissue necrosis (death) that accompanies tumour growth)
- extreme physical exercise
- pregnancy and labour of pregnancy.

Malignant cause of neutrophilia
Chronic myeloid leukaemia. The total white cell count is very high, usually greater than $> 50 \times 10^9/l$ and sometimes up to $500 \times 10^9/l$. These cells are predominantly of the myeloid series with greatly increased numbers of neutrophils.

Causes of increased lymphocyte count (lymphocytosis)
Infectious mononucleosis (glandular fever). This acute infectious disease caused by the Epstein–Barr virus is the most common cause of an isolated marked lymphocytosis. Most cases occur among teenagers and young adults. Symptoms include sore throat, fever, extreme tiredness, nausea and headache. Swollen and tender lymph nodes of the throat and neck are usual. Lymphocyte count rises a few days after symptoms appear and may peak very high (in the range $10–30 \times 10^9/l$) before gradually returning to normal over the following month or two

Viral infections. Other less common viral infections associated with lymphocytosis include cytomegalovirus, early stages of HIV infection, viral hepatitis, rubella, mumps and chicken pox.

Chronic bacterial infection. Although bacterial infections are usually associated with neutrophilia rather than lymphocytosis, bacterial infections which are long standing (chronic) in nature are characterised by lymphocytosis. The most common chronic bacterial infection is tuberculosis.

Other miscellaneous infections. These include whooping cough (caused by the bacterium *Bordella pertussis*), toxoplasmosis (caused by the protozoan, *Toxoplasma gondii*).

Chronic lymphatic leukaemia. The total white cell count is usually raised (often very high, in the range $50–100 \times 10^9/l$). Most of these cells are mature lymphocytes. Severe lymphocytosis (i.e. $> 50 \times 10^9/l$) in an older person is most likely due to CLL

Non-Hodgkin's lymphoma. This haematological malignant disease originating in lymph nodes accounts for some cases.

Cause of increase in eosinophil count (eosinophilia)

Eosinophilia is much less common than either neutrophilia or lymphocytosis. Principal causes are:

- parasitic worm infections (e.g. tapeworm, hookworm, strongyloides, schistosoma, etc.)
- allergic diseases (e.g. hay fever, eczema, allergic asthma, food sensitivity)
- (sometimes) Hodgkin's lymphoma.

Causes of increase in basophils and monocyte counts

An increase in the numbers of either of these cells is rare. Basophils numbers are raised in chronic myeloid leukaemia. Monocytosis may be a feature of TB, subacute bacterial endocarditis and other chronic bacterial infections.

Causes of a reduction in white cell numbers (leukopaenia)

General considerations

A reduction in total white cell numbers is much less common than an increase; it is never 'appropriate' in the same way an increase in white cell numbers often is. A reduced white cell count is almost always the result of decrease in either neutrophils or lymphocytes, or both.

Low neutrophil count (neutropaenia)

Viral infection. A slight neutropaenia is a feature of some viral infection (mumps, influenza, viral hepatitis, HIV, etc.). The combination of a low neutrophil count and raised lymphocyte count (see above) explains why in some viral illnesses the total white cell count may remain normal despite a reduction in neutrophils.

Overwhelming bacterial infection. In rare cases of extreme infection, the bone marrow is unable to replace neutrophils at a sufficiently rapid rate.

Aplastic anaemia. This condition of bone marrow stem cell failure results in life-threatening severe neutropaenia and failure to produce adequate numbers of all blood cell types (red cells, white cells and platelets). In many cases, there is no identifiable cause. However, aplastic anaemia is a known, although often unpredictable, side effect of some drug therapies. Among these are cytotoxic drugs used to kill malignant (cancerous) cells, some antibiotics (e.g. chloramphenicol) and gold therapy for treatment of rheumatoid arthritis. Exposure to radiation (e.g. radiation therapy for cancer treatment) can also cause aplastic anaemia. The risk of aplastic anaemia is one of the reasons for the health and safety policy of restricting the use of diagnostic X-rays.

Acute leukaemia. Malignant blood cells proliferate at the expense of normal blood cell development, with resulting neutropaenia. Many solid malignant tumours spread (metastasise) to the bone, where they infiltrate and suppress normal bone marrow blood cell production. Neutropaenia may therefore be a feature of advanced cancer.

Causes of reduced lymphocyte count

AIDS. Human immunodeficiency virus (HIV-1), which causes AIDS, exerts its devastating effects by specifically infecting T-lymphocytes. The virus replicates within the T-lymphocytes causing cell death, so AIDS is characterised by progressive T-lymphocyte destruction and resulting lymphocytopaenia.

Systemic lupus erythematosus (SLE) Autoimmune destruction of lymphocytes is the cause of the lymphocytopaenia which is a common feature of systemic lupus erythematosus (SLE).

Acute inflammatory conditions. A slight decrease in lymphocyte numbers often accompanies some acute inflammatory conditions; examples include pancreatitis, appendicitis and Crohn's disease.

Influenza virus infection.

Burns, surgery and severe trauma.

Congenital disorders. A profound deficiency of lymphocytes is a feature of several very rare congenital disorders discovered at birth. These include DiGeorge's syndrome, in which, due to failure of thymus development, babies are born with no T-lymphocytes. A lack of both B- and T-lymphocytes is a feature of severe combined immunodeficiency syndrome (SCID).

Clinical consequences of abnormal white cell numbers

Increased bone marrow production of white cells is a component of the body's normal inflammatory response to injury and infection, so an increase in white cell numbers is physiological and usually has no deleterious consequences. In some cases of leukaemia, however, the white cell count rises so high (> 100×10^9/l) that the sheer numbers of white cells reduces the fluidity of blood, making it more viscous. This increased viscosity of blood increases blood pressure causing headaches, confusion, visual disturbances and in the long term can contribute to development of congestive heart failure and thrombotic disease.

A reduction in white cell numbers leaves affected patients at risk of infection. This becomes clinically evident as neutrophil count drops below 1.0×10^9/l, when bacterial infections of the mouth and throat particularly occur. Without adequate numbers of protective neutrophils, these infections fail to resolve, causing ulceration. Those with neutrophil counts of less than 0.5×10^9/l are at high risk of death from uncontrolled bacterial infection. Even normally harmless bacteria, present on the skin or in the environment, pose a serious threat to life for these patients, who require careful barrier nursing to minimise the risk of infection.

A severe reduction in lymphocyte numbers compromises the immune response leaving affected patients also at high risk of infection from bacterial, viral and fungal infection. The life threatening opportunistic infections suffered by AIDS patients is a result of reduction in T-lymphocyte numbers.

Case history 15

James Herron, a 14-year-old boy, was admitted to the local hospital A&E department, via his GP, with severe central abdominal pain. James had been vomiting before admission and was slightly pyrexial (38°C) on admission. Physical examination and symptoms suggested that James was suffering acute appendicitis. The admitting doctor sampled blood for urgent urea and electrolytes (U&E) and full blood count (FBC).

The following FBC results were telephoned to A&E 30 minutes later.

Hb	13.1 g/l
PCV	42%
RBC	5.1×10^{12}/l
WBC (total)	18.1×10^9/l
Neutrophils 1	2.8×10^9/l
Lymphocytes	2.0×10^9/l
Monocytes	0.7×10^9/l
Eosinophils	0.2×10^9/l
Basophils	$< 0.1 \times 10^9$/l

Questions

(1) Are there any abnormalities in these results?
(2) Would you expect abnormalities in FBC results in a patient with acute appendicitis?

Discussion of case history

(1) Yes. There are two abnormal results. James has a slightly raised total white cell count due to an increase in neutrophil numbers (neutrophilia).

(2) Yes. Appendicitis is acute inflammation of the appendix. Any active inflammatory disease process is likely to be associated with an increase in neutrophil numbers. Such an increase is found in the vast majority of cases of acute appendicitis and therefore provides further evidence to support the provisional diagnosis made on the basis of physical examination, reported history and symptoms. A slight decrease in lymphocyte numbers is also sometimes a feature of acute appendicitis.

Further reading

Cavenagh J (2004) The white cell. *Medicine* **32**: 4–6.

Matules E & Deardon C (2004) Chronic lymphocytic leukaemia. *Medicine* **32**: 72–74.

Goldman J (2004) Chronic myeloid leukaemia. *Medicine* **32**: 70–71.

Shoentag R & Cangliarella J (1992) The nuances of lymphocytopaenia. *Clin Lab Med* **13**: 923–34.

Peterson L & Hrinsko M (1993) Benign lymphocytosis and reactive neutrophilia. *Clin Lab Med* **13**: 863–75.

Shapiro M & Greenfield S (1987) The complete blood count and leukocyte differential count. *Ann Intern Med* **106**: 65–74.

Chapter 17

TESTS OF HAEMOSTASIS: *PLATELET COUNT, PROTHROMBIN TIME (PT), ACTIVATED PARTIAL THROMBOPLASTIN TIME (APTT) AND THROMBIN TIME (TT)*

Blood loss following blood vessel injury is minimised by the capacity of the blood to coagulate or clot. The complex physiological process that ensures this life-preserving property of blood is called haemostasis. Blood must retain its ability to quickly form a 'plug' at the site of vessel injury, preventing undue blood loss, while remaining fluid and free of coagulated blood within undamaged vessels. Disturbance of this fine balance, a feature of many disease processes, can result either in an increased tendency to bleed if the coagulability of blood is less than normal; or formation of a blood clot (thrombus) within patent blood vessels, if coagulability is abnormally increased.

The four blood tests discussed in this chapter are the most commonly used tests in the first line investigation of patients who are suspected of suffering disease associated with an increased tendency to bleed. Two of the tests – prothrombin time (PT) and activated partial thromboplastin time (APTT) – are also used to monitor anticoagulation drug therapy, prescribed for those who are at risk of thrombus formation. A platelet count is usually included in a routine full blood count (FBC); the other three tests are usually requested together as 'coagulation screen'.

Normal physiology

The sequence of events that leads to formation of a stable fibrin plug and cessation of bleeding (haemostasis) following blood vessel injury is described in Figure 17.1.

Reduction in blood flow to the injured site minimises blood loss. Vessel injury also initiates two further physiological responses. The first is platelet adhesion and aggregation with formation of a physical plug of platelets, and the second is initiation of the so-called clotting cascade which results in production of the protein, fibrin. Fibrin strands form around and between the aggregated platelets, stabilising the somewhat fragile platelet plug.

Normal haemostasis is crucially dependent on two factors:

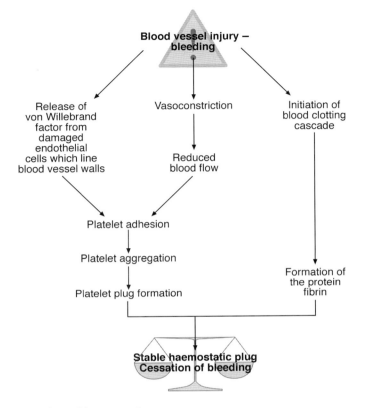

Figure 17.1 Overview of haemostasis.

- adequate numbers of normally functioning platelets
- normally functioning blood clotting cascade.

In order to understand the defects of haemostasis associated with disease and how the results of the four blood tests are applied, it is necessary to examine platelets and the clotting cascade in a little detail.

Platelet production, structure and function

Like the other formed elements that circulate in blood, platelets (alternative name thrombocytes) are derived from the stem cells of the bone marrow (Figure 15.1). A proportion of stem cells differentiate by stages within the bone marrow to megakaryocytes. Platelets are produced within the cytoplasm of these cells. Still within the bone marrow, platelets are released from mature megakaryocytes and pass from bone marrow to the blood. Each megakaryocyte produces around 4000 platelets. Platelets have a lifespan of only around 10 days in blood so constant bone marrow production is necessary. Having a diameter of between 1 and 2 μm, platelets are far smaller than either red cells or white cells. Like mature red cells, they have no nucleus.

The principal function of platelets is to plug 'holes' in vessel walls caused during injury. The first stage in this process is adhesion of platelets to the wall of the damaged vessel. This adhesion is facilitated in part by a protein called von Willebrand factor, which is released from injured endothelial cells that line the internal surface of blood vessels. Adhesion proteins present on the surface of passing platelets bind to von Willebrand factor, which itself is bound to proteins present on the surface of damaged endothelial cells. Following adhesion, platelets secrete many substances that modulate both the clotting cascade (see below) and further platelet function. Among these are substances (e.g. adenosine diphosphate (ADP) and thromboxane A_2) which both induce platelets to stick to each other and swell in size. This process, called aggregation, continues until the mass of aggregated swollen platelets is sufficiently large to plug the damaged vessel.

Blood clotting cascade

As platelets are aggregating at the site of vessel injury, fibrin is being produced locally by the blood clotting cascade. This is a series of reactions in which proteins present in blood plasma, called clotting factors, are activated in sequence. Each activated factor promotes activation of the next and so on down the cascade; the final product being fibrin. These reactions are enzymic in nature. In their inactive state factors are pro-enzymes (i.e. have no enzymic activity). Enzymic action converts proenzymes (unactivated factors) to active enzymes (activated factors). While most clotting factors are pro-enzymes/enzymes, some are not actually enzymes but substances required for enzymic action to occur. Thirteen clotting factors have been identified, numbered by convention in roman numerals in the order in which they were first discovered (Table 17.1). The once postulated Factor VI is no longer thought to exist.

A simplified account of current understanding of the blood clotting cascade is described in Figure 17.2. The cascade comprises the intrinsic and extrinsic pathway,

Table 17.1 Blood clotting factors.

Factor	Alternative Name(s)	Notes
Factor I	Fibrinogen	Glycoprotein precursor of fibrin synthesised in liver
Factor II	Prothrombin	Pro-enzyme synthesised in liver
Factor III	Tissue factor tissue thromboplastin	Protein present in most tissues initiates extrinsic pathway
Factor IV	Calcium	Inorganic ion co-factor
Factor V	Labile factor	Protein, co-factor synthesised in liver
Factor VI	Once proposed but no longer thought to exist	
Factor VII	Proconvertin stable factor	Pro-enzyme synthesised in liver
Factor VIII	Antihaemophillic factor	Protein, co-factor
Factor IX	Christmas factor	Pro-enzyme synthesised in liver
Factor X	Stuart factor	Pro-enzyme synthesised in liver
Factor XI	Plasma thromboplastin antecedent	Proenzyme
Factor XII	Hageman factor contact factor	Proenzyme
Factor XIII	Fibrin stabilising factor	Proenzyme

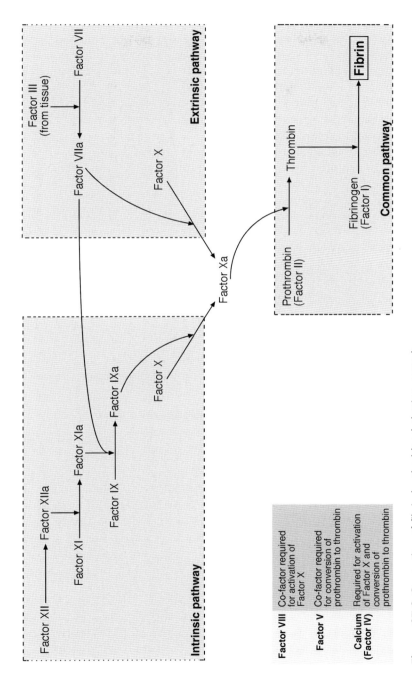

Figure 17.2 Generation of fibrin by the blood clotting cascade.

which both result in activation of Factor X. The route from activated Factor X to fibrin production is referred to as the common pathway.

The intrinsic pathway is initiated when Factor XII is activated by contact with a structural protein called collagen, exposed as a result of vessel wall injury. Activated Factor XII then activates Factor XI, which in turn activates Factor X. Co-factors, Factor VIII (antihaemophilic factor) and Factor IV (calcium) are required for this last reaction. The extrinsic pathway is initiated by Factor III. This is a substance called thromboplastin, found in most tissues and released to the blood during tissue injury. Factor III activates Factor VII, which in turn activates Factor IX. In the final common pathway, activated Factor X activates Factor II (prothrombin) to the active thrombin, which in turn converts fibrinogen (Factor I) to fibrin. Factor V is a co-factor required for conversion of prothrombin to thrombin.

Most of the factors of the blood clotting cascade including Factor I (fibrinogen), Factor II (prothrombin), Factors V, VII, IX, X, XI and XII are synthesised and released to the blood in their inactive form by the liver. The synthesis of Factors II (prothrombin), VII, IX and X is crucially dependent on vitamin K. Vitamin K is derived from two sources, diet and vitamin K-synthesising bacteria normally present in the gut.

The formation of fibrin by the clotting cascade depends on adequate plasma concentration of *all* clotting factors, which in turn is dependent on:

- normally functioning liver
- adequate dietary source of vitamin K
- normal bacterial flora in the gastrointestinal tract
- normal gastrointestinal absorption of dietary and non-dietary vitamin K.

What do tests of blood coagulation measure?

While it is clear that a platelet count is simply a measure of the number of platelets present in blood, it might be less obvious what is being measured by the other three tests considered in this chapter. Prothrombin time (PT) activated partial thromboplastin time (APTT) and thrombin time (TT) all test the ability of the blood to generate fibrin by the blood clotting cascade. In essence, they all measure the time taken for a sample of patient's blood plasma to form a fibrin clot in a test tube, after addition of a reagent that initiates the clotting cascade. Results are expressed in time (seconds). In the case of the prothrombin test, commercially produced thromboplastin (Factor III) is added to the plasma. This is the clotting factor that initiates the extrinsic pathway, so prothrombin time is a test specifically of the extrinsic and common pathways. A deficiency of any factor or factors of these two pathways (i.e. Factor X, VII, V, prothrombin and fibrinogen) will result in an abnormally prolonged time for a fibrin clot to form (i.e. PT will be raised).

In a similar way, by adding only an initiator of the intrinsic pathway to the patient's plasma, the APTT tests only the intrinsic and common pathways. In this case, an abnormally prolonged result indicates a deficiency of one or more of those factors required by the intrinsic and common pathways.

Finally, in the thrombin time test, thrombin is added to the patient's plasma. This is a test specifically of the final stages of the common pathway: fibrinogen to fibrin. An abnormally prolonged thrombin test indicates a deficiency of Factor I (fibrinogen).

If PT, APTT and TT are all within the reference range, the blood clotting cascade is assumed to be working normally.

Laboratory measurement of platelet count, PT, APTT and TT

A platelet count is one of the tests included in a full blood count. Laboratory measurement and sample requirements for full blood count are discussed in Chapter 15. This section is concerned only with PT, APTT and TT.

Patient preparation

No particular patient preparation is necessary.

Timing of sample

Blood for PT, APTT and TT may be sampled at any time. However, the proteins of the clotting cascade are not well preserved in a blood sample and falsely abnormal results can occur if blood is not tested within 4–6 hours of sampling. This period can be extended to 15 hours if the sample is stored in a refrigerator at 4°C. Samples more than 15 hours old are not suitable for analysis.

Sample requirements

The tests are performed on plasma, the fluid that remains when all cellular elements are removed from anticoagulated blood. The blood must be collected into a tube containing the anticoagulant sodium citrate (usually a light blue top), which also preserves blood clotting proteins (factors). The volume required (usually 5 ml) is indicated on the bottle; it is important that neither more nor less than the volume indicated is added to the bottle. Gentle inversion to mix blood with the anticoagulant is essential. It is inadvisable to sample blood for these tests via an indwelling catheter, since heparin flushes are often used to keep these lines patent; falsely abnormal results will be obtained if blood samples are contaminated with heparin.

Interpretation of results

Approximate reference ranges

Platelet count	$150–400 \times 10^9/l$
Prothrombin time (PT)	10–14 secs

Activated partial thromboplastin time (APTT)   30–40 secs
Thrombin time (TT)   14–16 secs

Critical values

Platelet count $< 40 \times 10^9/l$ or $> 1000 \times 10^9/l$
Prothombin time > 30 secs
Activated partial thromboplastin time > 78 secs

Terms used in interpretation

Thrombocytes   alternative name for platelet
Thrombocytopaenia   reduced platelet count, i.e. $< 150 \times 10^9/l$
Thrombocytosis   increased platelet count, i.e. $> 400 \times 10^9/l$
Haemophilia   a pathological state of decreased blood coagulability and therefore increased tendency to bleed
Thrombophilia   a pathological state of increased blood coagulability and therefore increased tendency to form blood clots inappropriately within patent blood vessels (thrombosis)

Causes of decreased platelet count

Reduction in platelet numbers can be caused by one of:

• reduced bone marrow production
• increased rate of platelet destruction
• increased rate of platelet consumption.

Reduced bone marrow production of platelets, with resulting severe decrease in platelet numbers (may be less than $50 \times 10^9/l$) is a feature of aplastic anaemia, acute leukaemia, cytotoxic drug therapy and radiotherapy. Megaloblastic anaemia, anaemia inavariably caused by deficiency of vitamins B_{12} or folate (Chapter 18), is also associated with decreased bone marrow production of platelets, although not usually severe. Secondary spread of primary cancer to the bone marrow can result in reduced platelet production, so a reduced platelet count is sometimes a feature of advanced cancer.

Immune thrombocytopaenic purpura (ITP), is the most common cause of increased platelet destruction. This relatively common disorder, affecting predominantly young to middle-aged women, results from production of autoantibodies against patient's platelets. The cause of this autoantibody production is not known. In most cases, the condition arises in otherwise well women, but it can arise as a secondary complication of some other primary disorder; these include systemic lupus erythematosus (SLE), infection with HIV and chronic lymphatic leukaemia. The antibodies bind to the platelets resulting in their premature removal and destruction within the reticuloendothelial system. Platelet lifespan is reduced from a normal 10 days to just a few hours in this condition. Bone marrow production cannot keep pace with this rate of destruction and the reduction in platelet numbers is severe, in the range $10–50 \times 10^9/l$. A similar disorder may complicate recovery from vaccination and some viral infections (e.g. chicken pox and measles) in childhood.

Increased platelet consumption is a feature of disseminated intravascular coagulation (DIC), a complication of many serious illnesses including severe infection of the blood (septicaemia), malignant disease, severe tissue damage during major surgery or trauma, some obstetric disorders and incompatible blood transfusion. DIC is characterised by abnormal (inappropriate) activation of clotting cascade and platelet aggregation within blood vessels. The result is depletion of both platelets and clotting factors leaving these already very sick patients at risk of severe, even fatal haemorrhage.

Many commonly used drugs sometimes induce production of antibodies directed at platelets with resulting increased platelet destruction. Drugs that may result in a reduction in platelet numbers include some anti-inflammatories, antibiotics (penicillin, sulphonamide) and some diuretics (frusemide, acetazolamide).

Causes of increased platelet count

An increase in platelet numbers, termed thrombocytosis, is a feature of those malignant disorders of the bone marrow, collectively called the myeloproliferative disorders, that are characterised by abnormal proliferation of myeloid stem cells. The myeloproliferative disorders in which an increase in platelet numbers can be expected include chronic myeloid leukaemia (around a third of all cases), polycythaemia vera (around a half of all cases) and essential thrombocythaemia (all cases).

A mild to moderate increase in platelet numbers (usually between 400 and 1000 $\times 10^9/l$) is a relatively common phenomenon among acutely ill patients. The raised platelet count reflects bone marrow stimulation induced by blood loss, infection, or tissue injury. It is termed secondary thrombocytosis to distinguish it from the thrombocytosis due to the primary bone marrow diseases described above. The conditions that might be associated with secondary thrombocytosis include: severe tissue injury due to major surgery or trauma; acute and chronic infection; malignancy; chronic inflammatory conditions such as rheumatoid arthritis or Crohn's disease and chronic iron deficiency anaemia. Surgical removal of the spleen (where platelets are sequestered when they are no longer viable) results in particularly high platelet count.

Consequences of abnormality in platelet numbers

Since platelets are required for normal haemostasis, patients with a reduced platelet count are at increased risk of excessive bleeding. Spontaneous bleeding may occur if platelet count falls below $50 \times 10^9/l$. Potentially fatal haemorrhage almost inevitably occurs if count falls below $5 \times 10^9/l$. An increased tendency to bleed due to platelet deficiency has several clinical manifestations, including increased menstrual blood loss (menorrhagia), easy or even spontaneous bruising, bleeding gums, nose bleeds (epistaxis), petechial (tiny pinpoint) haemorrhages into the skin giving a red rash-like appearance, and purpura. Widespread purple-brown discoloration of skin (ecchymosis), akin to bruising, occurs due to haemorrhage into tissues.

An increase in platelet numbers (thrombophilia) carries with it the risk of increased coagulability of blood and resulting thrombosis. In practice, this risk of thrombosis is not real until platelet count rises in excess of 1000×10^9/l.

Causes of increased PT, APTT and TT

An increase in any of these tests indicates a deficiency of one or more clotting factors. Deficiency may be congenital (i.e. inherited) or, much more commonly, acquired as a result of disease. Haemophilia A, which accounts for around 85% of all the many known inherited blood clotting defects, is the most common inherited blood clotting deficiency. The defect is in the gene that codes for production of Factor VIII (also called antihaemophilia factor). This is the co-factor required for activation of Factor X by Factor IXa (Figure 17.2). The result of the genetic defect is a marked deficiency or complete absence of Factor VIII and severely impaired blood clotting. Without Factor VIII replacement therapy, affected patients are at risk of life-threatening haemorrhage. The extrinsic and common pathways are intact in the patient with haemophilia A so PT and TT are normal. However, APTT (a test of the intrinsic pathway) is abnormally increased. Haemophilia B (Christmas disease), a less common but equally devastating inherited defect of the clotting cascade in which the deficiency is of Factor IX rather than Factor VIII, also causes raised APTT.

Since many clotting factors are synthesised in the liver, multiple factor deficiency is a feature of liver disease (acute and chronic hepatitis, cirrhosis, etc). PT, APTT and TT may all be increased in severe liver disease, although a raised TT is less usual. Of the three, PT is the most sensitive marker of liver disease and is routinely used as a test of liver function both in its detection and to monitor progress.

The production of several factors of both the intrinsic and extrinsic pathway is dependent on vitamin K, so deficiency of vitamin K is associated with an increase in both PT and APTT. Newborn babies, who are often deficient of vitamin K and therefore at risk of haemorrhage, are often given prophylactic vitamin K at the time of birth. Adult vitamin K deficiency usually only arises as result of impaired absorption from the gastrointestinal tract. Absorption of the fat-soluble vitamin K is dependent on the bile salts contained in bile, so diseases that may be associated with poor absorption of vitamin K include those that result in obstruction of the bile tract (e.g. gallstones, cancer of the head of pancreas) and pancreatitis.

Dietary deficiency of vitamin K may occur in malnourished adults. Antibiotic use can be associated with deficiency because it affects the balance of normal gut flora, and therefore bacterial production of vitamin K. Whatever the cause, vitamin K deficiency is associated with an increase in PT and APTT; TT is normal.

Consumption and resulting deficiency of several clotting factors is a feature of the abnormal coagulation within blood vessels that characterises DIC (see above). PT, APTT and TT are all raised in DIC. The increase in TT is particularly marked.

Clotting factors are not well preserved in stored blood, so those patients who receive massive blood transfusion (i.e. total blood volume replaced) are paradoxically at increased risk of haemorrhage because the blood that is being transfused is relatively deficient of clotting factors. Increased PT, APTT and TT may all be evident in the patient who has received massive blood transfusion.

Consequences of increased PT, APTT and TT

An increase in any or all of these tests implies a deficiency of one or more clotting factors and therefore an increased tendency to bleed.

Anticoagulation therapy

One of the major uses of the prothrombin time (PT) and activated partial thromboplastin time (APTT) tests is to monitor anticoagulation therapy.

The anticoagulant drugs warfarin and heparin are most widely used in the treatment and prevention of deep vein thrombosis (DVT) and its life-threatening complication, pulmonary thromboembolism. DVT is characterised by thrombi (plugs of coagulated blood and platelets) formation within veins, usually of the legs. Patients most at risk are those recovering from surgery, particularly of the hip and pelvis, and those who are immobile or obese. Old age and pregnancy also carries with it an increased risk of DVT. Some people inherit defects of blood coagulation that predispose to DVT. The most common of these is a condition called factor V Leiden (or activated protein C (APC) resistance), which affects around 5% of the UK population. In this condition, normal control of the clotting cascade is lost and patients have a resulting increased tendency to thrombosis.

The aim of anticoagulation therapy is to dissolve existing thrombi and prevent further thrombi formation by artificially reducing the coaguability of blood. Heparin, administered intravenously or subcutaneously for the treatment of existing DVT, functions by inhibiting the action of several activated factors of the extrinsic pathway; it also impairs platelet function. To prevent further DVT episodes in a patient who has suffered DVT, long-term oral anticoagulant warfarin is prescribed. Warfarin operates by inhibiting the action of vitamin K in production of vitamin K-dependent factors.

Reducing the coagulability of blood carries with it the risk of increased bleeding, so anticoagulation therapy must be carefully monitored to ensure the maximum level of anticoagulation consistent with minimum risk of excessive bleeding. Heparin is monitored using APTT and warfarin is monitored using the PT test. In the case of heparin use, dose is adjusted so that APTT is between 1.5 and 2 times the normal value.

Warfarin, prothrombin and INR

As we have seen when PT is used to investigate a suspected coagulation defect, results are expressed in time (seconds). This is not the case when PT is used to monitor warfarin therapy. Instead, the International Normalised Ratio (INR) is used. The INR provides a way of expressing PT results to take account of the differing activity of commercially prepared tissue thromboplastin used in the test. This ensures that prothrombin results are more directly comparable and provides a more accurate control of warfarin therapy. The INR is defined as the patient's PT in seconds, divided by the mean of the PT reference range, raised to the power of the international sensitivity index (ISI) of the particular thromboplastin being used:

$$\text{Patient's INR} = \left(\frac{\text{Patient's prothrombin time (secs)}}{\text{Mean normal prothrombin time (secs)}}\right)^{\text{ISI}}$$

Warfarin dose is adjusted so that the INR is maintained within a therapeutic range, which depends on the precise clinical reason for prescribing warfarin. For most patients, the INR must be maintained within the range 2.0–3.0. In some circumstances, increased level of anticoagulation is required, in which case the therapeutic INR range is 3.0–4.5. If INR rises above the prescribed range (i.e. 2.0–3.0 or 3.0–4.5), dose must be adjusted downwards. All patients on long-term warfarin therapy should have their INR checked at regular (2–3 weeks) intervals.

Advances in technology have allowed the development of portable analysers for monitoring warfarin therapy. These allow anticoagulant monitoring outside the laboratory, either in clinics or primary care centres, where analysis can be performed by nurses.[1] In some anticoagulant clinics, nursing staff are not only analysing patient samples but interpreting results and adjusting warfarin dose. The success of this arrangement has been demonstrated in several studies that have shown that an anticoagulant service run by nurse specialists is as effective as a haematology consultant-run service, in maintaining therapeutic control among patients receiving warfarin.[2]

Some studies[3,4] have demonstrated the feasibility of patients taking control of their own blood testing and dose management. Just as some diabetic patients monitor their own blood glucose and adjust insulin dose accordingly, so some patients can successfully self-manage their long-term anticoagulation therapy, thereby avoiding the inconvenience of frequent hospital appointments.

For more than 50 years, warfarin has been the only available oral anticoagulant and the mainstay for prophylaxis of DVT and other thromboembolic disease. Ximelagatran is a new oral anticoagulant that has only recently been licensed for limited use. Numerous large-scale clinical trials have demonstrated it is as effective as warfarin in a range of clinical settings,[5] and it has a major advantage over warfarin in that it requires no monitoring of blood coagulation. However, there are some safety concerns and it remains to be seen if this promising new drug will replace warfarin and end the inconvenience of frequent monitoring that so many patients currently have to endure.

Case history 16

Amy Waters, now aged 68 years, had to retire 10 years prematurely from her physically demanding work, because of rheumatoid arthritis. Two months ago, she was given a hip replacement to increase her mobility. Postoperative recovery was complicated by an infection and on the 10th day following surgery she suddenly became extremely breathless. Understandably panicked, Amy also reported chest pain. During physical examination, the orthopaedic senior house officer noted some swelling of the left calf, which Amy described as slightly tender when touched. A diagnosis of pulmonary embolus secondary to deep vein thrombosis in her left leg was eventually made. For the next few days, Amy was given a continuous intravenous infusion of heparin and the breathlessness quickly resolved. After heparin was withdrawn, Amy was prescribed warfarin tablets. She was eventually discharged home feeling well and delighted with her new hip. She was given a prescription to continue her daily dose of warfarin and asked to attend the haematology outpatients clinic every three weeks for a blood test.

Questions

(1) What blood test does Mrs Waters need?
(2) Why does she need this test?
(3) How long will she have to continue to attend outpatients for this test?

Discussion of case history

(1) The blood test required is prothrombin time (PT) reported as INR.

(2) Mrs Waters is receiving long-term anticoagulation therapy in the form of warfarin tablets to prevent recurrence of deep vein thrombosis (DVT) she suffered during postoperative recovery. This drug decreases the tendency of the blood to coagulate by inhibiting the production of several clotting factors (proteins) required for blood coagulation; in lay terms, it 'thins the blood'. The drug carries with it the risk of increased bleeding (haemorrhage) and so must be carefully monitored to ensure that the dose given continues to give the maximum protection against thrombus formation consistent with minimum risk of haemorrhage.

(3) Mrs Waters must continue to have her prothrombin time checked at regular intervals for the duration of time she is receiving warfarin. This may be for up to six months, after which time it may be considered not necessary. If she has a recurrence of DVT, then warfarin and regular testing would be resumed, most likely for a much longer period.

References

1. Hobbs F, Fitzmaurice D *et al.* (1999) Is the international normalised ratio (INR) reliable? A trial of comparative measurement in hospital laboratory and primary care settings. *J Clin Pathol* **52**: 494–97.
2. Connor C, Wright C & Fegan C (2002) The safety and effectivenss of a nurse-led anticoagulant service. *J Adv Nurs* **38**: 407–15.
3. Gardiner C, Williams K *et al.* (2005) Patient self-testing is a reliable and acceptable alternative to laboratory INR monitoring. *Br J Haematol* **128**: 242–47.

4. Heneghan C *et al.* (2006) Self-monitoring of oral anticoagulation: a systematic review and meta-analysis. *Lancet* **367**: 404–11.
5. Boos C, Hinton A & Lip G (2005) Ximelagatran: a clinical perspective. *Eur J Intern Med* **16**: 267–78.

Further reading

Casey G (2003) Haemostasis, anticoagulant and fibrinolysis. *Nurs Stand* **18**(7): 45–51.
Chines D, Bussel J *et al.* (2004) Congenital and acquired thrombocytopaenia. *Hematology* (Am Society of Hematology Education Program book) **1**: 390–406.
Glicksman H (2004) You're hurt and bleeding; How do you spell relief? *www.arn.org/ docs/glicksman/eyw_040501.htm*
Griesshammer M, Bangerter M & Sauer T (1999) Aetiology and clinical significance of thrombocytosis: analysis of 732 patients with an elevated platelet count. *J Intern Med* **245**: 295–300.
Hoyer L (1994) Haemophilia A. *New Eng J Med* **330**: 38–46.
Morris B (2004) Nursing initiatives for deep vein thrombosis prophylaxis. Pragmatic timing of administration. *Orthop Nurse* **23**: 142–47.
Pence C & McErlane K (2005) Anticoagulation self-monitoring. *Am J Nurs* **10**: 62–65.
Rempher K & Little J (2004) Assessment of red blood cell and coagulation laboratory data. *AACN Clin Issues* **15**(4): 622–37.

Chapter 18

LABORATORY INVESTIGATION OF ANAEMIA: *IRON, TOTAL IRON BINDING CAPACITY (TIBC), FERRITIN, B$_{12}$ AND FOLATE*

The means by which the results of full blood count (FBC) identify those patients who are anaemic was discussed in Chapter 15. It was emphasised that anaemia is not a disease but rather a symptom of disease with many possible causes. Successful treatment of anaemia depends crucially on identifying its cause. It will be remembered that tests included in the full blood count (most notably the mean cell volume, MCV) suggest possible causes of anaemia, but further testing may be necessary. The principal use of the five tests described in this chapter is to confirm the cause of anaemia.

Deficiency of iron is the most common cause of anaemia in the UK and around the world. World Health Organization (WHO) best estimates suggest that 2 billion people worldwide are anaemic and iron deficiency is the cause in around half of these cases.[1] Measurement of the serum or plasma concentration of serum iron, total iron binding capacity (TIBC) and ferritin together provide the means of confirming a diagnosis of iron deficiency anaemia. Similarly, measurement of the serum or plasma concentration of the vitamins B$_{12}$ and folate provides the means of identifying those patients who are suffering so called megaloblastic anaemia. As we shall see, anaemia is not the only condition in which abnormalities in results of these five tests can be expected.

Normal physiology

Function of iron and iron metabolism

The oxygen delivery function of haemoglobin contained within red cells is dependent on the presence of iron in the haem part of haemoglobin (Figure 15.3). Oxygen forms a reversible weak link with the single atom of iron in each of the four haem groups contained in the haemoglobin molecule. Iron is thus essential for haemoglobin production and function. The muscle protein, myoglobin and the

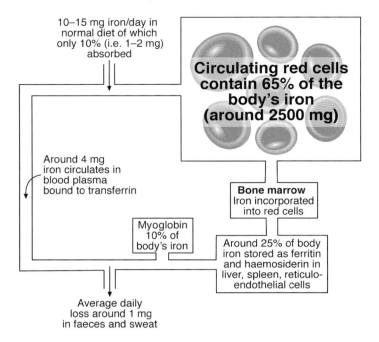

Figure 18.1 Distribution of iron in the body: daily intake and loss.

function of some enzymes are also dependent on iron, although compared with the role of iron in haemoglobin these are of much less clinical significance.

Around 70% of the approximately 4–5 g of iron present in the body is contained in the haemoglobin in circulating red cells (Figure 18.1). Most of the rest is stored in tissues (principally the liver but also the spleen and bone marrow). In these storage 'compartments', iron is contained within the proteins ferritin and haemosiderin. Some ferritin is present in the plasma part of blood and the concentration of ferritin in plasma is a reliable indicator of the body's total iron tissue stores. Just 3–4 mg (i.e. 0.1% of total body iron) circulates in blood plasma, bound to the transport protein transferrin. It is the concentration of this transferrin bound fraction of total body iron that is measured in the serum iron test.

Iron is well conserved by the body. When red cells die at the end of their 120-day life span, iron is returned to the body stores for bone marrow production of new red cells. Since iron is protein bound and therefore cannot be filtered out of blood at the glomerulus, very little iron is excreted in urine; the only significant loss is that contained in surface epithelial cells constantly shed from the body. Just 1 mg/day is lost from the body. Since most of the body's iron is contained within red cells, blood loss represents a potential route for significant iron depletion. For example, normal menstruation is associated with a loss of around 15 mg of iron every month. When this is taken into account, healthy premenopausal women lose on average 1.5–2 mg of iron a day. To replace these minimal losses and maintain normal iron stores, at least 1 mg of iron in the case of healthy children, adult men and postmenopausal women and up to 2 mg for premenopausal women, must be absorbed every day from diet. In fact, a normal well-balanced diet contains approximately 10 to 15 mg of iron per day. The principal sources of dietary iron are meat (particularly red meat) and fish, green leafed vegetables and breakfast cereals. Vitamin C increases the availability for absorption of the iron present in vegetables and cereals. Absorption of dietary iron occurs in the upper small intestine. Just 10% of available dietary iron is normally absorbed, sufficient to replace daily losses. It is vital for good health that iron stores remain replete but not overloaded with iron. Too much iron can be at least as damaging to health as too little iron. Since there is no control of the iron lost from the body, control of iron body stores depends crucially upon the control mechanisms of absorption of dietary iron. Absorption of dietary iron is minutely adjusted to meet the body's requirements at the time. Excess dietary iron is lost from the body in faeces.

Function and metabolism of vitamins B_{12} and folate

Vitamins are a group of organic substances of widely differing chemical structure that are essential, albeit in tiny amounts, for life. They cannot be synthesised by the human body and our only source is the food we eat. Most vitamins of the B group which includes both B_{12} (alternative name cobalamin) and folate (alternative name folic acid) function as essential co-enzymes or co-factors in the enzymic reactions of cellular metabolism.

Specifically B_{12} and folate are both required for the action of key enzymes in the synthesis of deoxyribonucleic acid (DNA) during cell division. Tissues characterised by rapid cell turnover and consequent unremitting cell division are particularly dependent on intact DNA synthesis and therefore vitamins B_{12} and folate. Bone marrow is one such tissue: blood cell production by the bone marrow continues minute by minute throughout life and an adequate supply of B_{12} and folate is essential for the continuing normal production of blood cells. Although essential for several other cellular enzyme reactions, the role of B_{12} and folate in the cell division required for normal production of blood cells is the one that is of prime clinical significance.

Both B_{12} and folate are synthesised in nature by bacteria, and we obtain them by eating animal and plant foods that are naturally contaminated with these bacteria. The principal dietary source of vitamin B_{12} is meat (animal liver is a particularly rich source), fish and dairy products. Vegetables do not contain B_{12}. Folic acid is present in green leafy vegetables; liver is a rich source. Most breakfast cereals are fortified with both B_{12} and folate. The minimum daily requirement for B_{12} is 1–2 µg and for folate 150 µg. A normal healthy diet provides well in excess of the minimum requirement of B_{12} but only just twice the amount of folate required.

Absorption of B_{12} (Figure 18.2)

The acid medium of the stomach is important for release of B_{12} from foods before absorption from the gastrointestinal tract. B_{12} is absorbed at the ileum but for this to occur, the vitamin must first be bound to so-called intrinsic factor, a peptide produced by the gastric parietal cells of the stomach. Absorbed B_{12} is transported in blood, to bone marrow and other cells, bound to the transport protein, transcobalamin.

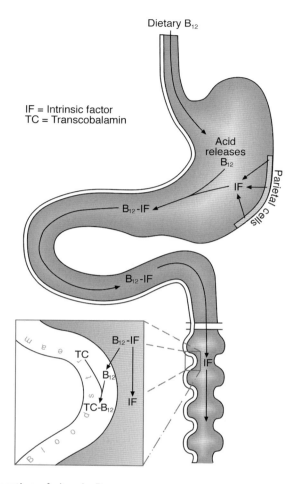

Figure 18.2 Absorption of vitamin B$_{12}$.

The body has considerable capacity to store large reserves of vitamin B$_{12}$ in the liver, sufficient in fact to remain in normal health for several years on an entirely vitamin B$_{12}$-free diet.

Absorption of folate

Absorption of folate is less complex. It is absorbed at the upper small intestine and is transported in blood to bone marrow and other folate requiring tissues either in its free form or bound to albumin.

Like vitamin B$_{12}$, folate is stored principally in the liver. However, folate stores are sufficient to last only a few months on a folate-free diet.

Normal production of red cells in the bone marrow is dependent on:

- a healthy diet containing sufficient B$_{12}$ and folate
- production of acid and intrinsic factor by the stomach for absorption of B$_{12}$

- normal absorption at the ileum (i.e. functioning gastrointestinal tract)
- adequate production of the transport protein transcobalamin.

Laboratory measurement

With few exceptions, the tests described in this chapter should be reserved for those patients in whom anaemia has been demonstrated by FBC (Chapter 15). The results of mean cell volume (MCV) indicate which of these tests are most appropriate. A reduced MCV indicates probable iron deficiency anaemia, in which case serum iron, total iron binding capacity and serum ferritin are appropriate. If MCV is raised, then B_{12} and folate should be measured first.

What is being measured

Serum/plasma iron. The concentration of the small proportion of total body iron that circulates in the plasma part of blood; it does not include the iron contained in red cells or that contained in ferritin.

Total iron binding capacity (TIBC). A test performed on plasma or serum, essentially a measure of plasma transferrin concentration. Transferrin is the protein to which iron in plasma is bound.

Serum ferritin. The concentration of ferritin in serum. Ferritin is a protein in which iron is stored in tissues. The concentration of ferritin in serum reflects total iron stores.

Serum B_{12} and folate. The concentration of vitamin B_{12} and folate in serum. A low result indicates deficiency.

Red cell folate. Concentration of folate in red cells. A low result indicates deficiency.

Patient preparation

No particular patient preparation is necessary.

Timing of sample

No particular timing is required. It is best practice to collect blood at a time to coincide with routine transport to the laboratory.

Sample requirements

Around 5 ml of venous blood is sufficient for iron, TIBC and ferritin. Most commonly serum is used, in which case blood should be collected into a plain tube containing no anticoagulant. Blood for red cell folate must be collected into a tube containing the anticoagulant EDTA (lavender coloured top) bottle. A further

5 ml of venous blood is required for serum B_{12} and folate (collected into a plain tube containing no additives).

Interpretation of results

Approximate reference ranges

Serum iron	10–30 μmol/l
Serum TIBC	40–75 μmol/l
Serum ferritin	10–300 μg/l
Serum B_{12}	of the order 150–1000 ng/l but values vary according to methodology – consult local laboratory
Red cell folate	of the order 150–700 μg/l but values vary – consult local laboratory

Conditions associated with abnormal results of serum iron, TIBC or ferritin

Conditions associated with abnormal results of serum iron, TIBC or ferritin are:

- iron deficiency anaemia
- chronic inflammation and infection (anaemia of chronic disease, ACD)
- iron overload.

Iron deficiency anaemia

Causes

In some patients, there may be more than one cause: iron deficiency anaemia is frequently multifactorial. The many possible causes can be addressed under the four main headings:

- insufficient iron in the diet, poor nutrition
- increased loss of iron (in blood) from the body
- inadequate absorption of dietary iron
- increased demand for iron.

It is unusual for poor diet to be the sole cause of iron deficiency in developed countries, although a diet relatively deficient of iron (e.g. high proportion of 'junk' food), may be a contributory factor in some cases. Poor nutrition is, however, a major cause of iron deficiency in most areas of the developing world.

The most common cause among adults in developed countries like the UK is chronic blood loss. Red cells contain 70% of the body's iron, and blood loss represents a significant iron deficit. As long as iron tissue stores are replete, a single acute episode of even severe blood loss will not cause iron deficiency. However, chronic blood loss, i.e. the continuous or regular loss of small amounts of blood over a prolonged period, will slowly exhaust iron stores. Excessive menstrual blood flow (menorrhagia) is the most frequent cause of iron deficiency among premenopausal women. Chronic blood loss from the gastrointestinal tract, which may go unrecognised for many months or even years, as blood is lost imperceptibly in faeces, is a feature of a number of relatively common but serious diseases of the gastrointestinal tract. These include ulcerative colitis; cancer of the oesophagus, stomach and colon; and stomach ulcers. Aspirin and some non-steroidal anti-inflammatory drugs irritate the gastric lining of the stomach sufficiently to cause low grade bleeding in some people. For this reason, long-term aspirin use is associated with a risk of iron deficiency anaemia. Together these gastrointestinal conditions associated with chronic blood loss account for most cases of iron deficiency anaemia among adult males and postmenopausal women.

Some diseases of the gastrointestinal tract cause iron deficiency by reducing absorption of dietary iron. Foremost among these is coeliac disease (gluten sensitivity) which is much more common than was previously supposed. In recent years, coeliac disease has emerged as a relatively common cause of iron deficiency. Chronic inflammatory bowel conditions (Crohn's disease and ulcerative colitis) are also associated with reduced iron absorption and consequent high risk of iron deficiency anaemia. Surgical removal of the stomach (gastrectomy) is associated with reduced absorption of iron. Colonisation of the stomach with the bacterium *Helicobacter pylori* is common and generally benign. In some people, however, it leads to gastritis and gastric ulcers. In others, it can cause iron deficiency anaemia. The mechanism is unclear but reduced absorption of iron is likely.

Increased red cell production is one of the many necessary physiological changes that occur during pregnancy. To accommodate this, around two to three times the normal amount of iron is required. This increased demand for iron can lead to iron deficiency if iron stores are not replete, and iron deficiency anaemia is a common complication of late pregnancy. Increased demand for iron during growth contributes to the iron deficiency that can occur in malnourished babies and children.

In all cases of iron deficiency anaemia, a cause should be sought no matter what the severity because it may be a presenting symptom of serious underlying gastrointestinal or gynaecological disease. Recently published guidelines[2] advise that all patients with unexplained iron deficiency anaemia, no matter what the severity, should be screened for coeliac disease and have urine tested for the presence of blood. In addition, gastrointestinal tract investigation (e.g. barium meal, endoscopic examinations) should be considered for all male patients and all female patients over the age of 50 (postmenopausal).

Symptoms

In addition to the general symptoms of anaemia listed on p 209, patients with iron deficiency anaemia may exhibit some other specific symptoms of iron deficiency, which include:

- glossitis (inflammation of the tongue)
- angular cheilosis (ulceration of lips at the corners of the mouth)
- changes to nails (unusually brittle; may become spoon-shaped (koilonychia)).

Results of blood testing

Serum ferritin concentration reflects iron stores, so a reduction in serum ferritin is evident before anaemia develops, during the period of progressive iron store depletion. By the time that iron stores are totally depleted, when signs and symptoms of iron deficiency anaemia begin to occur, serum ferritin concentration is extremely low or undetectable. Serum iron is usually reduced, but may remain at the low end of the reference range. Serum total iron binding capacity is always raised.

Typical blood results in iron deficiency anaemia are:

- Serum iron usually reduced, in the range 5–10 µmol/l (may be at the low end of the reference range)
- Serum TIBC raised (i.e. greater than 75 µmol/l)
- Serum ferritin greatly reduced (usually undetectable, i.e. < 5 µg/l).

Chronic inflammation and infection

As outlined in Chapter 15, many patients with chronic infectious or inflammatory disease, as well as those with malignant disease, may become mildly to moderately anaemic (it is unusual for Hb to fall lower than 9 g/dl in such cases).

This is called anaemia of chronic disease (ACD). Although the anaemia of chronic disease is not the result of iron deficiency (iron stores are not depleted), it is associated with disturbances of iron metabolism that are reflected in blood test results. Serum iron concentration is usually reduced, as it is in iron deficiency anaemia. However, in contrast to iron deficiency anaemia, serum TIBC is reduced and serum ferritin is either normal, or in some cases increased. Since a deficiency of iron is not the problem, iron supplements are of no use to these patients. Indeed, such treatment may be harmful by putting them at risk of iron overload. Instead, treatment is directed at the underlying condition; as this resolves, anaemia disappears.

To summarise, patients with chronic infections (e.g. tuberculosis, bacterial endocarditis, pneumonia, etc.) and chronic inflammation (e.g. rheumatoid arthritis, systemic lupus erythomatosus, Crohn's disease, etc.) as well as some cancer patients may be anaemic. The severity of anaemia reflects the severity of the underlying disorder.

Anaemia of chronic disease (ACD) is associated with:

- reduced serum iron concentration
- reduced serum TIBC
- normal or raised serum ferritin concentration.

Iron overload

In the physiological state, all iron is bound to a protein (haemoglobin in red cells, ferritin in storage compartments and transferrin in blood plasma). In this state, it is non-toxic. However, free (unbound) iron is toxic. There is a finite amount of each of the 'protective' binding and storage proteins, and once they are saturated with iron, any additional iron in cells exists in its toxic free (unbound to protein) state. Free iron is toxic because it promotes production of highly reactive free radicals that disrupt normal cell structure and function. Unchecked, this can lead to tissue damage. Tissues affected in disease caused by chronic iron overload include:

- pancreas   fibrosis of pancreas leading to diabetes
- liver   cirrhosis and eventual liver failure, liver cancer
- heart   arrhythmias, heart failure
- gonads   impotence
- joints   severe joint pain (similar to arthritis)

Causes

Hereditary haemachromatosis. Those with this genetically determined disease absorb increased amounts of available iron in diet, 3 to 4 mg per day instead of the normal 1–2 mg. There is no physiological means of increasing iron excretion, so iron accumulates at the rate of 0.5–1.0 g per year. In late middle age when first clinical effects of iron overload occur, total body iron may be in the range 20–40 g rather than normal 4–5 g. Around 1 in 10 of us carry a single copy of the defective gene (it is the most common inherited genetic defect). Only inheritance of the defective gene from both parents (i.e. two copies of the defective gene) results in the most severe form of haemachromatosis which leads to diabetes, cirrhosis, etc.

Other causes of iron overload include repeated blood transfusion and inappropriate iron therapy. One unit of blood contains around 250 mg of iron in red cells, 100 times the daily requirement. Patients whose treatment includes repeated blood transfusion over a prolonged period (e.g. those suffering thalassaemia and sickle cell anaemia) are particularly at risk of iron overload.

Blood test results

The blood test results of those with iron overload are, as might be expected, the opposite of those associated with iron deficiency. No matter what the cause, iron overload is associated with:

- raised serum iron
- reduced serum TIBC
- raised serum ferritin.

Conditions associated with reduced B$_{12}$ and folate results

Megaloblastic anaemia

Megaloblastic anaemia is a term applied to all those anaemias in which, due to impaired DNA synthesis, there is abnormal development of blood cells in the bone marrow. Impaired DNA synthesis results in production of large (mega) immature (blast) red cells, many of which do not develop to maturity and die within the bone marrow. There is thus a marked reduction in the number of circulating red cells, hence the anaemia. Those red cells that do survive and appear in peripheral blood are larger than normal, often characteristically oval in shape. Large red cells in peripheral blood are called macrocytes, so the term macrocytic anaemia is sometimes used as an alternative name for megaloblastic anaemia, although the terms are not, strictly speaking, synonymous. The effect of impaired DNA synthesis is not confined to red cells; numbers of both white cell and platelets may be reduced in those with severe megaloblastic anaemia. With a few very rare exceptions, the cause of the impaired DNA synthesis that leads to megaloblastic anaemia, is either vitamin B_{12} and/or folate deficiency.

Causes of vitamin B_{12} or folate deficiency

The causes can be summarised under the following headings:

- dietary deficiency
- failure to absorb B_{12} due to inadequate production intrinsic factor
- failure to absorb either B_{12} or folate due to gastrointestinal disease
- increased demand for B_{12} and folate during pregnancy.

Dietary deficiency of B_{12} is rare except among strict vegetarians (vegans) who eat no dairy products. Dietary deficiency of folate is more common; in fact, it is the most common cause of folate deficiency. Unlike vitamin B_{12}, folate in food can be destroyed by cooking, and the normal dietary intake is close to the minimum required. Dietary deficiency of folate is quite common among chronic alcoholics; this combined with the effects of alcohol on folate metabolism, render this group particularly susceptible to folate deficiency. The infirm elderly, whose diet is often not well balanced and may be deficient of folate, are considered another group at risk of folate deficiency.

The most common cause of vitamin B_{12} deficiency is failure to absorb the vitamin due to lack of intrinsic factor. This specific type of megaloblastic anaemia is known as pernicious anaemia. Those with pernicious anaemia are unable to produce intrinsic factor because of damage (autoimmune in nature) to the cells of the stomach, where intrinsic factor is produced. The condition tends to run in families and is often associated with other autoimmune disease (e.g. thyroid disease and Addison's disease). Absorption of folate is not affected in pernicious anaemia. Patients with pernicious anaemia must be given B_{12} by injection, as that given by the oral route cannot be absorbed.

Partial and total gastrectomy can of course also result in reduced production of intrinsic factor.

A number of gastrointestinal diseases associated with inflammatory or other damage to areas where B_{12} and folate are normally absorbed can result in reduced absorption and vitamin deficiency. Surgical removal of areas of the gastrointestinal tract (e.g. jejunal or ileal resection) can lead to either B_{12} or folate deficiency.

Patients receiving such surgery may be given regular injections of B_{12} and folate to prevent anaemia developing.

Symptoms of megaloblastic anaemia

Whether it is caused by dietary deficiency or poor absorption of B_{12} or folate, the resulting symptoms of megaloblastic anaemia may include:

- general symptoms of all anaemias (page 209)
- mild jaundice
- glossitis (inflamed tongue)
- angular cheilosis (sores at the corner of the mouth).

Patients with B_{12} deficiency but less commonly, those with folate deficiency may also suffer neurological symptoms including:

- paraesthesia (abnormal sensation, e.g. numbness, tingling in fingers and toes)
- gait ataxia, resulting in difficulty in walking
- increased irritability
- memory loss
- rarely, personality change and other overt psychiatric problems.

The neurological symptoms of B_{12} deficiency may be present without any signs or symptoms of anaemia.

Blood test results

Serum B_{12} is usually reduced in pernicious anaemia and all other cases of megaloblastic anaemia and neuropathy caused by deficiency of B_{12}. In some cases, the serum level remains at the low end of the reference range, causing some diagnostic difficulty. Serum folate is usually normal but may be slightly raised. Red cell folate, by contrast, is either normal or low in cases of B_{12} deficiency.

In cases of megaloblastic anaemia caused solely by folate deficiency, serum B_{12} is normal, but as might be expected both serum and red cell folate are reduced. Red cell folate is considered a more reliable test of folate status because serum folate may be low in some illnesses (e.g. severe liver and kidney disease) despite normal folate status.

Case history 17

Jane Baker is a 32-year-old solicitor who is being investigated by her GP because of increasing tiredness of several months' duration (see Case history 14). The results of an FBC demonstrate that she is anaemic and that the anaemia may be due to iron deficiency. Jane's GP prescribes a course of iron tablets and takes a further sample of blood for iron studies. Four days later, the following laboratory report is received at the GP surgery:

Serum iron	9 μmol/l
Serum TIBC	113 μmol/l
Serum ferritin	< 5 μg/l

Questions

(1) Are results normal?
(2) What is ferritin and why is its concentration in blood serum measured in patients who are suspected of being iron deficient?
(3) What do the results indicate?
(4) Why might further investigation be necessary?

Discussion of case history

(1) No. Serum iron and ferritin are abnormally reduced and serum TIBC is raised.

(2) Ferritin is a water-soluble molecule composed of an outer protein shell enclosing an iron core. Each molecule contains 4000–5000 atoms of iron and this iron constitutes around 20% of its weight. Most of the body's ferritin is in tissue cells (liver, spleen, bone marrow) where its function is iron storage. A small fraction circulates in blood plasma where its concentration reflects total iron body stores. Reduction in serum ferritin concentration as iron stores become progressively depleted, is the first objective evidence of iron deficiency.

Reduction in serum ferritin concentration occurs before iron is sufficiently depleted to affect haemoglobin production and therefore occurs before symptoms of iron deficiency anaemia occur. Serum ferritin remains low or undetectable until iron stores are replete.

(3) Reduced serum iron and increased serum TIBC in association with undetectable levels of ferritin in blood serum is the typical pattern of results expected in iron deficiency. There can be no doubt that Mrs Baker is iron deficient and requires the iron supplements prescribed.

(4) A diagnosis of iron deficiency should be followed by investigation of its cause. Why has Mrs Baker become iron deficient? In a woman of reproductive age like Mrs Baker, the most common cause is menorrhagia (increased loss of iron in menstrual blood) but this is by no means the only cause of iron deficiency. Current guidelines[2] suggest that a woman of Mrs Baker's age should be offered, in the first instance, a blood test to screen for coeliac disease. Her urine should also be tested for the presence of blood to screen for malignancy of the renal tract.

References

1. World Health Organization (2004) Focusing on anaemia. *www.who.int/topics/anaemia/en/who_unicef-anaemiastatement.pdf*
2. Goddard A, James M, Mcintyre A *et al.* (2005) Guidelines for the management of iron deficiency anaemia. *www.bsg.org.uk/pdf_word_docs/iron_def.pdf*

Further reading

Gasche C, Lomer M *et al.* (2004) Iron, anaemia and inflammatory bowel disease. *Gut* **53**: 1190–97.

Chanarin I (2000) A history of pernicious anaemia. Historical review. *Br J Haematol* **111**: 407–15.

Weiss G & Goodnough L (2005) Anemia of chronic disease. *N Eng J Med* **352**: 1011–23.

Burke W, Thomson E *et al.* (1998) Hereditary haemochromatosis. *JAMA* **280**: 172–78.

Yates J, Logan E & Stewart R (2004) Iron deficiency anaemia in general practice: clinical outcomes over three years and factors influencing diagnostic investigations. *Postgrad Med J* **80**: 405–410.

Chapter 19

ERYTHROCYTE SEDIMENTATION RATE AND C-REACTIVE PROTEIN

The principal function of the two tests that are the focus of this chapter is detection and monitoring of inflammatory and infectious disease. They both serve essentially the same purpose. Erythrocyte sedimentation rate (ESR), the older and more established of the two, is performed in the haematology laboratory using a whole blood sample. C-reactive protein (CRP) is an alternative test to the ESR, usually performed in the immunology or clinical chemistry laboratory using a plasma or serum sample. The newer test has some advantages over the ESR. The diagnostic information that the two tests provide can sometimes be complementary; under these circumstances, it is useful to have the results of both tests. We begin with consideration of the ESR.

Erythrocyte sedimentation rate (ESR)

The ESR test is one of the oldest and simplest tests still performed in clinical laboratories, and is based on a very visible phenomenon, familiar to all those who have collected blood. If a blood sample collected into a tube containing an anticoagulant is left undisturbed, the red cells (erythrocytes) gradually fall or sediment to the bottom of the container, leaving the clear, straw-coloured, plasma fluid above. At the end of the last century, physicians investigated this phenomenon and discovered that the red cells in a blood sample taken from healthy volunteers sediment slowly, but that the cells in a blood sample taken from those suffering a range of disease, sediment much faster. From these observations the erythrocyte sedimentation rate (ESR) test was born.

Despite minor modifications, measurement of ESR has remained essentially unchanged since its introduction nearly 90 years ago. A narrow bore tube of standard length is filled with anticoagulated blood and placed in a vertical position. The tube is left undisturbed for a defined time (usually one hour). During that time, the erythrocytes sediment, leaving an increasingly large column of clear plasma above. After one hour has elapsed, the distance from the top of the tube to the interface between clear plasma and red cells is measured. This distance is the ESR expressed in millimetres per hour (mm/hr).

Normal physiology: what affects red cell sedimentation?

Although apparently simple, the rate at which erythrocytes sediment is a complex phenomenon, which even now is not entirely understood. Clearly red cells fall because they have a greater density than the plasma in which they are suspended. Red cells have a net negative charge due to the presence of membrane bound proteins on their surface. This electrostatic force tends to make red cells repel each other. This is the situation in health; red cells are for the most part separate and fall individually. If for any reason this tendency of cells to repel each other is overcome, they aggregate together to form 'rouleaux' (red cells stacked together rather like a pile of coins). Since an aggregation of red cells has greater density than single cells, aggregated cells sediment faster. It is this abnormal tendency for cells to overcome their natural repulsion for each other, and aggregate, which explains the increased ESR found in disease. The crucial question is: what makes red cells aggregate? The answer lies in the plasma in which red cells are suspended. Certain proteins in plasma, most notably fibrinogen and immunoglobulins, act as molecular bridges between red cells. When present in high concentration, the effect of these proteins is a marked increase in the aggregation of red cells. As will become clear, disease states associated with abnormally high concentration of these proteins in plasma most commonly result in a raised ESR.

In addition to the composition of the plasma in which they are suspended, the rate at which red cells sediment is also affected by both numbers and shape of red cells themselves. For example, a significant decrease in the number of red cells as occurs in anaemia is associated with an increase in ESR, while an abnormal increase in red cell numbers (polycythaemia) reduces ESR. The shape of red cells of those suffering sickle cell anaemia is abnormal; these so-called sickle cells sediment slower than normal red cells.

Laboratory measurement

Patient preparation

No particular patient preparation is necessary.

Sample timing

Depending on the method being used, a delay of more than a few hours in processing samples can affect results. Samples stored overnight may be unsuitable for analysis. It is therefore best practice to take samples at a time that coincides with routine transport to the laboratory.

Sample requirements

A sample of venous blood is required. Most laboratories provide a specific tube for ESR only (black top) which contains the anticoagulant sodium citrate. The required volume is printed on the label. It is essential that anticoagulant in the bottle is mixed with the blood by gentle inversion.

Interpretation of results

Approximate reference range

Males	1–10 mm/hr
Females	5–20 mm/hr

Causes of a raised ESR

General considerations
ESR increases gradually with age, rising at the rate of around 0.8 mm/hr every five years. From the fourth month of pregnancy, ESR usually rises to a peak of 40 to 50 mm/hr, returning to normal after parturition.

ESR is one of the least specific of all laboratory tests. Like a raised temperature or heart rate, a raised ESR occurs in many different sorts of illness. The changes in plasma proteins which give rise to increased red cell aggregation and raised ESR are a feature of any illness associated with significant tissue injury, inflammation, infection or malignancy. Unfortunately from a diagnostic point of view, in most of these disease states it is possible for the ESR to be normal. Furthermore it is clear that ESR is occasionally raised in normal healthy individuals. Despite these awkward anomalies that tend to confound interpretation of an ESR result, the ESR continues to be used in clinical practice. In general, the higher the ESR the greater is the likelihood of a significant inflammatory, infectious or malignant disease.

Inflammatory disease
The inflammatory response to tissue injury results in abnormal increase in the synthesis of plasma proteins including fibrinogen, which tend to promote rouleaux formation and raise ESR. Potentially, any disease with an acute or chronic inflammatory component may be associated with an increase in ESR. In clinical practice, the test is used as supportive evidence of inflammation in the diagnosis of disease associated with chronic inflammation such as rheumatoid arthritis, Crohn's disease and ulcerative colitis. It is frequently used to monitor disease activity in these conditions. A rising ESR in a patient with a known chronic inflammatory condition, such as rheumatoid arthritis, implies that disease activity is continuing or increasing and therefore not responding to current therapy. Conversely, a falling ESR indicates reduced inflammation and therefore response to therapy.

Although the ESR has a limited diagnostic role for most diseases with an inflammatory component, because there are other more reliable and specific tests available, there are two related conditions in which ESR is the only investigation that is abnormal. These are temporal arteritis (sometimes called giant cell arteritis) and polymyalgia rheumatica. The first is an inflammatory disease of arteries, usually in the head and neck. The condition is relatively common in the elderly causing general feeling of malaise and tiredness along with severe headaches; sudden blindness may occur if the optic artery is affected. The second is an inflammatory condition affecting muscles causing severe muscle pain and stiffness particularly after resting. The two conditions often appear together in the same patient and both are associated with very high ESR, usually greater than 75 mm/hr, often higher. The ESR gradually returns to normal during treatment with steroids and the test is used to monitor response to therapy. These are the only conditions in which diagnosis depends on the ESR test.

Infectious disease

Infection may be associated with an increased ESR. In general, bacterial infections tend to result in an increased ESR more frequently than those caused by viruses. Particularly high ESR (i.e. greater than 75 mm/hr) is most frequently found in those suffering chronic infections, e.g. tuberculosis and subacute bacterial endocarditis (infection of valves of the heart), but any bacterial infection, if sufficiently severe, may be associated with very high ESR.

Malignant disease

Many patients suffering cancer of all types have a raised ESR. However, since a significant proportion of cancer patients do not have a raised ESR, the test has no place in cancer diagnosis. In the absence of infectious or inflammatory disease a significant increase in ESR (i.e. greater than 75 mm/hr) might suggest that further investigation to detect cancer is warranted. Some authorities believe that a particularly raised ESR (i.e. greater than 100 mm/hr) in a patient with cancer is reliable evidence of tumour spread beyond the primary site (metastasis).

The only widely accepted use of the ESR as far as malignant disease is concerned is in the diagnosis of multiple myeloma, a malignant disease of bone marrow in which uncontrolled proliferation of plasma cells within the bone marrow causes bone pain and bone destruction. These malignant plasma cells synthesise huge quantities of abnormal immunoglobulin at the expense of normal immunoglobulin (antibody) production. Since immunoglobulin is one of those proteins which increase rouleaux formation and thereby the ESR, multiple myeloma is usually associated with an increase in ESR (often greater than 100 mm/hr). So consistent is this finding that a raised ESR is among the criterion required for diagnosis of multiple myeloma.

Finally, ESR is usually raised in patients with Hodgkin's disease (malignant tumour of lymph nodes). The ESR is not used to make a diagnosis, but is frequently used to monitor disease progress and therapeutic effectiveness.

Other common causes of raised ESR

Myocardial infarction (heart attack) involves tissue injury to heart muscle (myocardium). The consequent inflammatory response to this injury includes increased synthesis of plasma proteins (fibrinogen) which causes increased red cell aggregation, and therefore raised ESR. Thus myocardial infarction is a common cause of raised ESR. Typically ESR rises after an infarct, peaking one week later. A gradual return to normal is usual over the next few weeks. A raised ESR is also common in patients suffering renal disease.

Causes of reduced ESR

A reduced ESR is far less common than an increased ESR and actually of little clinical significance. An abnormally high red cell count (polycythaemia) is the most frequent cause. Rare causes include sickle cell anaemia and hereditary spherocytosis; both conditions are associated with abnormally-shaped red cells which slow the rate at which they sediment.

Normal physiology: C-reactive protein (CRP) synthesis and function

C-reactive protein (CRP) is so called because the first of its properties to be identified at the time of its discovery in 1930 was its ability to react with (precipitate) C-polysaccharide, a constituent of the wall of streptococcal bacteria. CRP is synthesised in the liver and is one of a number of proteins present in blood plasma that are collectively called the acute phase proteins. Fibrinogen, a protein already discussed for its significance in the ESR test, is another of these acute phase proteins. In health, acute phase proteins are present in blood plasma at low concentration. However, following any tissue injury, infection or acute inflammation, blood concentration rises. This acute phase reaction, as it is called, is one part of the body's overall complex protective response to tissue injury or microbial attack. The ESR test owes its clinical utility to the acute phase reaction because the increase in plasma concentration of the acute phase protein fibrinogen accounts for the increased rate of red cell sedimentation associated with disease.

CRP is considered the archetypal acute phase protein. Under the influence of a chemical messenger called interleukin 6 (IL-6) released from macrophages at the site of infection or tissue injury, liver cells are stimulated to increase synthesis of CRP. Within 5–6 hours of the initial insult, plasma CRP concentration begins to rise rapidly to a maximal peak concentration at around 48 hours. In the case of bacterial infection concentration can increase up to 10 000 fold.[1] As the stimulus for increased production ceases, plasma CRP concentration falls rapidly to normal concentration; CRP has a half-life in plasma of 19 hours, meaning plasma concentration is halved every 19 hours, once the stimulus for increased production is removed.

The physiological function of CRP is as a contributor to the body's overall innate defences against microbial attack. In this regard, it is potent activator of the complement cascade, which leads to phagocytosis and bacterial destruction.

Laboratory measurement

Patient preparation

No particular patient preparation is necessary.

Sample timing

Blood for CRP may be taken at any time of the day, ideally at a time that allows immediate transport to the laboratory. However, CRP is stable and samples can be stored at room temperature or in a sample fridge for up to 48 hours before being processed in the laboratory.

Sample requirements

Around 5 ml of blood is required for CRP measurement. Analysis can be performed on either serum or plasma. If local policy is to use serum, the blood must be collected into a plain tube (without additives). If local policy is to use plasma, blood must be collected into a tube containing the anticoagulant lithium heparin.

Interpretation of results

Approximate reference range

Adults and children	< 10 mg/l
Pregnancy	< 20 mg/l
Neonates	< 4 mg/l (a high sensitivity assay (hs-CRP) is required to reliably distinguish normal and abnormal plasma CRP concentration in neonates)

Causes of increased CRP

General considerations

Increase in both CRP and ESR are due to an acute phase reaction (APR) to tissue injury, infection, inflammation or malignancy. ESR is an indirect measure of APR (because it measures an effect of APR, namely the increased rate of red cell sedimentation) whereas CRP is a more direct measure. Still, in general terms, the conditions that give rise to a raised ESR also give rise to an increase in CRP; like ESR, CRP is a non-specific indicator of tissue injury, infection, inflammation and malignancy.

CRP has some advantages over ESR.

Rapidity of response. CRP rises within hours of an insult (e.g. infection); ESR is slower to respond over a period of days and weeks rather than hours.

Sensitivity. CRP is generally a more sensitive test of inflammation – minimal inflammation might not be detected if only ESR was measured.

Specificity. CRP is not affected – as ESR is – by abnormality in red cell numbers and shape. For example, CRP remains normal in patients whose sole problem is anaemia. ESR is raised in this condition, giving false evidence of inflammation or infection, etc.

Infection

CRP is raised following infection. Bacterial infection is associated with highest concentration (in the range 80–1000 mg/l). The rise is more modest during viral infection (10–20 mg/l). This difference has been utilised clinically, for example in identifying the cause of meningitis (bacterial versus viral). Measurement of CRP has proven useful for early identification of bacterial infection in a variety of clinical contexts. For example, detection of postoperative infection and infection among patients being cared for in intensive care (a group at particularly high risk of hospital-acquired infection).

Inflammation

CRP is a very sensitive indicator of severity of inflammation. Highest concentration (> 200 mg/l) indicates acute inflammation, for example, during the active phase of chronic conditions such as rheumatoid arthritis and Crohn's disease. With few exceptions all conditions with an inflammatory component are associated with increase in CRP concentration; the magnitude of the increase reflecting severity. The test is very helpful in providing objective evidence of the therapeutic effect (or the lack of it) of treatment for inflammatory disease.

Tissue injury

Tissue injury, whatever its cause, is associated with increased CRP concentration. Severity correlates with concentration so that particularly high concentrations (> 500 mg/l) might be evident following severe trauma or major surgery. The necrosis of heart muscle associated with myocardial infarction causes increase.

Clinically useful anomalies

As we have seen, the normal response to active inflammatory disease is an increase in plasma CRP concentration. For reasons that remain unclear, that response is either significantly lower in magnitude or entirely absent in a few inflammatory conditions. This has proven diagnostically useful because there are very few inflammatory conditions in which ESR is significantly raised (reflecting an inflammatory process) but plasma CRP is only slightly raised or even normal. Systemic lupus erythematosus (SLE or lupus), a relatively common chronic autoimmune disease that predominantly affects women of childbearing age, is one of these conditions. Joint inflammation similar to that seen in rheumatoid arthritis is a common feature of lupus. When this inflammation occurs in the lupus patient it is accompanied as expected by a marked increase in ESR. However, in contrast to most other inflammatory conditions the plasma CRP remains resolutely normal. The combination of raised ESR and normal CRP is a useful diagnostic feature of SLE.

A similar combination of results (raised ESR and normal or only slightly raised CRP) is typical of the inflammatory bowel disease ulcerative colitis. This feature distinguishes it from the only other inflammatory bowel disorder, Crohn's disease, in which the increase in ESR and CRP are equal. The difference can be diagnostically helpful.

CRP and cardiovascular disease

The development of highly sensitive assays for CRP measurement that are capable of detecting concentration well below 10 mg/l has revealed that the mean concentration of plasma CRP in apparently healthy individuals is around 0.8 mg/l with a range of 0.01 mg/l to 10 mg/l. Many studies conducted over the past decade have demonstrated that CRP within this range predicts future risk of cardiovascular disease. The higher the plasma CRP concentration, the greater the risk of cardiovascular disease.[2] The only blood test currently used to assess risk of cardiovascular disease is blood cholesterol measurement. In the future, measurement of plasma CRP might also be used in this way.

Case history 18

Alex Manson was a cheerful, healthy five-year-old until he first became acutely ill just over six months ago. His first complaint was a sore throat. Over the next two weeks he had a spiking fever almost every day and a recurring rash on his trunk. His knee joints became painful making him uncharacteristically tearful. He was often tired and spent long periods just lying on the couch. After a course of antibiotics prescribed by his GP failed to have any effect and during a particularly severe fever, Alex was admitted for investigation to his local hospital nearly three weeks after the first sign of illness. Among the blood tests performed was an ESR, which was reported as 89 mm/hr. A diagnosis of Still's disease (a form of juvenile chronic arthritis) was eventually made and the intensity of symptoms resolved with administration of the anti-inflammatory drug, naprosyn. After three weeks in hospital, Alex was discharged home with prescriptions for naprosyn and methotrexate. At his most recent rheumatology outpatients clinic, blood was collected from Alex for ESR. The result on this occasion was 18 mm/hr.

Questions

(1) Was Alex's ESR normal at the time of admission to hospital?
(2) Was this ESR result consistent with a diagnosis of Still's disease?
(3) What is the significance of the ESR result at Alex's recent outpatient appointment?
(4) What is meant when ESR is described as a non-specific test?

Discussion of case history

(1) No. Alex's ESR was grossly elevated.

(2) Yes. Like many other forms of arthritis, Still's disease is a chronic condition characterised by inflammation of the joints. A raised ESR is usually a feature of active inflammatory disease.

(3) The most recent ESR shows a marked reduction, reflecting a reduction in disease activity. The result provides objective evidence that the prescribed drug

regime (naprosyn and methotrexate) is, for the moment at least, keeping this chronic disease under control.

(4) A non-specific test like ESR is one that is abnormal in a wide range of pathological conditions. By contrast, a specific test is one that is abnormal in one or a few related conditions. There are few tests that are absolutely specific for a single disease, but nearly all are more specific than ESR. In the context of this case history, the non-specificity of the ESR means that although ESR is usually raised in patients with Still's disease, it is not useful to make the diagnosis, there are many other conditions in which a raised ESR is equally likely.

References

1. Pepys M & Hirshfield G (2003) C-Reactive Protein: a critical update. *J Clin Invest* **111**: 1805–12.
2. Ridker P, Rifai N *et al.* (2002) Comparison of C-Reactive protein and low density lipoprotein cholesterol levels in the prediction of first cardiovascular events. *New Eng J Med* **347**: 1557–65.

Further reading

Bedell S & Bush B (1985) Erythrocyte sedimentation rate. *Am. J Med.* **78**: 1001–1007.

Dinant G, Knottnerus J & Van Wersch J (1991) Discriminating ability of the erythrocyte sedimentation rate: a prospective study in general practice. *Br J Gen Pract* **41**: 365–70.

Fincher R & Page M (1986) Clinical significance of extreme elevation of the erythrocyte sedimentation rate. *Arch Intern Med* **146**: 1581–83.

Kanfer E & Nicol B (1997) Haemoglobin concentration and erythrocyte sedimentation rate in primary care patients. *J Roy Soc Med* **90**: 16–18.

PART 4

Blood transfusion testing

Chapter 20

BLOOD GROUP, ANTIBODY SCREEN AND CROSSMATCH

Blood transfusion is such a commonplace procedure that it is perhaps easy to underestimate the dangers involved. Although often of life-saving benefit, transfusion of donated blood is associated with considerable potential risk to the recipient patient. The two most significant risks are: transmission of serious blood-borne infection and the potentially fatal haemolytic transfusion reaction that can occur if patients receive incompatible blood. The risk of infection is virtually eliminated[1,2] by careful donor selection and rigorous screening of all blood donations for evidence of infection (Table 20.1). This screening procedure, which ensures supply of the safest possible blood to local hospital blood transfusion laboratories, is the responsibility of the four national blood transfusion services in the UK. Prevention of the second major risk associated with blood transfusion, i.e. incompatible

Table 20.1 Some of the selection criteria for blood donors and mandatory blood tests to prevent transmission of infectious diseases.

Blood donors must:

- be aged between 18 and 56 years
- be in good health
- have a haemoglobin (Hb) greater then 13.1 g/dl (men) or 12.5 g/dl (women)

Blood donors must not:

- be pregnant or have been pregnant during previous 12 months
- ever have suffered from cancer, syphillis or brucellosis
- have a recent history of malaria, hepatitis, jaundice, or glandular fever
- be in a high-risk group for HIV infection
- donate blood more than twice in one year

All donated blood units tested for the presence of:

- hepatitis B surface antigen ⎫
- antibody to hepatitis C antibody ⎬ To prevent transmission of viral hepatitis
- antibody to Trepanoma pallidium To prevent transmission of syphillis
- antibody to HIV-1 ⎫
- antibody to HIV-2 ⎬ To prevent transmission of HIV

transfusion reaction, begins with the pre-transfusion tests of donor and recipient blood conducted in local hospital blood transfusion laboratories. Of crucial importance are the three tests that are the subject of this chapter: determination of blood group, antibody screen and crossmatch. In order to understand what is meant by an incompatible blood transfusion and the significance of these tests for its prevention, a little background immunology is required.

Background immunology

What are antigens and antibodies?

Our ability to withstand attack from invading micro-organisms such as bacteria and viruses, depends in part on antibodies produced by plasma cells, derived from white blood cells called B-lymphocytes. Antibodies are immunoglobulin proteins. They bind to, and neutralise, bacteria and viruses. Each antibody is very specific in its action, so an antibody that binds and neutralises one sort of bacterium will have no effect on another. This specificity is due to the specific nature of the molecular target on the surface of each sort of bacterium. This molecular target is called the antigen. Recognition by B-lymphocytes of specific bacterial or viral antigens induces specific antibody production.

This ability of the body to produce destructive antibodies to 'foreign' antigens is not confined to those antigens present on the surface of bacteria or viruses. Proteins and other molecular substances present on the surface of any foreign (i.e. non-self) cell are 'seen' as antigens and provoke a similarly destructive specific antibody response. It is, for example, this same antibody response to foreign antigens that accounts in part for the tissue rejection that occurs following organ transplantation.

To summarise:

An **antigen** is any substance (most commonly a protein, but may be a carbohydrate), which causes production of antibodies by plasma cells (B-lymphocytes). Antigens are found usually, although not exclusively, on the surface of cells.

An **antibody** is a protein (immunoglobulin) that circulates in blood plasma and binds only with the antigen that provoked its production.

When an antibody binds with an antigen present on the surface of a cell, be it a bacteria, virus or tissue cell, a sequence of events follows which invariably leads to that cell's disruption or destruction.

One of the characteristics of the immune system is its ability to remember. On the first occasion lymphocytes 'meet' a foreign antigen; antibody production is low and therefore not very effective. However, the immune system is now primed. Specialised lymphocytes (called memory lymphocytes) 'remember' the antigen, so that when it is encountered on subsequent occasions, both speed and intensity of antibody production are greatly increased. This is the basis of the concept of acquired immunity: we have little protection (immunity) against a particular bacteria or virus until our immune system has been primed by initial exposure.

Clearly, it is vital for health that we do not produce antibodies to our own antigens, and the immune system has a means of preventing this occurring. However, it is worth mentioning in passing that there are a large group of pathological conditions, collectively known as the autoimmune diseases, in which this ability to distinguish 'self' from 'non-self' antigens is lost. These diseases are characterised by the production of antibodies directed at self-antigens. Common diseases with an autoimmune component include rheumatoid arthritis, type 1 diabetes, most thyroid disease and systemic lupus erythematosus (SLE); there are many others.

Notwithstanding these pathological exceptions, it is important to remember that it is normally not possible to produce antibodies to one's own antigens.

Red cell antigens and blood group

The surfaces of red cells, like all other cells, are covered with inherited antigens. These red cell antigens (or the lack of them) determine an individual's blood group. More than 700 different red cell antigens (most very rare) have been identified, which make up the 28 blood group systems so far described. Fortunately, only a tiny minority of these antigens are of significance in transfusion medicine. Of those that do have significance, the antigens of the ABO and Rh blood group system are of prime importance.

ABO blood group system

We all belong to one of four groups of the ABO blood group system determined by the inheritance or non-inheritance of two red cell antigens A and B. Those who inherit neither A nor B red cell antigens belong to group O; those who inherit the A red cell antigen belong to group A, those who inherit the B red cell antigen belong to group B and those inherit both the A and the B red cell antigen belong to group AB. Most (88%) of the UK population belong to either group O or group A.

Rh blood group system

The Rh blood group system, so called because early research was conducted on rhesus (Rh) monkeys is the only other blood group system of major significance to blood transfusion. There are five red cell antigens in the Rh system: C, c, D, E and e but only the D antigen is of major significance. Around 85% of the UK population have the D antigen on their red cells and are said to be RhD positive, the remaining 15% do not have the D antigen and are RhD negative.

Other less significant red cell antigens

A routine blood group means determination of the ABO group and RhD typing (either positive or negative). Of the remaining 700-plus red cell antigens that may or may not be present on the surface of an individual's red cells, a few have occasional significance for transfusion medicine. Among these are the remaining antigens of the Rh blood group system (i.e. the c, C, e and E antigens) and the antigens of the Kell (K), Duffy (Fy), Kidd (Jk), MNS and Lewis (Le) blood group systems.

These antigens are rare causes of transfusion reaction either because they are themselves rare, or because they are relatively weakly immunogenic.

Antibodies to red cell antigens: incompatible blood transfusion

The significance of red cell antigens for blood transfusion medicine lies in the specific antibodies to these red cell antigens, which may or may not be present in the recipient's plasma. An incompatible transfusion reaction occurs when antibodies present in the patient's (recipient) plasma bind to its complementary antigen present on the red cells of transfused blood. Such antibody-antigen binding can result in the destruction of the donated red cells; this destruction is called haemolysis, so the term immune haemolytic transfusion reaction is used to describe this complication of blood transfusion. As long as the patient's plasma contains no significant antibodies to the antigens present on the red cells of donated blood, the patient and donor blood are said to be compatible and donor blood can be safely transfused.

Production of red cell antibodies

It was stated above that antibodies are only produced when B-lymphocytes come into contact with the relevant 'foreign' antigen. There are two situations in which an individual's antibody producing lymphocytes may come into contact with 'foreign' red cell antigens. The first is blood transfusion, and the second is pregnancy. During pregnancy, fetal blood leaks to maternal circulation. If fetal blood red cells bear antigens inherited from the father, which are not present on the mother's red cells, they are 'seen' as foreign by the mother's lymphocytes, which then proceed to manufacture antibody.

As with any other immune response, initial antibody production during the first immunising blood transfusion or pregnancy is low and usually has no effect. But the immune system is now primed to synthesise large quantities of antibody the next time the 'foreign' red cell antigen is encountered. Antibodies produced in this way are called immune red cell antibodies. The clinically most significant immune red cell antibody is anti-D, the antibody to the RhD antigen. Of course, only those who lack the RhD antigen (i.e. the 15% of the population who are RhD negative), can be immunised to produce anti-D in this way. In fact, around 1% of the population have anti-D in their plasma, all the result of previous immunising transfusion or pregnancy. If such people were transfused with RhD positive blood, the anti-D in their plasma would bind to the D antigen on the surface of donated red cells, resulting in a haemolytic transfusion reaction.

If immune red cell antibodies were the only red cell antibodies present in plasma, only those who have a history of previous blood transfusion or pregnancy would be at risk of incompatible blood transfusion; this is not the case.

The overriding clinical significance of the ABO blood group system lies in the fact that antibodies to these antigens are naturally occurring, i.e. they do not arise as a result of previous immunisation by foreign red cells. All of us have antibodies to the A or B antigen that we lack. Thus all those who:

Table 20.2 The ABO blood group system and RhD type.

ABO Blood group	Antigen present on red cells	Naturally occurring antibody in plasma	Relative frequency in UK population
O	Neither A nor B	anti-A and anti-B	47%
A	A	anti-B	42%
B	B	anti-A	8%
AB	A and B	None	3%

RhD antigen present on the red cells of 85% of UK population; these are RhD positive. RhD antigen not present on the red cells of 15%; these are RhD negative.
For a routine blood group- only ABO group and RhD status (i.e. negative or positive) is determined.

- belong to group O and lack both the A and B antigen have antibodies to both antigens (i.e. anti-A and anti-B) in their plasma
- belong to group A and have the A antigen on their red cells have antibodies to the B antigen (i.e. anti-B) in their plasma
- belong to group B have the antibody to the A antigen (i.e. anti-A) in their plasma.

Only the 3% of the UK population belonging to group AB, who have both the A and B antigen on their red cells, have no naturally occurring anti-A or anti-B in their plasma. The antigens and antibodies associated with the four groups of the ABO blood group system are summarised in Table 20.2.

It is the relative ubiquity and potency of naturally occurring anti-A and anti-B that determines the prime clinical importance of the ABO blood group system. Like anti-D, practically all other clinically significant red cell antibodies are immune antibodies so they cannot be present in the plasma of a person who has not been immunised by a previous transfusion or pregnancy. Thus the only significant red cell antibodies present in a patient who has never received a blood transfusion or been pregnant is naturally occurring anti-A or anti-B. It has been estimated that if only ABO compatibility were ensured, and no other tests were performed, blood transfusion would still be immunologically safe in 97% of cases.

Immune haemolytic transfusion reaction: ABO incompatibility

The consequences of transfusing ABO incompatible blood are described in Figure 20.1. Such a reaction can occur after only a few millilitres of blood have been transfused; such is the potency of anti-A and anti-B. In this example, blood from a donor who is blood group A is transfused to a patient who is blood group B. Anti-A present in the patient's plasma binds to the A antigen on the surface of donated red cells. The red cells clump together (agglutinate). Antigen-antibody binding activates the so-called complement pathway; it is the complement proteins (by convention denoted by the letter C followed by a number), produced as a result of this activation, which accounts for many of the signs and symptoms of a haemolytic transfusion reaction.

Complement proteins C5, C6, C7, C8 and C9 are all involved in the process of red cell destruction (haemolysis), in which holes are made through the red cell

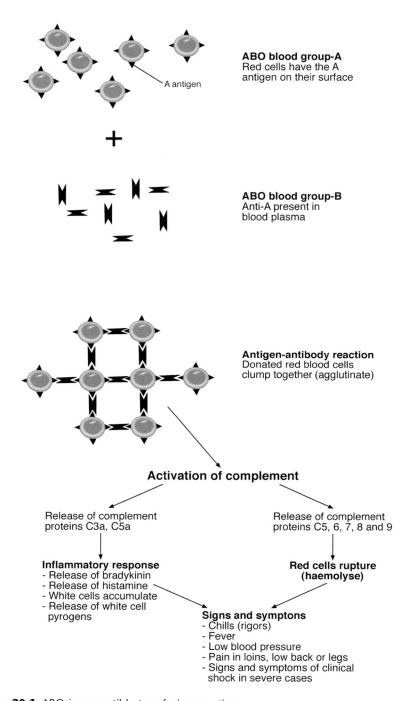

Figure 20.1 ABO incompatible transfusion reaction.

membrane. By this complement-mediated haemolysis, all donated red cells are destroyed in the most severe cases of ABO incompatibility. Complement proteins C3a and C5a initiate an inflammatory response that includes release from activated mast cells of various potent chemicals (e.g. histamine, bradykinin) that causes a sudden fall in blood pressure (hypotension) and other very visible symptoms. The fall in blood pressure leads to symptoms of clinical shock and reduced flow of blood to the kidneys with the onset of acute renal failure, in the most severe cases. Other complications of severe haemolytic transfusion reaction include disseminated intravascular coagulation (DIC), and jaundice, as haemoglobin released from damaged red cells is metabolised to bilirubin.

Other immune haemolytic transfusion reactions

Even if donated blood is ABO compatible with recipient blood, there remains a risk of immune haemolytic transfusion reaction if there are other significant red cell antibodies present in the patient's plasma. Since these are all immune antibodies, they can only be present in the plasma of those patients who have been immunised by previous blood transfusion or pregnancy. The most important of these is anti-D. Others include anti-C, anti-c, anti-E, and anti-e (i.e. remaining antibodies to Rh blood group antigens); anti-K (antibody to the Kell (K) blood group antigen); anti-Fy^a and anti-Fy^b (antibodies to two of the Duffy (Fy) blood group antigens); and anti-Jk^a and anti-Jk^b (antibodies to two of the Kidd (Jk) blood group antigens). Symptoms of haemolytic transfusion reaction that result from these antibodies are, generally speaking, less severe than those associated with ABO incompatibility. The reaction may be delayed for up to 10 days after the transfusion, when chills and fever develop. Red cell destruction may cause anaemia and mild jaundice.

Laboratory testing: blood group, antibody screen and crossmatch

Sample collection

When a patient requires a blood transfusion, 10 ml of venous blood must be collected into a plain tube containing no additives; this is sufficient for all three tests. Most blood transfusion laboratories supply designated tubes (usually pink top) that are to be used only for these tests.

Because of the potentially fatal consequences of giving donated blood to the 'wrong' patient, scrupulous attention to the detail of patient identification and documentation is vital when collecting blood for any of these tests. Before taking blood, ensure beyond any doubt the identification of the patient, preferably by asking the patient his name and crosschecking with his identification armband.

The following minimum information must be written legibly on the sample label and accompanying request card:

- patient's first and last name (taken from the patient's armband)
- hospital number (taken from the patient's armband)
- patient's ward or department
- date and time of collection
- initials of person taking the blood.

The request card should also include the following details:

- the nature of donated blood required (whole blood, packed red cells, etc.)
- number of units required
- when the blood is required: level of urgency
- why the blood is required (acute blood loss, chronic anaemia, elective surgery, etc.)
- ABO and rhesus blood group (if known)
- any relevant transfusion or obstetric history (if known)
- signature of the medical officer making the request.

These are guidelines only; healthcare workers involved in the collection of blood for pre-transfusion testing must adhere scrupulously to protocol contained in the local blood transfusion policy document, which should reflect best practice as defined by the British Committee for Standards in Haematology (BCSH) in collaboration with the Royal College of Nursing and the Royal College of Surgeons.[3,4]

Principles of the three tests

The purpose of the three tests is to prevent immune haemolytic transfusion reaction by issuing only donated blood that is immunologically compatible with the blood of the patient who is to receive the transfusion. In essence, this means first determining which antibodies to red cell antigens are present in the patient's plasma and then selecting donated blood that has none of the relevant red cell antigens. The only significant antibody which can be expected with certainty to be present in most patient's plasma are the naturally occurring antibodies to the red cell antigens of the ABO group system, so determination of the patient's ABO blood group is the prime test. At the same time as the ABO group is determined the RhD status (either negative or positive) is also determined. Together these are the blood group.

The binding of red cell antibody to its complementary antigen results in agglutination (clumping together) of cells. This visible phenomenon is exploited in all blood banking tests and is reflected in the alternative name for red cell antibodies and antigens. In many texts, red cell antibodies are referred to as agglutinins and antigens as agglutinogens.

Blood grouping

The patient's ABO blood group is determined by simply mixing a sample of patient's red cells with sera containing anti-A and sera containing anti-B. The red cells either

	Patient 1	Patient 2	Patient 3	Patient 4
Anti-A				
Anti-B				
Result	No agglutination when either anti-A or anti-B is added	Agglutination only when anti-A added	Agglutination only when anti-B added	Agglutination when both anti-A and anti-B are added
Interpretation of result	**Group O**	**Group A**	**Group B**	**Group AB**
Per cent frequency in UK population	47	42	8	3

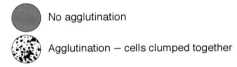

No agglutination

Agglutination – cells clumped together

Figure 20.2 Determination of ABO blood group.

agglutinate or stay separate in suspension (Figure 20.2). As an additional check, a reverse group is performed in which the patient's serum is added to red cells of known ABO group. RhD type is determined by mixing patient's cells with a solution of anti-D. Agglutination indicates the presence of the D antigen on patient's cells (RhD positive). No agglutination indicates the patient's blood is RhD negative.

Antibody screen

By performing an ABO blood group, we know that patient's plasma contains either anti-A or anti-B or both of these or neither of these. In around 97% of cases, no further antibody is present. With a few rare exceptions, all other significant red cell antibodies, including antibody to the RhD antigen, are present in the patient's serum only as a result of previous immunising blood transfusion or pregnancy. However, since the presence of these red cell immune antibodies may provoke a haemolytic reaction if the red cells to be transfused bear the relevant antigen, a search for the presence of any significant atypical antibodies is performed on the serum of all patients who are to receive donated blood. This is the antibody screening test.

Essentially the antibody screening test is performed by adding a drop of patient's serum to a panel of different group O red cells each bearing a different and known combination of the most common red cell antigens known to cause immune reactions. Since group O red cells do not have the A or B antigen on their surface, any agglutination when the patient's serum is added to this panel of red cells must be due to the presence of an atypical antibody in the patient's serum. No agglutination indicates no atypical antibodies and the result antibody screen negative is reported. The antibodies tested for in the antibody screening test usually include at least all of the following:

- anti-D, anti-C, anti-c, anti-E, and anti-e (antibodies to Rh blood group antigens)
- anti-K, anti-k (antibodies to Kell (K) blood group antigens)
- anti-Fy^a and anti-Fy^b (antibodies to two of the Duffy (Fy) blood group antigens)
- anti-Jk^a and anti-Jk^b (antibodies to two of the Kidd (Jk) blood group antigens)
- anti-S, anti-s, anti-M, anti-N (antibodies to four of the MNS blood group antigens).

If the screen is positive, the identity of the antibody causing the positive result can usually be deduced from the pattern of reactions displayed by the panel of O red cells.

Selection of donor blood

Having established what significant red cell antibodies are present in the patient's plasma, the next step is selection of a suitable donor unit. What is required is blood whose red cells do not bear any of the antigens that react with any significant antibodies present in the recipient patient's serum. For those patients whose antibody screen is negative (the vast majority), the only consideration is ABO and RhD compatibility. In most instances, this simply means selecting blood that has the same ABO and RhD blood group as the patient. However, if ABO or RhD identical blood is not available, there is some room for manoeuvre.

- A patient whose blood group is AB has no ABO antibodies in his plasma, so can receive red cells of any ABO group. Under these circumstances, however, consideration must be given to the naturally occurring antibodies (i.e. anti-A and anti-B) present in the plasma of donated blood. There is the potential for a haemolytic reaction caused by binding of these to A and B antigens present on the surface of the patient's AB red cells. In practice, this is not usually a major problem because most of the donor plasma and therefore most of the offending antibody has been removed in the case of packed red cells. The effect of any remaining anti-A or anti-B is diluted in the patient's blood plasma.
- Around 5% of the population (which includes those who donate blood) have particularly high amounts of anti-A and anti-B. They are said to be high titre positive. All donated blood units have a label indicating whether the blood is high titre negative or high titre positive. If donated blood of group O, A or B is being selected for patients whose blood group is AB, then only packed cells which are high titre negative are selected.

- The red cells of blood group O have no A or B antigens on their surface, so can be safely transfused to all patients. The risk of reaction between anti-A and anti-B present in the donated plasma and A or B antigens present on the red cells of group A, B and AB recipient patients is removed by selecting packed red cells that are high titre negative.
- Patients who are RhD positive cannot have antibodies to the D antigen and can therefore be given blood which is either RhD positive or negative.
- Patients who are RhD negative may or may not have antibodies to the D antigen but whether they do or not, transfusion of RhD positive blood almost invariably invokes anti-D production. For this reason, only RhD negative blood should be selected for transfusion to RhD negative patients.

Table 20.3 summarises the criteria for selection of donor unit for transfusion, based on the ABO group and RhD type of the patient. It will be noted that O RhD negative red cells can be safely transfused to all patients, so long as they are high titre negative. In the rare event of life-threatening haemorrhage, where the clinical need for a blood transfusion is so urgent that it does not allow time for laboratory testing, O RhD negative (high titre negative) blood is transfused. It will also be noted from Table 20.3 that patients with the blood group AB RhD positive can be safely transfused with red cells of any blood group, again as long as they are high titre negative.

For those patients whose antibody screen is positive, a further step is required. First, ABO RhD identical or compatible donated blood units are selected as described above. The red cells of these are then tested for the presence of red cell antigens that react with the atypical antibody found in the patient's serum. For example, suppose the antibody screen revealed that the patient had the antibody that reacts with the Rh C antigen (i.e. anti-C), the red cells of donated blood must be tested for the presence of the C antigen. Only blood that is negative for the C antigen can be transfused.

Crossmatch

Having selected a unit of donated blood whose red cells have no antigens that could react with antibodies present in the patient's plasma, one final checking test must be performed to ensure compatibility. This is the crossmatch in which transfusion is simulated in a test tube. Essentially a sample of donor red cells is mixed with a sample of the recipient patient's serum and inspected for agglutination. No agglutination indicates there is no red cell antigen/antibody reaction, that the donor red cells are compatible with patient's plasma, and can be safely transfused.

Pre-transfusion checks on the ward

Severe acute immune haemolytic reactions (invariably caused by ABO incompatibility) are rare events but when they do occur the cause is usually transfusion of blood to the 'wrong' patient due to clerical error or error in patient identification.[5]

Table 20.3 Selecting blood for transfusion.

		Recipient (patient) blood group						
Donor blood group	O RhD Pos	O RhD Neg	A RhD Pos	A RhD Neg	B RhD Pos	B RhD Neg	AB RhD Pos	AB RhD Neg
O RhD Pos	✓	✗	✓R	✗	✓R	✗	✓R	✗
O RhD Neg	✓	✓	✓R	✓R	✓R	✓R	✓R	✓R
A RhD Pos	✗	✗	✓	✗	✗	✗	✓R	✗
A RhD Neg	✗	✗	✓	✓	✗	✗	✓R	✓R
B RhD Pos	✗	✗	✗	✗	✓	✗	✓R	✗
B RhD Neg	✗	✗	✗	✗	✓	✓	✓R	✓R
AB RhD Pos	✗	✗	✗	✗	✗	✗	✓	✗
AB RhD Neg	✗	✗	✗	✗	✗	✗	✓	✓

✓ ABO compatible. No risk of Rh sensitisation. Safe to transfuse if patient antibody screen is negative.

✗ ABO incompatible or risk of Rh sensitisation. Not safe to transfuse.

✓R ABO compatible red cells. No risk of Rh sensitisation. Safe to transfuse high titre negative packed red cells if patient antibody screen negative.

The most common single error is failure to check at the bedside that the right blood is being given to the right patient.

Adherence to the agreed protocol for pre-transfusion checks, contained in the local blood transfusion policy document, is vital. Local protocols must reflect best practice as defined by the British Committee for Standards in Haematology (BCSH) in collaboration with the Royal College of Nursing and the Royal College of Surgeons.[3,4]

Pre-transfusion checks, which ideally should be made by two nurses, one of whom is state registered, should include:

- confirmation of patient's identity, preferably by asking the patient and cross-checking with identity armband
- confirmation that the patient details on the blood compatibility report match in every detail the identity of the patient to be given blood
- confirmation that the identifying unit number printed on the unit of blood to be transfused matches the unit number on the compatibility report
- confirmation that the ABO blood group and rhesus D type printed on the blood unit is the same as, or compatible with the patient's ABO and RhD blood group or compatible with it
- confirmation that the unit of blood to be transfused has not passed its expiry date and that no more than 30 minutes have elapsed since the unit was removed from the blood bank refrigerator
- baseline measurement of patient's blood pressure, temperature, pulse and respiration rate must be recorded immediately before the start of blood transfusion.

Other transfusion reactions

The laboratory tests discussed in this chapter are designed solely to prevent immune haemolytic transfusion reactions but these are not the only adverse reactions that a patient can suffer during a blood transfusion.

Febrile reactions

Patients who have received previous blood transfusions may have developed antibodies to antigens present on the surface of white cells. If blood whose white cells bear these antigens is transfused to such patients, a febrile reaction characterised by shivering and fever may develop. The symptoms are due to potent chemicals (cytokines) released from damaged white cells. Although quite common among patients who have previously received multiple transfusions, febrile reactions are usually mild and self-limiting.

Transfusion-related acute lung injury (TRALI)

This is a much more serious condition with a mortality rate of around 10%. It is caused by the presence of antibodies in donor plasma directed at antigens present on recipient patient's white cells. Agglutinated white cells, sequestered in the microvasculature of the lungs, release a range of toxic products that damage the endothelial lining of these vessels. The most significant consequence is pulmonary oedema and acute respiratory distress, which can be either rapidly fatal or resolve almost as quickly. Symptoms, which begin within an hour or so of transfusion, include breathlessness, coughing, rigors and fever. Severe hypoxaemia is usual.

Allergic reaction

Mild allergic reactions to a variety of donated plasma constituents are common, occurring in 1–2% of all transfusions. They are manifest as a red itchy skin rash within an hour of starting transfusion; antihistamine treatment is effective in such cases. Rarely, potentially fatal systemic allergic (anaphylactic) reactions occur; patients with IgA deficiency are particularly vulnerable. Dramatic effect may be seen after transfusion of just a few millilitres. Signs and symptoms include flushing of the skin, hypotension, nausea, abdominal pain, respiratory distress and cyanosis. Rapid treatment response is vital for survival in these extreme, but rare, allergy cases.

Bacterial infection

Scrupulous aseptic technique during donor blood collection and care that donated blood is stored at a temperature (+ 4°C) that minimises bacterial growth, ensures that donated blood is free from bacteria at the time of transfusion. Additional safeguards include the disposal of blood which has passed its expiry date and protocols which ensure that donated blood is not left at room temperature for longer than absolutely necessary before it is transfused. Although rare, reactions due to transfusion of bacterially contaminated blood can occur. Depending on the nature of the contaminating bacteria, symptoms vary. In the most severe cases, symptoms can develop within a few minutes of starting the transfusion. These include fever, sudden chills and shivering (rigors), nausea and vomiting. Sudden fall in blood pressure can herald severe sepsis and risk of multi-organ failure. Transfusion of blood contaminated with bacteria is potentially fatal.

Patient monitoring during transfusion

Most blood transfusions are uneventful, but because of the potentially serious adverse effects, careful observation of the patient is necessary during blood transfusion. Locally agreed protocol for the monitoring and management of patients receiving a blood transfusion must reflect best practice as defined by the BCSH in collaboration with the Royal College of Nursing and the Royal College of Surgeons.[3,4] Some general points are made here. Monitoring is particularly important during the early stages when most severe reactions develop. Temperature, pulse, respiration and blood pressure should be checked at 15-minute intervals during the first hour and at hourly intervals thereafter. Patients should be observed for signs and symptoms of all adverse reactions. In the event of a suspected reaction, the transfusion should be stopped immediately and medical staff summoned. The management of a patient suffering a transfusion reaction depends on its cause and severity. Mild febrile reactions may require only the administration of an antipyretic drug (e.g. aspirin) to control temperature. The transfusion can be restarted, only at a slower rate. Mild allergic reactions may be treated with antihistamine drugs. For severe reactions, i.e. immune haemolytic reactions, severe allergic reactions and those caused by bacterial infection, the principal first objective is to maintain blood pressure in order to preserve blood flow to the kidneys. Adrenalin and steroids may be administered to control allergy and shock. Diuretics may be administered to increase urine flow. In the case of suspected bacterial infection, broad-spectrum antibiotics are administered.

Laboratory investigation of transfusion reaction

In all cases of severe reaction, the laboratory must be informed as soon as possible, so that the cause of the reaction can be investigated. A fresh sample of patient's blood collected into a plain tube, along with the donor blood pack must be sent to the laboratory for this purpose. Blood group, antibody screen and crossmatch will be repeated. Because of the risk of disseminated intravascular coagulation (DIC) and resulting excessive bleeding, associated with severe immune haemolytic reaction and reaction due to transfusion of bacterially contaminated blood, a sample of blood for haemoglobin estimation and a further sample of blood for coagulation studies should also be sent to the laboratory. Finally blood from the donor pack and blood from the patient must be cultured for the detection of bacteria.

Post-transfusion reactions

For the vast majority of patients, blood transfusion passes uneventfully. There remains a small risk of a delayed immune haemolytic reaction (usually mild) during the hours and days that follow a blood transfusion. Sudden onset of chills, rise in temperature, anaemia and jaundice at any time during the 10-day period following a transfusion may signal such a reaction.

Incidence of serious adverse events: how safe is transfusion?

Transfusion transmitted infection

Measures taken to minimise the risk of hepatitis B and C viruses (HBV and HCV), human immunodeficiency virus (HIV) and human T-cell lymphotropic virus (HTLV) infection during transfusion have been highly successful. The blood supply has never been safer and the theoretical risk of contracting these viral infections during red cell transfusion is now extremely small. The chance that a unit of donated blood might transmit HIV in the UK is estimated at 0.014 per 100 000 units. The relevant figure for HCV is 0.024 and for HBV 0.176.[6]

Incidents of blood transfusion adverse events are collated in an annual Serious Hazards of Transfusion (SHOT) report. For the five-year period 1999–2004

SHOT identified just 24 cases of probable transfusion transmitted infection for all blood products, of which six were viral (2 HBV, 2 HIV, 1 HTLV and 1 case of hepatitis E). There was one case of malarial transmission and the remaining 16 were bacterial (15 during platelet transfusion and just one during red cell transfusion).

In recent years, there has been much concern about whether the prion agent that causes new variant Creutzfeldt–Jacob (nvCJD) disease is transmissible during transfusion. As a precautionary measure, white cells (where these agents are presumed to reside) are now removed from donated blood. No cases of proven transmission via transfusion have occurred, but to date there have been two cases of possible transfusion transmitted nvCJD.[7,8]

ABO incompatibility

The transfusion of ABO incompatible red cells is avoidable and each case represents system failure invariably involving human error. Every year in the UK, around 2.6 million red cell units are transfused and on average there are around 24 cases of ABO incompatible red cell transfusions (19 cases in 2004). In most cases these result in minor or no ill effects, but in up to third, patients suffer serious morbidity requiring admission to intensive care and rarely (0–2 cases per year in the UK over the past 10 years), patients die as a direct result of receiving ABO incompatible red cells. The risk of an ABO incompatible transfusion is currently estimated to be 1 : 100 000 and the risk of death caused by transfusing incompatible red cells 1 : 1 800 000.[5]

Transfusion-related lung injury (TRALI)

Over the past 5–10 years, TRALI has emerged as a significant cause of transfusion-related morbidity and mortality and in this respect ranks second only to ABO incompatibility. In 2004, SHOT identified 13 TRALI cases in the UK. Of these, just two involved transfusion of red cells. The remainder were due to transfusion of other blood products.[9]

Haemolytic disease of the newborn (HDN)

Both determination of blood group and the antibody screening test are important not only for the prevention of immune haemolytic transfusion reactions but also for the diagnosis and prevention of haemolytic disease of the newborn (HDN). As part of their antenatal care, all pregnant women have a sample of blood taken, usually at their first antenatal appointment, for blood group determination and antibody screen in case a blood transfusion is required either during pregnancy or in the postpartum period. Another purpose of this testing is to identify those women whose developing baby is at risk of HDN, a condition which at best threatens wellbeing of the baby and at worst, the life of the baby.

What is HDN?

Some red cell antibodies (most notably antibodies to the antigens of the Rh blood group system, e.g. anti-D) can pass from the mother's blood across the placenta to the fetal circulation. If the baby has inherited red cell antigens from the father that these maternal antibodies react with, an immune haemolytic reaction occurs and fetal red cells are destroyed.

Pregnancies most at risk are those in which the mother is RhD negative and the father is group RhD positive. There is a one in four chance that the baby of such a union will be RhD positive. If the baby is, in fact, RhD positive then when fetal red cells, as they do in all pregnancies, pass from fetal circulation to the mother's blood, the mother's lymphocytes 'see' the D antigen present on the baby's red cells as foreign and produces anti-D.

During the first such pregnancy the titre (amount) of anti-D in the mother's plasma is usually insufficient to have any effect. But the mother's immune system is now primed to produce massive quantities of anti-D the next time it encounters RhD positive red cells. In subsequent pregnancies, if the baby is once again RhD positive, large amounts of anti-D pass from the mother to fetal circulation, bind to the D antigen on fetal red cells, provoking a massive haemolytic reaction, with destruction of the developing baby's red cells.

The effects of HDN are variable; some babies are unaffected but in the most severe cases, the anaemia that results from red cell destruction can lead to death in *utero*. More often babies are born anaemic and jaundiced. The jaundice is due to increased production of bilirubin from haemoglobin released from haemolysed (destroyed) red cells. If haemolysis is particularly marked and serum bilirubin concentration rises very high, there is a risk of permanent brain damage caused by the deposition of bilirubin in the cells of the brain, a condition called kernicterus. Affected babies may need exchange transfusion, in which O RhD negative blood (which, because it lacks the RhD antigen, cannot be destroyed by any anti-D present) is transfused, as the baby's O RhD positive blood, containing the damaging antibody and bilirubin, is removed. This transfusion corrects the anaemia and prevents further red cell damage; the severe jaundice resolves. If the developing fetus is severely affected, consideration may be given to intrauterine transfusion from as early as 18 weeks into the pregnancy.

Prevention of RhD HDN

To prevent HDN caused by RhD incompatibility, all RhD negative women who have not been previously immunised to produce anti-D are offered an injection of anti-D at 28 and 34 weeks of pregnancy. This administered anti-D destroys any fetal cells before the mother can mount an immune response, thus preventing maternal production of anti-D which could jeopardise subsequent pregnancies.

HDN can be caused by other red cell antibodies

Although RhD incompatibility between mother and baby is the most significant cause of HDN, other red cell antibodies that may or may not be present in the mother's serum can cause HDN. It is rare for ABO incompatibility to cause HDN because anti-A and anti-B, unlike anti-D, cannot normally cross the placenta so therefore does not come into contact with fetal red cells. When HDN is caused by ABO incompatibility, it is usually mild and of much less clinical significance than that due to RhD incompatibility. Other antibodies of significance are the antibodies to other rhesus group antigens (i.e. anti-C, anti-E and anti-e), anti-K (antibody to Kell blood group antigens) and anti-Dfy (antibody to Duffy blood group antigens). An antibody screen performed early in pregnancy is designed to detect if any antibodies capable of causing HDN are present in the mother's blood plasma.

Case history 19

Mrs Greenwood, a 24-year-old mother, attends surgical outpatient department to have blood taken for various tests before surgery, scheduled later in the week. Among the blood tests requested is 'group, screen and save'.

Questions

(1) What sample is required?
(2) What is the purpose of the tests?
   Mrs Greenwood's blood group is found to be AB RhD negative. During surgery, Mrs Greenwood suffers a significant haemorrhage and a request for two units of crossmatched packed red cells is sent urgently to the laboratory. During the pre-transfusion checks in the recovery room, before administration of the first unit, it is noted that the blood to be transfused is A RhD negative.
(3) In view of the ABO blood group discrepancy between the donor and Mrs Greenwood, is it safe to go ahead with the transfusion?
(4) Why is it important that Mrs Greenwood does not receive RhD positive blood?

Discussion of case history

(1) A 10 ml sample of venous blood collected into a plain bottle specially designated for blood transfusion tests.

(2) These tests are performed to reduce delay should Mrs Greenwood require a blood transfusion during surgery. Her ABO group and RhD type will be determined. The term 'screen' refers to the antibody screening test in which her plasma is tested for the presence of any atypical red cell antibodies, which may complicate the selection of a suitable donor unit. 'Save' simply means store the sample. Should a blood transfusion become necessary, the only remaining test to be performed is the crossmatch test in which Mrs Greenwood's stored sample of plasma is mixed with the red cells of a selected ABO and Rh compatible donor unit. If Mrs Greenwood were scheduled for major surgery in which excessive bleeding were a routine and expected complication, blood would be crossmatched before surgery.

(3) Although the ABO blood group of the donated unit is not identical, it is compatible with Mrs Greenwood's group. The cells of the donated blood group bear the A antigen; it is imperative that this blood is not given to a patient whose serum

anti-A or anti-B, so she can be given group A red cells. The donor plasma contains anti-B, which can react with the B antigen present on Mrs Greenwood's red cells. This is not a problem, however, because the unit requested is packed red cells, that is a donor unit from which most of the plasma (and therefore most of the anti-B) has been removed. Any anti-B remaining in the small volume of plasma will be diluted in the patient's own plasma and have no adverse effect. Only 3% of the population belong, like Mrs Greenwood, to group AB so it is often difficult to find ABO identical blood for such patients; Group A or Group B packed red cells are a suitable alternative.

(4) Mrs Greenwood belongs to the 15% of the population whose red cells do not bear the RhD antigen. She is RhD negative. If she were given blood whose red cells did bear the antigen (i.e. RhD positive blood) she would 'see' these cells as foreign and invoke an immune response with production of anti-D. This would be significant for future transfusions. If in any subsequent transfusion she were given RhD positive blood, her primed immune system would produce large quantities of anti-D, which would bind to the D antigen on transfused red cells and initiate an acute immune haemolytic reaction. There is also a greatly increased risk that if Mrs Greenwood became pregnant, her pregnancy would be complicated by severe RhD haemolytic disease of the newborn. For these reasons it is imperative that patients who are RhD negative, particularly women of childbearing age, are only given RhD negative blood.

References

1. Coste J, Ressnik H *et al.* (2005) Implementation of donor screening for infectious agents transmitted by blood by nucleic acid technology: update to 2003. *Vox Sanguinis* **88**: 289–303.
2. Soldan K, Barbara J *et al.* (2003) Estimation of risk of hepatitis B virus, hepatitis C virus and human immunodeficiency virus infections entering the blood supply in England, 1993–2001. *Vox Sanguinis* **84**: 274–286.
3. NHS Executive (2002) Better blood transfusion. *Health Services Circular* 2002/9. London: HMSO.
4. British Committee for Standards in Haematology (1999) Guidelines for the administration of blood and blood components and the management of the transfused patient. *Transfus Med* **9**: 227–38.
5. Stainsby D, Russell J *et al.* (2005) Reducing adverse events in blood transfusion. *Br J Haem* **131**: 8–12.
6. McClelland D & Contreras M (2005) Effectiveness and safety of blood transfusion; have we lost the plot? *J R Coll Physicians Edinb* **35**: 2–4.
7. Llewelyn C, Hewitt PE *et al.* (2004) Possible transmission of variant Creutzfeldt–Jakob disease by transfusion. *Lancet* **363**: 411–12.
8. Peden A & Head H (2004) Pre-clinical v CJD after blood transfusion in a codon 129 heterozygous patient. *Lancet* **364**: 527–29.
9. SHOT (2004) *Serious Hazards of Transfusion*, Steering Group Annual Report. Manchester: SHOT office, Manchester Blood Centre. ISBN 09532 789 7 2.

Further reading

Atterbury C & Wilkinson J (2000) Blood Transfusion. *Nurs Stand* **14** (13): 47–52.

British Committee for Standards in Haematology (2001) Guidelines for the clinical use of red cell transfusions. *BrJ Haem* **113**: 24–31.

Contreras M (1998) *ABC of Transfusion*. London: BMJ Publishing Group.

Dellinger E & Anaya D (2004) Infectious and immunologic consequences of blood transfusion. *Critical Care* **8** (suppl 2): 18–23.

Glover G & Powell F (1996) Blood transfusion. *Nurs Stand* **10**: 49–54.

Royal College of Nursing (2004) Right blood, right patient, right time. RCN guidance for improving transfusion practice. London: RCN. *www.rcn.org.uk/members/downloads/rightblood.pdf*

Useful website

www.shotuk.org Serious Hazards of Transfusion (SHOT) website: contains annual reports.

PART 5

Microbiology testing

Chapter 21

URINE MICROSCOPY, CULTURE AND SENSITIVITY

In this chapter and the next, attention is focused on the work of the clinical microbiology laboratory. Of all microbiological tests conducted in clinical laboratories, urine microscopy, culture and sensitivity (MC&S) is the most frequently requested. The test is used to help make or exclude a diagnosis of urine tract infection (UTI) among patients who exhibit signs and symptoms of UTI, and among patients who are asymptomatic, but at high risk of UTI. After the respiratory tract, the urine tract is the most frequent site of bacterial infection.

Normal physiology

The urine tract: formation of urine

The urinary system (Figure 21.1) comprises the kidneys and ureters (the upper urine tract), and bladder and urethra (lower urine tract). Urine formation occurs in the kidney. The functional unit of the kidney is a microscopically small tube called a nephron (Figure 5.1); there are around 1 million nephrons in each kidney. Urine formation begins when blood delivered to the kidney via the renal artery is filtered at the glomerulus of each nephron. The fluid that passes through the glomerular filter is called the ultrafiltrate and is essentially blood from which all cells and large protein molecules have been removed. During its passage through the nephron, the volume and composition of this ultrafiltrate is adjusted. By the time the ultrafiltrate has passed to the end of the nephron, only waste products of the body's metabolic processes dissolved in a little water are left; this is urine. The urine from each nephron flows into a system of collecting ducts. These ducts join at the pelvis of the kidney, where urine leaves the kidney.

Urine is conducted from the pelvis of each kidney to the bladder, via tubes called ureters. The walls of the ureters contain smooth muscle. Peristaltic contractions of this muscle wall, occurring around three times per minute, propel urine towards the bladder. The ureters are joined obliquely to the bladder at its base, and urine enters the bladder in continuous spurts due to the peristaltic action of the ureters. The oblique entry of ureters to bladder ensures that the opening to the bladder is kept closed, except during peristaltic contraction when urine enters.

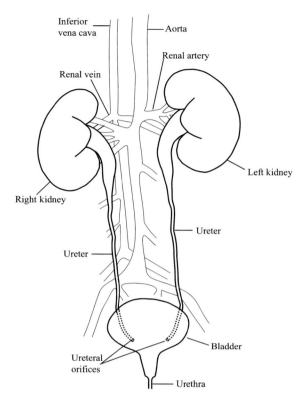

Figure 21.1 Urine tract.

This effectively prevents urine passing from the bladder in the reverse direction up the ureters.

The bladder is an innervated muscular bag whose function is to store urine, before urination (micturition) and expel all the urine it contains at the time of micturition. The volume of the bladder increases as it fills with urine. Between 150 and 400 ml of urine are collected in the adult bladder before the desire to urinate arises. When 700 ml of urine are present, the desire to urinate becomes urgent and painful. A sphincter muscle (the external urethral sphincter), situated where the urethra joins the bladder, prevents accumulating urine leaving the bladder. At the time of micturition, this sphincter is relaxed; the detrusor muscle in the wall of the bladder contracts, forcing urine out of the bladder and urine flows from the bladder down the urethra.

The urethra is the tubular structure through which urine flows on the final part of its journey from the bladder out of the body. In the female, the opening of the urethra (called the meatus) is in front of the vaginal orifice and in the male is at the tip of the penis. The male urethra is thus significantly longer than the female urethra.

Bacteria in the urine tract

The urine tract, from kidney to the final distal third of the urethra, normally contains no bacteria, so in health the urine present in the bladder is sterile. Bacteria normally present on the skin of the perineum and in faeces can find their way up the urethra, so bacteria may be present without any untoward effect in the lower third of the urethra. The normal flushing effect of urine as it passes down the urethra and other non-immune and immune defence against bacterial invasion serve to keep this bacterial contamination of urethra under control. In health, normally voided urine is either sterile (contains no bacteria) or contains low numbers of bacteria, flushed from the urethra during micturition.

Urine tract infection

Route of infection

Urine tract infection (Figure 21.2) most often results from ascending infection by bacteria that constitute part of the normal bacterial flora of either the gastrointestinal tract or skin. Bacteria normally present in the gastrointestinal tract are present in faeces. These bacteria find their way from the perianal region via the perineum to the urethra and up into the bladder. The skin of the perineum is also a source of urine tract pathogens. Bacteria that are normally present specifically in the female genital tract are a less common cause of UTI.

Infection and resulting inflammation of the bladder is called cystitis. This is the most common form of UTI. In a minority of individuals, infection spreads on up the urine tract, infecting the kidney. Although far less common than infection of the lower urine tract, infection of the kidney (pyelonephritis) is more serious than cystitis. Scarring of kidney tissue can, in the long term, reduce kidney function. Chronic infection of the kidney may result in renal failure. Pyelonephritis is associated with increased of risk of infection spreading to the blood causing septicaemia.

Although the ascending route of infection is the most usual, urine tract infection may be caused by septicaemia. In this case, bacteria present in blood may initiate descending infection of the urine tract affecting first the kidneys and then the lower urine tract.

Predisposing factors

Gender
The relatively short female urethra is considered one of the principal reasons for the particular susceptibility of women to ascending UTI. Around a third of all women have a UTI before the age of 65,[1] while for men under the age of 50, UTI is relatively rare. The incidence of UTI infection among men increases significantly

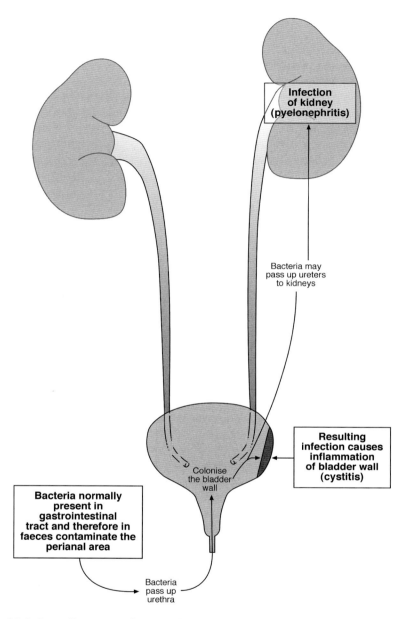

Figure 21.2 Ascending route of urine infection.

with age past 50 years, so there is no gender difference in UTI among elderly patients.[1] Among children, girls are more prone to UTI than boys.

Sexual activity
Women who are sexually active are more likely to suffer UTI than those who are not.

Pregnancy

Changes in the urine tract early in pregnancy increase the risk of UTI spreading up the urine tract with resulting pyelonephritis. For this reason, all pregnant women are screened for UTI at least once during the first half of pregnancy.

Urine stasis

One of the principal physiological processes which prevents UTI is the flushing effect of sterile bladder urine through the lower urine tract. Any disease process that inhibits urine flow or complete bladder emptying increases the risk of UTI. Obstruction of the urine tract by stones (urinary calculi) or tumour and disease of the prostate, which all impair urine flow, contribute to the increased incidence of UTI in older men compared with younger men.

Immunosuppression

A suppressed immune system reduces host defence against bacterial invasion of the urine tract. This explains the increased incidence of UTI among HIV patients and those who have been given immunosuppressive drugs (e.g. transplant patients).

Diabetes mellitus

Diabetics are more likely to suffer infections than non-diabetics. Urine tract infection is a particular complication of long-standing diabetes.

Vesicoureteral reflux

Anatomy of the normal urine tract prevents urine from passing from the bladder back into the ureters. Vesicoureteral reflux is a pathological condition in which reflux of infected urine from bladder to ureters greatly predisposes to ascending infection with resulting pyelonephritis. This is a particular problem among children and is a major cause of pyelonephritis among this age group. Other congenital abnormalities of the urine tract cause UTI in babies and young children. If not identified and treated these anomalies, and associated recurrent UTI, can lead to renal failure later in life. For this reason, UTI in childhood warrants intensive urological investigation.

Hospitalisation

Illness that necessitates a stay in hospital is quite commonly associated with a temporary state of reduced immune defence against infectious disease. Furthermore the hospital environment is one in which the risk of coming into contact with infectious organisms is high. It is perhaps not surprising that many patients acquire an infection as a direct result of being admitted to hospital. Around half of all patients in hospital who are suffering an infection, acquired the infection after admission. The principal site of hospital-acquired (nosocomial) infection is the urine tract; around 40% of all nosocomial infections are UTIs.[2] Patients at particularly high risk of nosocomial UTI are those who require urine catheterisation or cystoscopy (endoscopic examination of the urine tract). Urological surgery is also associated with an increased risk of UTI. All patients who require long-term catheterisation, i.e. for more than a month, whether in hospital or the community, almost inevitably contract a urine tract infection, though most are asymptomatic[3] (i.e. they have significant bacteriuria, but do not feel unwell).

Signs and symptoms

Lower urine tract infection (cystitis)

The principal signs and symptoms of cystitis are:

- frequent urge to urinate even when there is not much urine in the bladder (frequency and urgency)
- burning pain during and immediately after urination (dysuria)
- fever may be a feature.

Upper urine tract infection (acute pyelonephritis)

Those with upper urine tract infections are usually significantly more unwell than those with uncomplicated cystitis. Principal signs and symptoms include:

- fever and rigors (fits of shivering)
- general malaise with nausea and vomiting
- renal (i.e. low back) pain
- symptoms of lower urine tract infection may also be present.

Microbiological examination of urine

Specimen collection: MSU

The sample required is a 'clean catch' midstream specimen of urine (Table 21.1). It is important that the sample is taken before antibiotics are given, as these can reduce the numbers of any bacteria present, resulting in a falsely negative result. If antibiotics have been given, this should be stated on the accompanying request card.

Specimen collection: CSU

The once widely adopted practice of catheterising patients simply to obtain a specimen of bladder urine for microbiological testing was abandoned when it was realised that the process of catheterisation itself increases the risk of UTI. However, the collection of a catheter specimen of urine (CSU) is necessary for the investigation of catheterised patients. Any bacteria present in bladder urine will quickly multiply as it stands in a catheter drainage bag. Urine should not therefore be sampled from the drainage bag; it will give a false impression of the bacterial content of bladder urine. Urine should instead be sampled using scrupulous aseptic technique by syringe and needle from the self-sealing sleeve of the drainage tube. Aseptic technique reduces the risks of:

Table 21.1 Collection of a 'clean catch' midstream urine specimen (MSU).

Object:
To collect a specimen of bladder urine uncontaminated by bacteria which may be present on

● skin
● external genital tract
● perianal region
● distal third of urethra

and in the environment (on surfaces, outside of collection bottle etc.)

Principle:
Any bacteria present in the urethra is washed away in the the first portion of urine voided. This is not collected. All other potential contamination is avoided by thorough cleansing and good clean aseptic technique.

Protocol for women:
1. Wash hands thoroughly with soap and water and dry.
2. With one hand spread the labia.
3. Area around the urinary meatus must be cleansed from front to back with soap and water and dried.
4. Still with labia separated, the patient voids the first 20 ml or so of urine into the toilet bowl and then collects a portion of the remaining urine into a *sterile* universal container.
5. Screw on cap of urine bottle immediately taking care not to touch either the rim of the bottle or inside of the bottle cap.

Protocol for men:
1. Wash hands thoroughly with soap and water and dry.
2. Retract foreskin and clean around the urinary meatus with soap and water.
3. Patient passes the first 20 ml or so into the toilet bowl and collects a portion of the remaining urine into a *sterile* universal container.
4. Screw on cap of bottle immediately taking care not to touch either the inside rim of the bottle or inside of the cap.

● infecting the catheterised patient
● cross-infection from the catheterised patient to staff and other patients
● the specimen being contaminated with bacteria in the environment.

Specimen collection bottle

Urine (either MSU or CSU) must be collected into a sterile bottle. It is not necessary to fill the bottle; 5–10 ml is all that is required.

Transport to the laboratory

Urine is a good medium for bacterial growth. Any bacteria present in the urine at collection will continue to multiply in the specimen bottle, giving falsely positive results. It is important that the urine is examined within a few hours of collection. The time of sample collection should be recorded on the accompanying request card. If there is to be any delay in transportation to the laboratory, urine is best stored in a designated refrigerator, as low temperature slows bacterial growth. Some laboratories provide sterile universal bottles that contain boric acid, a chemical that inhibits bacterial growth. The dip-slide culture method is designed for immediate culture of urine the moment the sample is voided. The slide, which is covered with a culture medium, is dipped into freshly voided urine, drained and then sent to the laboratory.

In the laboratory

As with any specimen submitted for microbiological examination, urine is:

- examined macroscopically
- examined microscopically
- cultured to detect and identify any bacteria present

Any potential pathogenic bacteria discovered are tested for sensitivity or resistance to a range of antimicrobial drugs.

Macroscopic examination

Normal urine is a clear straw-yellow coloured fluid. Although by no means diagnostic, the appearance of urine can sometimes provide suggestive evidence of UTI. Like any other bacterial infection, UTI is associated with recruitment of phagocytic white blood cells (WBC) to the site of infection. Dead and dying white cells are removed from the site of any infection in an inflammatory exudate called pus. Pus in urine (pyuria) turns clear urine turbid (cloudy). The absence of cloudiness, however, does not rule out an infection and turbid urine does not necessarily mean the urine is infected; there are other benign causes of urine turbidity. Infection with some bacteria can make urine foul smelling.

Microscopical examination

A measured volume of urine is examined under the microscope, principally for the presence of white and red blood cells. Urine normally contains a few white and red blood cells but a significant increase in white cell numbers, is strong evidence of an infective process. However, an increased white cell count is occasionally seen in urine, which when cultured is found to contain no bacteria. Conversely a small minority of urines from patients suffering UTI contain no increase in the number of white cells. Infection is sometimes associated with an increase in red cell numbers (haematuria). There are other pathological causes (mostly renal disease) for an increase in urine red cell numbers.[4] Epithelial (skin) cells naturally shed from the surface of the female genital tract may be seen in urine; these have no pathological significance but rather indicate that the urine was not collected properly and may contain contaminating bacteria from the genital tract. Bacteria if present in large enough numbers may be seen during microscopical examination of urine.

Culture

The only sure way of confirming the presence or absence of bacteria and identifying the species is to culture the urine. Culture in this context means grow. A measured volume of urine is placed on a sterile solid culture medium in a petri dish. The culture medium contains all the nutrients necessary for bacterial growth. The petri dish is then covered and placed in an incubator at 37°C (optimum temperature for bacterial growth) and left for 24 hours. Any bacterial growth is seen as visible colonies on the surface of the solid medium. Each colony contains many thousands of bacteria, all derived from a single bacterium present in the urine sample. The number of these visible colonies is directly related to the number of organisms in the urine sample. If the urine were sterile (i.e. contained no bacteria) there would be no visible colonies and the culture medium would appear unchanged.

As previously stated, it is quite normal for urine to contain small numbers of bacteria, mostly derived from the distal third of the urethra, so the mere presence of bacteria in urine (bacteriuria) is not sufficient to make a diagnosis of UTI. The term 'significant bacteriuria' was first used by Kass in 1956[5] to diagnose UTI. He determined that, with some provisos, a bacterial count of more than 10^5 (i.e. 100 000) organisms per ml of urine was diagnostic of UTI. Although it has been demonstrated since that symptoms of UTI can occasionally occur when bacterial count drops as low as 10^3/ml and that some patients have no symptoms when their bacterial count is above 10^5/ml, Kass' dictum is still widely applied and a bacterial count of greater than 10^5/ml remains a working definition of urine tract infection. By counting the number of colonies in culture grown from a known volume of urine, it is possible to deduce the original concentration of bacteria in the urine specimen.

Each colony is the product of division of a single bacterium, so each colony is pure (i.e. contains only one sort of bacterium). The macroscopic appearance of the colony provides some evidence of the sort of bacteria it contains but further testing is required for positive identification.

Although several types of bacteria are known to cause UTI, the commonest being *Escherichia Coli (E. Coli)* (Table 21.2), it is very rare for the infected urine tract of any one patient (except catheterised patients) to be colonised by more than one sort of bacteria. Thus the finding of many sorts of bacteria and no single one predominating (called a mixed bacterial growth), tends to indicate, not that the urine tract is infected, but rather that the urine has been contaminated with the mixture of bacteria normally present in the lower third of the urethra or genito-anal area. In other words, the sample was not collected properly. A pure growth (i.e. growth of one type of bacteria) with a bacterial count of greater than 10^5 organisms/ml of urine is virtually diagnostic of urine tract infection.

Sensitivity

The results of this final test inform the decision about which antibiotic is to be prescribed in cases of bacterial infection. It is therefore a test which would not be performed if the results of urine culture revealed that the urine was sterile or

Table 21.2 Most common causes of urine tract infection.

Bacteria	Normally present in	% of UTI acquired in community	% of UTI acquired in hospital
Escherichia Coli (E. Coli)	GI tract: faeces	75–80%	50–60%
Staphylococcus epidermis (S. epidermis)	Skin External genital tract	5–10%	< 5%
Staphylococcus saprophyticus (S. saprophyticus)	GI tract: faeces	5–10%	< 5%
Proteus species	GI tract: faeces Hospital environment	< 5%	10–15%
Klebsiella species	GI tract: faeces External genital tract	< 5%	10–15%
Pseudomonas aeruginosa (P. aeruginosa)	GI tract: faeces (rarely) Hospital environment	< 5%	5–10%
Other (many species)		< 5%	5–10%

contained insignificant numbers of bacteria. The object of the test is to determine the resistance or sensitivity of the particular strain of bacteria causing the UTI, to a range of antibiotics. A bacterium is said to be resistant to an antibiotic if that antibiotic fails to kill the bacteria in culture. If prescribed, that particular antibiotic would not be effective in eradicating the infection. Conversely, a strain of bacteria that is sensitive to a particular antibiotic will be killed by that antibiotic.

The test takes colonies of bacteria previously grown by culture of the urine specimen and re-inoculates them on a culture medium as before, this time in the presence of a range of antibiotics. After a period of incubation, the culture medium is inspected. If the strain of bacteria is resistant to the antibiotic being tested, no effect on bacterial growth is seen; the culture appears as it would if the antibiotic were not present. If, however, the bacteria are sensitive to the antibiotic being tested, there is no evidence of bacterial growth; the bacteria are killed and the culture medium appears as if no bacteria had been applied.

Since sensitivity testing involves a further period of incubation, there is an inevitable delay of up to 24 hours before the final report can be issued. If there is strong evidence of UTI at microscopy, i.e. there is a high white cell count and bacteria are visible, some laboratories perform sensitivity tests on urine directly, without waiting for the bacteria to grow in culture.

Interpretation of results

- Pure growth of bacteria with bacterial count of $> 10^5$ organisms/ml urine *indicates urine tract infection*. Increase in number of white cells (i.e. > 10 per mm^3 urine) provides supportive evidence.

- Pure growth of bacteria and bacterial count of between 10^3 and 10^5 organisms/ml urine *indicates equivocal result*. May or may not be UTI. The presence of increased numbers of white cells (i.e. greater than 10 per mm^3 urine) supports a diagnosis of UTI. The higher the white cell count, the stronger is the possibility of infection.
- Mixed bacterial growth indicates *probable contamination*, especially if epithelial cells are present. However, this mixed growth may be masking urine tract infection caused by one type of bacteria within the mixed growth, particularly if the bacterial count is high (i.e. > 10^5 organisms/ml urine.) A carefully collected repeat sample may be indicated. A normal white cell count tends to suggest there is no UTI, whereas a raised white cell count suggests there might be.
- Sterile urine (no bacteria detected) or bacterial count of < 10^3/ml urine indicates *no evidence of UTI*. A white cell count of < 10 per mm^3 urine also indicates no evidence of UTI.

Post-treatment testing

Symptoms of UTI may disappear within a few days of beginning a course of antibiotic therapy, but the only sure way of ensuring that a cure has been elicited, is microbiological examination of urine. An MSU should be examined at around 1 week and 4 weeks after the course of antibiotics has been completed. If the bacterial species that caused the infection cannot be isolated from urine by culture at these times, a cure can be assumed.

Dipstick testing for UTI

Rapid dipstick tests to screen for UTI are commercially available. The tests are discussed in Chapter 24.

Although extremely convenient, these rapid dipstick methods have limitations. The number of false positive results associated with their use is unacceptably high to make a definitive diagnosis of UTI.[6] In any case, without culture of the urine, it is not possible to identify the bacteria and perform sensitivity studies. All urines found to be positive by urinalysis dipstick testing should be submitted to the laboratory for full urine culture and sensitivity.

Many studies have concluded, however, that a negative result using urinalysis dipstick testing is reliable.[6,7] So long as the manufacturers' instructions are followed to the letter, the finding of no bacteria, white cells, blood or protein in urine is robust evidence that the patient is not suffering a UTI. Unless there is particularly strong clinical evidence suggestive of UTI, most authorities agree that such negative urines need not normally be submitted for full microbiological examination.

Case history 20

Hayley Smith is a 24-year-old mother of two who is 16 weeks pregnant. At her most recent routine antenatal care appointment she was asked to provide a mid-stream specimen of urine (MSU) for microscopy, culture and sensitivity (M, C&S).

A few days later, the laboratory report of this test is received. The report includes the following results:

WBC	< 5/mm^3
RBC	< 5/mm^3
Urine culture	< 10^3 bacteria/ml 'mixed coliform growth'

Questions

(1) Why is microbiological examination of MSU a routine part of antenatal care?
(2) Do the results suggest Hayley is suffering a urine tract infection?

Discussion of case history

(1) Pregnancy is normally associated with changes in the gross structure of the urine tract, in part caused by compression of the growing uterus on the kidneys and lower urine tract. The ureters are elongated, widen and become more curved. One effect of these changes is a relative urine stasis (urine flow is not as efficient as usual) and resulting higher than normal risk of infection of the lower urine tract spreading upwards to the kidneys with resulting infection of the kidney (pyelonephritis). An estimated 20–40% of pregnant women with signific-ant bacteriuria early in pregnancy, even if asymptomatic, will go on to develop pyelonephritis later in pregnancy if the bacteria are not quickly eliminated with antibiotic therapy. Pyelonephritis is a serious infection that may lead to renal failure. Babies of mothers suffering pyelonephritis during pregnancy may be born pre-maturely or have a low birthweight. To prevent pyelonephritis, all pregnant women are screened for evidence of urine tract infection. Since significant bacteriuria may occur without any symptoms, testing in this context should not be confined to those who have symptomatic UTI.

(2) Despite the finding of bacteria in Hayley's urine, there is no evidence of infec-tion. The numbers of bacteria are not significant and those discovered are a mixed growth of many bacterial species, suggesting contamination of the specimen with bacteria normally present in the lower part of urethra or the perianal region. There is also no increase in the number of white blood cells in Hayley's urine, providing further evidence that her urine tract is not infected.

References

1. Neu H (1992) Urinary tract infections. *Amer J Med* **92** (suppl 4A): 63–69.
2. Kalsi J, Arya M & Wilson P (2003) Hospital-acquired urinary tract infection. *Int J Clin Prac* **57**: 388–91.
3. Tambayah P & Maki D (2000) Catheter-associated urinary tract infection is rarely symp-tomatic – a prospective study of 1497 catheterized patients. *Arch Intern Med* **160**: 678–82.
4. Cohen R & Brown R (2003) Clinical practice. Microscopic haematuria. *N Engl J Med* **348**: 2330–38.

5. Kass EH & Finland M (1956) Asymptomatic infection of the urinary tract. *Trans Assoc Am Physicians* **69**: 56–64.
6. Patel H, Livsey S, Swann R *et al.* (2005) Can urine dipstick testing for urinary tract infection reduce laboratory workload? *J Clin Pathol* **58**: 951–54.
7. Whiting P, Westwood M, Watt I *et al.* (2005) Rapid tests and urine sampling techniques for the diagnosis of urinary tract infection (UTI) in children under 5 years: a systematic review. *BMC Pediatr* **5**: 4–17.

Further reading

Foxman B (2002) Urinary tract infections: incidence morbidity and economic costs. *Am J Med* **113**(1) Suppl 1A: 5S–13S.

Gould D & Brooker C (2000) *Applied Microbiology for Nurses*. Basingstoke: Palgrave Macmillan. ISBN: 0333714253.

Loanne V (2005) Obtaining urine for culture from non-potty trained children. *Paediatr Nurs* **17**(9): 39–42.

Marklew A (2004) Urinary catheter care in the intensive care unit. *Nurs Crit Care* **9**(1): 21–27.

Saint S & Lipsky B (1999) Preventing catheter-related bacteriuria. *Arch Intern Med* **159**: 800–808.

Winn W (1993) Diagnosis of urine tract infection – a modern Procrustean Bed. *Amer J Clin Pathol* **99**: 117–19.

Chapter 22
BLOOD CULTURE

In this second of two chapters devoted to the work of the clinical microbiology laboratory, attention is focused on blood culture, a test used to confirm the presence of bacteria or fungi in blood (bacteraemia or fungaemia). Blood culture is useful in three broad clinical contexts. The first is among patients who are suspected of suffering sepsis (systemic disease caused by bacterial, and much more rarely, fungal infection). Secondly, there are several infectious diseases that are caused by spread of bacteria via the bloodstream. These diseases include endocarditis (infection of the valves of the heart), osteomyelitis (infection of bone), and infective arthritis (infection of joints). A positive blood culture provides supportive evidence for diagnosis of these conditions. The third group of patients who are likely to have their blood cultured are those with PUO (pyrexia of unknown origin). This is usually defined as a raised body temperature for more than ten days, with no immediate explanation. The clinical investigation of a patient with PUO routinely includes a blood culture in the search for an infective cause of pyrexia.

Normal physiology

Blood is normally sterile (contains no bacteria or other microbes). However, normal life is associated with the risk of bacteria coming into contact with circulating blood, and transient bacteraemia may occur from time to time without ill effect. For example, bacteria normally present in the mouth have access to the bloodstream during dental surgery; transient bacteraemia invariably follows dental surgery. Even vigorous chewing has been shown to facilitate entry of bacteria, normally present in the mouth, to the bloodstream. Likewise, a 'dirty' cut allows environmental bacteria, and bacteria normally present on the skin, access to the bloodstream. Small numbers of bacteria or fungi may enter the bloodstream from an existing infection site (e.g. the urinary tract, the respiratory tract, a wound infection etc). Despite scrupulous aseptic technique, any surgical procedure may be associated with passage of bacteria from sites (e.g. the skin and bowel), where bacteria are normally present in abundance, to the bloodstream. The innate and acquired immune defences of the blood maintain its sterility, and prevent transient bacteraemia, which inevitably occurs from time to time, developing to clinically significant bacteraemia, sometimes referred to as bloodstream infection.

Innate immune defences in blood

Innate immunity is the sum of the protective mechanisms against infection that we are born with. One of the principal functions of the skin, for example, is to act as a physical barrier to invading organisms; in this way, skin contributes the body's innate immune defence. The most significant innate immune defence against microbial invasion within blood is neutrophils, phagocytic white blood cells. These cells engulf invading bacteria by the process of phagocytosis. Once phagocytosed, bacteria are killed by enzymes and highly reactive 'free radical' chemicals produced within the neutrophil. The process of phagocytosis is greatly enhanced by the so-called complement proteins, which also make a significant contribution to innate immunity. The production of these blood proteins is activated by some species of invading bacteria. One of the complement proteins, known as C3b, binds to bacteria. Bacteria that are coated with C3b are much more easily phagocytosed by neutrophils. Other complement proteins (C6, C7, C8 and C9) kill or damage some species of bacteria directly by insertion in bacterial membranes, and some (e.g. C5a) act by attracting neutrophils towards bacteria, thus enhancing phagocytosis.

Acquired immune defence in blood

Acquired immunity is very specific and can only arise after initial exposure to an invading organism; we are not born with this form of immune defence. Acquired immunity against bacterial invasion of blood depends on lymphocytes, another type of white blood cell. Bacterial invasion results in production of specific antibodies (immunoglobulins) to bacteria by plasma cells, which are derived from B-lymphocytes. An antibody binds to the specific bacterial antigen that induced its plasma cell production. This antibody binding of bacteria has two major effects: firstly, it enhances neutrophil phagocytosis of bacteria and secondly it enhances the bactericidal effect of complement proteins. Many bacteria produce chemical toxins; specific antibodies bind to these toxins, effectively neutralising them. Finally, antibodies can activate production of the protective complement proteins by an alternative pathway to that induced by bacteria.

Thus by a complex synergy of action of innate and acquired immune effects, any bacteria present in blood are destroyed and blood remains essentially sterile.

Bacteraemia and fungaemia

Predisposing factors

If bacteria (or fungi) invade the bloodstream and the normal defences against invasion are overwhelmed, they multiply causing infection.

Contributory factors include:

- reduced host defence
- an existing focus of infection
- the virulence of invasive organism
- invasive hospital procedures that facilitate entry of bacteria to the bloodstream.

Reduced host defences
Any condition associated with reduced immune (either innate or acquired) defence against bacterial infection, predisposes to bacteraemia. Severe immunosuppression associated with conditions such as AIDS and the use of immunosuppressive and cytotoxic drugs (which result in a marked reduction in production of white blood cells by the bone marrow) greatly predispose to bacterial infection of the blood by opportunistic bacteria and fungi (i.e. bacteria or fungi of low virulence which in healthy individuals would cause no problem). In fact, any severe debilitating illness (e.g. cancer, renal failure, heart failure, etc.) or major trauma, including surgery, is associated with some degree of reduction in the normal immune response to infection. Premature babies have an underdeveloped immune system and are particularly prone to infection during the first few months of life. Response to infection is less effective in the very elderly. Finally, diabetic patients are more at risk of some bacterial infections spreading to the bloodstream, than non-diabetics.

Existing focus of infection
In most cases of bacteraemia, there is a pre-existing infection at some site (called the focus of infection) in the body. Bacteria from this primary site invade the blood. If the organisms are not susceptible to the bactericidal (bacterial killing) action of blood, or the numbers of organisms are overwhelming, bacteria multiply within the bloodstream. The most common foci of infection in patients with bacteraemia is the lower respiratory tract, but bacteria may enter the blood from any site of infection and if the conditions are 'right', multiply within the bloodstream.

Virulence of invading organism
The vulnerability of bacteria to blood defences varies between species, so for example, Gram-positive bacteria are, generally speaking, resistant to the bactericidal properties of antibody and complement, although they are vulnerable to phagocytosis. This variation determines that invasion by some species of highly virulent bacteria is more likely to result in bacteraemia than others of low virulence. However, if there is an established focus of infection in the body and/or the patient's defences are severely impaired, any bacterial species, no matter what its virulence, can cause bacteraemia. In fact, although only a few species of bacteria cause most cases, all species of pathogenic (disease-causing) bacteria and even some normally non-pathogenic species can cause clinically significant bacteraemia if present in large enough numbers, and host (patient) immune defences are sufficiently debilitated.

Hospital procedures that facilitate entry of bacteria to the bloodstream

Around 60% of all patients with bacteraemia acquire the infection while in hospital.[1] Patients at greatest risk of hospital-acquired (nosocomial) bacteraemia are those who are subjected to surgical procedures, intravenous or urinary catheterisation, cystoscopy and other operative invasive interventions. An infected intravenous catheter is the focus of infection in around 20% of all patients suffering hospital-acquired bacteraemia and most of those patients with hospital-acquired bacteraemia whose focus of infection is the urinary tract have been catheterised, or have had their urinary tract investigated using a cystoscope. Surgery of areas that are normally heavily contaminated with bacteria (e.g. the mouth, the colon, genital area) carry the highest risk of postoperative bacteraemia.

Causative bacteria

Usually a single species of bacterium is the cause of bacteraemia, but in around 8% of cases, more than one bacterial species is found in blood.[2] All pathogenic (disease-causing) bacteria and more rarely, some usually non-pathogenic (opportunistic) bacteria, have been implicated as the cause of bacteraemia in particular cases. There, are however, a few species of bacteria that account for the majority of cases.

The two most common causes of bacteraemia are the Gram-positive bacteria *Staphylococcus aureus* ('Staph' or *S. aureus)* and *Escherichia coli* (*E. coli*) a Gram-negative bacterium.[2,3] They each account for around 10–15% of all cases of bacteraemia, so together account for close to third of all cases.

Staph aureus, a Gram-positive coccus, is present without ill effect in the nose of between 20 and 30% of the population; it may also be found on the moist skin of 5–10% of healthy individuals. It is, however, also a common pathogen of the skin, being responsible for superficial skin infections, like boils and carbuncles. Surgical and trauma-induced wound infections are frequently caused by *Staph aureus* and the organism is responsible for most (> 80%) cases of bone infection (osteomyelitis) and joint infection (septic arthritis). The most common foci of infection in cases of *Staph aureus* bacteraemia are infected wounds and infected intravenous catheters. In around 40% of cases caused by *Staph aureus*, the particular strain is resistant to methicillin and related antibiotics[4] – it is an MRSA strain.

E. Coli is present as part of the normal bacterial flora of the gastrointestinal tract and many cases of bacteraemia associated with this organism result from disease or trauma of the abdominal area and resulting blood invasion of bacteria from the gut. Abdominal surgery, for example, is associated with risk of *E. Coli* bacteraemia. *E. coli* is responsible for most cases of urinary tract infection so the focus of infection in some cases of *E. Coli* bacteraemia is the urinary tract, particularly the upper urinary tract.

More than 300 species of bacteria are the causes in the remaining two thirds of cases. Most are rare – but the following are relatively common, together accounting for around another third of cases: *Streptococcus pneumoniae, Streptococcus pyogenes*, *Staphylococcus epidermis*, *Pseudomonas aeruginosa*, enterococcal species, klebsiella species, proteus species and *Neisseria meningitidis*.

Strep pneumoniae is a Gram-positive coccus which may be present in the mouth and nose of healthy people, but is the most significant bacterial cause of the common lower respiratory tract infection, pneumonia. It is the causative organism in around 2–5% of cases of bacteraemia; most of these are the result of spread of the organism to blood from infected respiratory tract, in patients suffering pneumococcal pneumonia.

Strep pyogenes is a common pathogen of the upper respiratory tract: responsible for pharyngitis ('strep throat'); skin infections (e.g. impetigo, cellulitis) and serious invasive tissue infection (necrotising fasciitis). Bacteraemia can be associated with toxic shock syndrome. This is usually a community-acquired infection.

Staph epidermis is the most significant of a group of staphylococcal bacteria known collectively as coagulase negative staphylococci (CNS). In common with all other species in the group, *Staph epidermis* is abundantly present on the skin and inside the nose of healthy individuals and this determines that it is a common contaminant of blood culture. However, it can also be a causative organism in cases of bacteraemia, most particularly among immunocompromised patients who have undergone some invasive procedure (e.g. intravenous catheterisation). Bacteraemia caused by this organism is invariably hospital acquired.

Pseudomonas aeruginosa is a Gram-negative bacillus (rod-shaped). It is a common environmental bacterium that thrives on moist surfaces and can be found contaminating hospital environment, surfaces, equipment, etc. Most cases of bacteraemia caused by this organism are related to infected venous or urinary catheters, so it is usually hospital acquired.

Enterococcal species. These are Gram-positive cocci (sphere-shaped) normally present in the gastrointestinal tract. Clinically, the most significant species are *Enterococcus faecium* and *Enterococcus faecalis*, which can be the causative organism in cases of abdominal infections (e.g. peritonitis) and urine tract infection. Spread from these sites of infection to blood can occur in severely debilitated patients.

Klebsiella and proteus species. These are a common cause of urine tract infection and much more rarely, lower respiratory tract infection (pneumonia). The urine tract or infected wounds are usually the focus of infection among those with bacteraemia associated with these organisms.

Neisseria meningitidis is a Gram-negative diplococcus, present without harmful effect in the nose and throat of up to a fifth of the population. However, it is the most common cause of bacterial meningitis (infection of the central nervous system). If the causative organism is *N. menigitidis*, the condition is known as meningococcal meningitis. In most cases of meningococcal meningitis, the organism spreads via the bloodstream from nose and throat to meninges and can thus be isolated from blood. Infection with this organism is community-acquired, largely confined to children and young adults.

Causative fungi

Fungi are the cause in < 2% of cases of blood infection.[3] Almost all of these occur in patients who are severely immunosuppressed. The causative organism in almost all cases of fungaemia is *Candida albicans*, a fungus that is present in low numbers on the skin of healthy individuals. It is the cause of common superficial skin and nail infections and vaginal candidosis, a superficial infection of the vagina.

Consequences of bacteraemia

The symptomatic and potentially life-threatening consequences of bacteraemia and fungaemia are due in large part not to the invading organism, but to dysregulation of the body's normal physiological response to infection, which was very briefly outlined above. The detail of the dysregulation is complex, only partially understood and the object of intensive current research.[5,6] It is manifest clinically as sepsis, which can quickly progress to severe sepsis, septic shock and death. An outline understanding of the clinical significance of bacteraemia depends crucially on defining the following terms:

- systemic inflammatory response syndrome (SIRS)
- sepsis
- severe sepsis
- septic shock.

Systemic inflammatory response syndrome (SIRS)

Inflammation is the normally protective response to injury that ensures limitation and resolution of the injury (healing). In health, the inflammatory response is limited to the site of injury and is exquisitely controlled by an opposing anti-inflammatory process. Systemic inflammatory response syndrome (SIRS) is defined as an abnormal (dysregulated) inflammatory response that has effect in organs or sites removed from the site of injury. It is thus inappropriate and harmful. SIRS can be caused by any major insult to the body, e.g. severe trauma and major surgery; burns; diseases like acute pancreatitis that are associated with extensive tissue damage; and infection. A diagnosis of SIRS is made if patients exhibit at least two of the following abnormal signs of systemic inflammation:

High or low body temperature	< 36°C or > 38°C
Tachycardia	heart rate > 90 bpm
Hyperventilation	respiratory rate > 20 bpm or PCO_2 > 4.2 kPa
High or low white cell count	> 12.0×10^9/l or < 4.0×10^9/l

Sepsis

Sepsis is defined as infection in the presence of SIRS. Thus the finding of bacteraemia in a patient exhibiting two or more of the qualifying SIRS signs allows a diagnosis of sepsis. Since bacteraemia is a systemic infection, eliciting a blood-borne systemic inflammatory response, sepsis is usual in those with bacteraemia. However, bacteraemia is not, as was once supposed, necessary for a diagnosis of sepsis; it is now clear that infection at any site can elicit SIRS, so a diagnosis of sepsis can be made even if blood is sterile, as long as there is evidence of infection somewhere in the body in association with systemic inflammation. The term septicaemia (bacterial infection of blood) is often used as a synonym for sepsis, but since sepsis can occur in the absence of blood infection they are not synonyms. Experts now argue that because of this confusion, use of the term septicaemia should be discouraged.

Severe sepsis

The dysregulated response to infection that sepsis represents is associated with inappropriate release of a host of potent chemicals (cytokines) to blood from a range of cells involved in the immune process. Unchecked pro-inflammatory cytokines cause damage to the endothelial cells that line the microvasculature, making capillaries leaky with loss of fluid to the interstitial space, hypovolaemia and fall in blood pressure (hypotension). Inappropriate inflammation and damaged endothelium activates the clotting cascade as well as platelets, and a pro-coagulant state ensues in which microthrombi (small blood clots) form inappropriately within capillaries. The damaging cascade continues as the reduced blood pressure, presence of microthrombi and endothelial damage combine to reduce blood flow through the microvasculature. This leaves tissues deficient of the oxygen required for cells to survive and ischaemic tissue damage progresses to organ dysfunction; it is this organ dysfunction that defines severe sepsis.

Progression to severe sepsis occurs unpredictably in around a third of sepsis cases, but may be prevented by early recognition and prompt antibiotic therapy. It is defined as sepsis with evidence of organ dysfunction, hypotension or poor tissue perfusion. The damaging effects on the microvasculature are widespread so any or all organ systems can be affected.

Septic shock

The most severe presentation of sepsis is septic shock, characterised by acute circulatory failure and persistent hypotension (systolic pressure < 90 mm Hg), despite adequate fluid resuscitation. Reduced tissue perfusion can lead to multiple organ failure and death.

Sepsis, severe sepsis and septic shock are not separate conditions but rather represent a continuum of severity of the same condition, namely an abnormal systemic response to bacterial infection. Patients with bacteraemia or fungaemia may present at any stage. Severity is reflected in mortality rates: sepsis is associated with around 25% mortality, severe sepsis with 40% mortality and septic shock with 60% mortality.[7] Sepsis remains the most common cause of death among patients being cared for in intensive care units.

Summary of the general symptomatic effects of bacteraemia

Infection caused by particular bacterial species may be associated with specific symptoms. The most common general symptoms are:

- fever (body temperature > 38°C)
- rigors (shivering chills)
- tachycardia (heart rate > 95 beats/min)
- increased respiratory rate
- alteration of mental state (confusion, apprehension)
- hypotension (reduced blood pressure)

Signs and symptoms associated with organ dysfunction include

- jaundice (liver)
- increased tendency to bleed – haemorrhage (coagulation defects)
- reduced urine output (kidney)
- cyanosis – reduced PO_2 (respiratory system).

Principles of microbiological examination of blood

The primary objective of the laboratory is to determine if the patient's blood contains bacteria (or fungi). It is not possible to confirm or exclude the presence of bacteria in blood by simply examining a sample under the microscope: there simply are not sufficient numbers present. Instead, bacteria must first be grown (cultured) in a liquid (called the culture medium) that contains the nutrients necessary for bacteria to multiply. The culture medium containing the blood sample is incubated at 37°C, the optimum temperature for bacterial growth, until there is evidence of bacterial growth. This usually takes between 6 and 18 hours, but may take days for particularly slow growing species. In practice, if there is no evidence of bacterial growth after three days incubation, it is highly unlikely that the culture (and therefore the blood sample added to the culture medium) contains any bacteria. However, the culture may continue to be monitored for longer to allow for the possibility that rare, slow-growing species were present in the blood sample.

As soon as there is evidence of bacterial growth, a sample of the culture, now rich in bacteria, is stained and examined under the microscope. This provides the first evidence of the identity of the species of bacteria present (e.g. whether Gram-positive or negative, cocci or bacilli, etc). More precise identification may require that the liquid culture be further grown (subcultured) on a solid culture medium in a petri dish. This allows the growth of visible, pure colonies of bacteria, each colony being the product of multiplication of a single bacterium. A sample of the visible colony is then subjected to a range of chemical tests that finally determine the identity of the bacteria it contains.

Having isolated and identified the bacteria present in the culture, the final step is sensitivity testing. This involves testing the bacteria isolated in culture for reaction with a range of antibiotics, to establish which antibiotic is likely to be most effective in combating this particular infection.

Bacteraemia and fungaemia are potentially life-threatening conditions which demand immediate antibiotic treatment. It is often not practicable, therefore, to wait for the results of laboratory tests before starting treatment, and initial antibiotic therapy must be based on the clinical history, which provides important clues as to the likely nature of the invading bacterial species. However, when the results of laboratory tests, particularly sensitivity testing become available (usually within a day or two) antibiotic therapy can be altered if necessary.

Sample collection

Objective: to introduce a sample of patient's blood into culture bottles without *any* bacterial contamination (e.g. from environment, operators or patient's skin, etc.).

Timing of sampling

Blood for culture should be sampled before administration of antibiotic therapy as antibiotics may delay or prevent bacterial growth, causing falsely negative results. For patients with intermittent fever, blood should ideally be taken while temperature is rising, or as soon after the spike of temperature as is possible, when the bacteria are present in blood at highest concentration. Most laboratories recommend taking a second or third sample, not less than one hour after the first, to increase the chances of recovering bacteria and to distinguish true bacteraemia (which would be present in all culture sets) from bacterial contamination.

Blood culture bottles

Blood must be collected into specially designated blood culture bottles. There are several commercially available blood culture systems, but they all contain a sterile liquid mixture of nutrients (called the culture medium) necessary for bacterial growth. Most laboratories supply two blood culture bottles per blood culture set. The first has oxygen in the space above the culture medium to allow growth of those species of bacteria that require oxygen. The second bottle has a mixture of gases without oxygen. This bottle is required for culture of anaerobic bacteria (i.e. bacteria which only grow best in an oxygen-free environment). A sample of blood must be introduced into both bottles.

Volume of blood required

In a patient with bacteraemia there may be as few as one bacterium per millilitre of blood, so a falsely negative result can occur if insufficient blood is introduced into the culture bottle. Paradoxically, a false negative result can also occur if too much blood is introduced. This is because blood continues to have a bactericidal effect in culture. This effect is diluted out in the liquid culture medium. A compromise must be sought between too small a volume of blood, which might well contain insufficient bacteria, and too large a volume, which would remove the dilution effect of the culture medium on bactericidal property of blood. An approximate 1:10 dilution of blood in culture medium is optimal but the actual volume required (usually between 5 and 10 ml) depends on the blood culture system being used. It is vital that no less than the local laboratory recommended minimum volume of blood is sampled for each culture bottle.

Technique

Aseptic technique is essential throughout to ensure that no bacterial contamination of the culture occurs. If successful, only bacteria present in the patient's blood will transferred to the culture bottle.

- Blood should be sampled from a peripheral vein, not via an indwelling catheter, which might itself be contaminated with bacteria.
- With sterile gloved hands, the venepuncture site must be cleansed with 2% tincture of iodine, or some other suitable disinfectant. The iodine should be removed after a minute or two with 70% alcohol, ensuring that the site is dry. The top of both blood culture bottles, through which the sample is introduced, must be similarly disinfected.
- Taking care not to touch the venepuncture site, blood is collected using sterile syringe and needle.
- Blood is inoculated into the blood culture bottle via the rubber septum in the blood culture top. Never remove the top of a blood culture bottle. This would expose the culture to environmental bacteria.
- If blood is being collected for other tests, always inoculate blood culture bottles first, to prevent bacteria present on other specimen bottles being transferred to the culture.
- Blood culture bottles must be carefully labelled with patient details and sent along with the appropriate request card to the laboratory without delay. If blood is collected out of normal laboratory hours, blood cultures must be placed in a specially designated 37°C incubator so that bacterial growth can begin. It is important to record on the request card outline clinical details and any antibiotic therapy if given before blood sampling.

Blood culture reports

Interim reports of progress in examination of a blood culture are issued daily. A final report will include the identity of any bacteria recovered from the culture, along with a report of the sensitivity or resistance of that particular strain to a range of antibiotics.

Results of blood culture fall into one of three main groups:

- blood culture negative: no bacterial growth
- blood culture positive: pure growth
- blood culture positive: mixed bacterial growth.

Blood culture negative

This is a normal result, i.e. one that would be obtained from a person whose blood was sterile (contained no bacteria). Before a negative culture result is interpreted in this way, it is important to consider the possibility that the result is falsely negative, i.e. the patient has bacteraemia but the test has failed to detect it. Causes of false negative results include:

- insufficient blood added to culture bottle
- antibiotic therapy administered before blood sampled
- incubation period insufficient for growth of rare, slow-growing organisms.

Blood culture positive: pure growth

This means that a pure growth of a single identified species of bacteria (e.g. *E. Coli*, *Strep pneumoniae*, *Staph aureus*, etc.) was isolated from the culture. This is the result that would be expected from a patient with sepsis. However, in around 10 to 20% of positive blood cultures, the bacteria isolated and identified are derived not from the patient's blood but are present as a result of bacterial contamination of the culture, due most often to poor aseptic technique at the time of sample collection. Since all species of bacteria have been implicated in bacteraemia, and as a cause of sepsis at one time or another, it is sometimes difficult to decide whether a positive blood culture is due to contamination (false positive) or reflects bacteraemia and possible sepsis (true positive).

To illustrate this, suppose a blood culture yields a pure growth of the organism *Staph epidermis*. This organism, which is normally present in abundance on the skin of us all, could quite easily be transferred from the skin of patient or staff to blood culture during the process of blood collection. In fact, it is one of the most common organisms to contaminate blood cultures. However, *Staph epidermis* is also a quite common cause of sepsis among debilitated patients whose focus of infection is an infected catheter. It is also the most significant cause of endocarditis among patients who have received heart surgery. The finding may reflect contamination, but in some circumstances can be of clinical significance.

It is bacteria like *Staph epidermis* that are part of the normal resident flora of skin that usually contaminate blood cultures. A pure growth of any organism in blood culture is more likely to be due to bacteraemia than contamination, if:

- the same organism has been isolated from the same patient at some other infected site
- the same organism is isolated from repeated blood cultures.

Blood culture positive: mixed growth

This result indicates that more than one species of bacteria was isolated from the blood culture. It is rare for blood to be infected by more than one species of bacteria although it may occur. A mixed growth of bacteria suggests that the culture was contaminated, particularly if the bacterial species isolated are common contaminants. Interpretation may be difficult and frequently requires the expert help of a microbiologist.

Case history 21

Until the evening before admission to hospital, 18-year-old Kevin Thomas was a fit and healthy student. On that evening, he went to bed early complaining of a headache; he was also feverish. The next morning his mother, a nurse, went to check on him. He was clearly very ill, moaning quietly, with a very high temperature. He had vomited during the night. Mrs Thomas was so alarmed by Kevin's condition that she took him straight to the local A&E department where she worked, believing that he may be suffering from meningitis. On admission, Kevin's temperature was 40°C, his heart rate was 126 and he was becoming increasingly drowsy. A rash was noted on Kevin's legs. Blood was sampled for among other tests, blood culture. In view of his rapidly deteriorating condition Kevin was given a broad-spectrum antibiotic intravenously and admitted to the intensive care unit. Later that day the laboratory reported the presence of Gram-negative bacteria in the culture of Kevin's blood which was subsequently identified as *Neisseria meningitidis*.

Questions

(1) What was the diagnosis?
(2) What other serious infectious disease is caused by the bacteria isolated from Kevin's blood?
(3) Is it possible to isolate the bacteria causing Kevin's illness from normally healthy individuals?

Discussion of case history

(1) Kevin was suffering meningococcal sepsis, a life-threatening infection of the bloodstream caused by the bacterium *Neisseria meningitidis*. A diagnosis of sepsis depends on two elements: infection and systemic inflammation. Raised body temperature and heart rate provided sufficient evidence of systemic inflammation and the positive blood culture (bacteraemia) was evidence of infection.

(2) The same bacterium is one of two main causes of bacterial meningitis; the other is *Streptococcus pneumoniae*. When the causative bacteria is *N. meningitidis*, the condition is known as meningococcal meningitis. Usually meningococcal meningitis and meningococcal infection of the blood coexist in the same patient, but in recent years there has been an increase in the number of patients whose infection is confined to blood and have, like Kevin, no infection of the meninges.

(3) Yes. *Neisseria meningitides* is present in the nose and throat of around 10–20% of the healthy population.

References

1. Eykyn S, Gransden W & Phillips I (1990) The causative organisms of septicaemia and their epidemiology. *J Antimicrob Chemother* **25** (suppl C): 41–58.
2. Health Protection Agency (2005) Polymicrobial bacteraemias and fungaemias England, Wales and Northern Ireland. *Communicable Diseases Report Weekly (CDR weekly)* **15**(50). Available at: *www.hpa.org.uk/cdr/archives/2005/cdr5005.pdf*
3. Reacher M, Shah A, Livermore D *et al.* (2000) Bacteraemia and antibiotic resistance of its pathogens reported in England and Wales between 1990 and 1998: trend analysis. *Br Med J* **320**: 213–16.
4. Health Protection Agency (2005) The fourth year of regional and national analyses of the Department of Health's mandatory *Staphyolococcus aureus* surveillance scheme in England: April 2001–March 2005. *Communicable Diseases Report Weekly (CDR weekly)* **15**(24). Available at: *www.hpa.org.uk/cdr/archives/2005/2505_MRSA.pdf*
5. Riedemann N, Guo R-F & Ward P (2003) The enigma of sepsis. *J Clin Invest* **112**: 460–67.
6. Tsiotou A, Sakorafus G *et al.* (2005) Septic shock; current pathogenetic concepts from a clinical perspective. *Med Sci Monit* **11**(3): RA76–85.
7. Alberti C, Brun Busisson C *et al.* (2003) Influence of systemic inflammatory response syndrome and sepsis on outcome of critically ill infected patients. *Am J Respir Crit Care Med* **168**: 77–84.

Further reading

Cheek D *et al.* (2005) Sepsis: taking a deeper look. *Nursing 2005* **35**(1): 38–42.
Gould D & Brooker C (2000) *Applied Microbiology for Nurses*. Basingstoke: Palgrave Macmillan. ISBN: 0333714253.
Robson W & Newell J (2005) Assessing, treating and managing patients with sepsis. *Nurs Stand* **19**(50): 56–64.
Seaton R & Nathwani D (2000) Rationale for sepsis management in immunocompetent adults. *Proc R Coll Physicians Edinb* **30**.
Williams E (2006) Taking blood for culture. *Br J Hosp Med* **67**(2): M22–23.

PART 6

Cytopathology testing

Chapter 23

CERVICAL ('PAP') SMEAR TEST

The purpose of most clinical laboratory tests is to aid clinical diagnosis and monitor the progress of disease or effectiveness of therapy. By contrast, the purpose of the test that is the subject of this chapter is to *prevent* disease. The cervical smear test involves the microscopical examination of cells recovered by scraping the surface of the cervix. Abnormal changes in the appearance of these cells occur up to 10–15 years before cancer of the cervix develops. Since early treatment of these changes prevents cervical cancer developing, all women are actively encouraged to have the test at regular intervals. In the UK around 4.5 million cervical smears are examined in clinical laboratories every year.[1,2,3] This work accounts for a significant proportion of the total workload of cytopathology departments.

The cervix

Anatomy

The cervix (from the Greek meaning neck or neck like) is part of the female genital tract. It is a tubular structure around 4 cm in length that forms the lower part or neck of the uterus, connecting the uterus to the vagina. Four main anatomical features can be identified (Figure 23.1). The ectocervix is the lower part of the cervix, which extends into the vaginal canal. At the centre of the ectocervix is the external os, the tiny opening to the endocervical canal. The endocervical canal is the tubular structure of the cervix, which opens at the internal os to the uterus.

As the connection between uterus and vagina, the endocervical canal is the first part of the birth canal. Late in pregnancy, the normally tough and fibrous cervix softens or 'ripens', allowing it to dilate to several times its normal diameter, for passage of the developed fetus from uterus to vagina during birth.

Cervical epithelium

The surface of the cervix is covered with a protective layer of epithelium. The cervical smear test samples the epithelial cells that make up this protective layer. In the case of the cervix, there are two sorts of epithelium: squamous epithelium

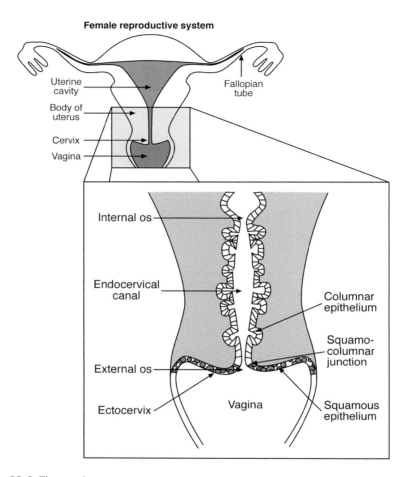

Figure 23.1 The cervix.

covers the ectocervix, while columnar epithelium lines the endocervical canal. Four distinct layers of squamous epithelium can be distinguished on the surface of the ectocervix. The deepest of these is the basal layer, which comprises one row of immature squamous (basal) epithelial cells. Above this is the parabasal layer: two rows of immature squamous (parabasal) cells, which are constantly dividing to maintain the epithelium above. The intermediate layer comprises four to six rows of more mature cells, and the most mature squamous epithelial cells are those within the five to eight rows of the superficial layer. Cells in this superficial layer become increasingly less attached to each other and are continuously cast off from the surface of the ectocervix by a process called desquamation or exfoliation.

Constant regeneration of squamous epithelial cells in the basal layers is required to replace those that are lost from the surface of the ectocervix, by exfoliation. Most of the squamous epithelial cells recovered in a cervical smear are from the superficial and intermediate layers. Cells from the parabasal layer constitute only around 5% of all squamous epithelial cells in a normal smear from young women. The cells in a smear from older women contain slightly more parabasal cells, and disease of the cervix is associated with a significant increase in the number of parabasal cells in a cervical smear. Because of their relative depth, basal cells are rarely seen in a cervical smear.

The mucous secreting columnar epithelium of the endocervical canal is composed simply of one row of columnar epithelial cells; some are mucous secreting and others have cilia on their surface. The mucous and cilia are thought to facilitate the passage of spermatozoa through the endocervical canal. When columnar epithelial cells are seen in a cervical smear, they are referred to as endocervical cells.

The squamo-columnar junction and transformation zone

The point where the squamous epithelium of the ectocervix meets the columnar epithelium of the endocervical canal is called the squamo-columnar junction (Figure 23.1). This junction is of great pathological significance because it is in this area that most cases of cervical cancer originate. Before puberty the junction lies at the external os (Figure 23.2) but in response to the normal hormonal changes that occur at puberty, the lower end of the endocervix everts somewhat, so that

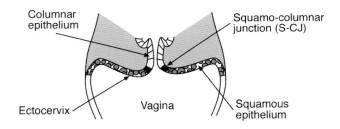

Before puberty S-C junction at the external os

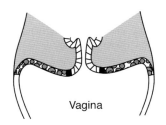

During reproductive age the S-C junction moves on to the ectocervix with formation of transformation zone (ectropion)

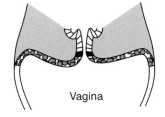

At the menopause S-C junction retreats into the endocervical canal

Figure 23.2 Location of the squamo-columnar junction at different stages of a woman's life.

the junction moves outwards from the external os on to the ectocervix. A second important physiological change occurs as a result of eversion of the endocervix. The columnar epithelium that covers the everted part of the endocervix is now exposed to the acidic vaginal environment and this environmental change, in combination with other factors, induces the exposed columnar epithelial cells to undergo transformation to squamous epithelial cells, a process called metaplasia. The area around the external os of the ectocervix where this transformation of columnar to squamous epithelium occurs is called the transformation zone. Epithelial cells undergoing transformation are called squamous metaplastic cells. As the transformation occurs, throughout a woman's reproductive years, the squamo-columnar junction moves back towards the external os. After the menopause the junction usually retreats into the endocervical canal.

Cancer of the cervix

Almost all (85–90%) cervical cancers originate in the squamous epithelial cells of the transformation zone on the ectocervix. This is known technically as cervical squamous cell carcinoma. The rest originate in the columnar epithelial cells of the endocervix; this is known as cervical adenocarcinoma. Generally speaking, the second of these two kinds of cervical cancer is considered to have the worse prognosis.

With an annual incidence of just under 3000, cervical cancer is currently the 11th most common cancer to affect women in the UK.[4] Cervical cancer can arise at any age but it is most often diagnosed between the ages of 40 and 60 years. Younger women, as long as they are of reproductive age, are also at risk; around 1.7% of cases occur before the age of 25.[5] There are often no symptoms during the early stages of cervical cancer. The only common symptoms are abnormal vaginal bleeding and discomfort during sexual intercourse. Postcoital bleeding is fairly common.

The prognosis for a woman with invasive cancer of the cervix depends, as with most other cancers, on the extent of cancer spread at the time of diagnosis. As long as the cancer is confined to the cervix, the prognosis is good; treatment can effect a cure. Untreated, invasive cervical cancer spreads from the cervix first to the upper part of the vagina, then to the ureters and lower part of the vagina. In the most advanced cases, invasion of the bladder wall and rectum may be evident at diagnosis. Such advanced disease is associated with a poor prognosis; only 10% of patients with the most advanced disease survive more than five years. The annual UK death toll due to cervical cancer is close to 1100.[6] There is now overwhelming evidence that infection with the human papilloma virus (HPV) is the cause of cervical cancer.

HPV and cervical cancer

Early epidemiological studies suggested that a sexually transmitted agent might have role in cervical cancer. These studies demonstrated that early age of first sexual intercourse, increasing number of sexual partners and sexual intercourse with a man who himself has had many sexual partners, all independently increase the risk of cervical cancer. Cervical cancer is very rare among virgins. By the end of the 1970s, human papilloma virus (HPV) had emerged as the most likely of several candidate sexually transmitted agents. The more recent observation that HPV is present in all cervical cancers and infection predates cancer development has allowed the now widely held view that HPV is a necessary, but not sufficient cause for cervical cancer.[7] Thus only those who have been infected with HPV can develop cervical cancer. HPV is, incidentally, the only necessary cause of any cancer to be identified. Cervical cancer is by no means an inevitable consequence of HPV infection. Up to 75% of sexually active women become infected with HPV at some point in their life.[8] The vast majority eradicate the virus without even knowing they have been infected and with no long-term consequences; only a very small proportion develop cervical cancer.

There are around 100 different HPV types, which have been broadly categorised to those that infect skin (the cutaneous types) and those that infect the mucosal surface of the mouth and genital tract (mucosotropic types). The cutaneous HPV types are responsible for common, invariably benign, wart infection of hands and feet. The mucosotropic group includes 40 different HPV types that, following transmission by sexual contact, infect the genital tract. These are divided into low-risk types that can cause benign genital warts and high-risk types that can, after many years of clinical latency, cause cervical cancer. Seventeen high-risk types have been identified but just six types (HPV 16, 18, 31, 33, 45 and 46) account for 95% of all cervical cancers. The two most common high-risk types, HPV 16 and HPV 18, account for 70% of cases. It remains unclear why in a small proportion of women infected with high-risk HPV, the virus is not eradicated but persists for many years, eventually causing cervical cancer. Some risk factors have been identified and include cigarette smoking, the use of oral contraceptives and immune suppression (e.g. co-infection with the human immunodeficiency virus (HIV) that causes AIDS).

Natural history of cervical cancer

The preventative value of the cervical smear test is due to the usually long natural history of cervical cancer. Identifiable pre-cancerous changes occur up to 10–15 years before invasive cancer develops. If these are identified and treated, cervical cancer can be prevented.

Many years before cervical cancer develops, microscopical changes to the squamous epithelial cells in the transformation zone occur. These changes are known technically as cervical intra-epithelial neoplasia (CIN). CIN is a potentially progressive lesion, caused by HPV infection, which may, if not treated, ultimately lead to cervical cancer. Three grades of severity of CIN have been identified. If the cellular changes which characterise CIN are confined to the lowest third of epithelium, a diagnosis of CIN 1 is made, if such changes are seen in the lower two thirds, CIN 2 is diagnosed. The most severe form of CIN, CIN 3, is diagnosed when abnormal cells are seen throughout the full thickness of the epithelium; this is also called carcinoma *in situ*. The level of CIN determines the risk of invasive cervical cancer developing. For example, patients with CIN 1 have a relatively low risk of cancer developing; in around 50% of cases the abnormality resolves spontaneously. However, CIN 1 may persist without any untoward effects, or for an unpredictable small minority of patients, may progress through CIN 2 to CIN 3. Around 30% of patients with CIN 3, if left untreated, would progress to invasive cancer within 10 years. There is currently no way of predicting with any certainty which patients with CIN will progress to invasive cancer, or how speedy that progression will be. All that can be said is that there is an increased risk of cervical cancer for women with CIN and that the risk is highest in those with CIN 3.

Treatment of CIN prevents cancer developing in nearly all cases. The definitive diagnosis of CIN depends on microscopical examination of a piece of cervical tissue. However the microscopical appearance of cells scraped from the surface of the cervix reflect the abnormalities that constitute CIN. This is the rationale for the cervical smear test as a screening test for prevention of cervical cancer.

Cervical screening

History

The cervical smear test is often referred to as the Pap smear test. This alternative name celebrates the research of George Papanicolaou, a Greek physician who worked in the USA. In the 1920s, Papanicolaou first observed that cancerous cervical cells could be found in vaginal smears. To enhance the appearance of these cells he developed a staining technique using the Papanicolaou stain, which is used to this day to stain cervical smears. In the late 1940s, Ayre demonstrated that scraping the surface of cervix was a more reliable means of recovering cancerous cervical cells. He developed the Ayre spatula for this purpose. At around this time, the concept of pre-cancerous disease of the cervix was introduced, allowing the rationale for the use of the cervical smear test to screen for early evidence of cervical cancer.

A screening programme using the cervical smear test was first introduced in the UK during 1964. However, the organisation of the scheme was not nationally co-ordinated and evolved in an *ad hoc* fashion. The result was that the scheme had much less impact in reducing the incidence of cervical cancer than expected. Experience of cervical screening in other European countries, particularly Denmark, Iceland, Sweden and Finland had demonstrated that a well-organised scheme in which all women at risk are regularly given a cervical smear test, can be successful. In these countries there had been a huge steady reduction in the incidence of cervical cancer from the time screening was introduced in the 1960s. In recognition of the relative failure of the *ad hoc* screening programme then in operation in the UK, a nationally co-ordinated cervical screening programme was introduced in 1988. With some changes to the scheme in 1990 and 2003, this is the scheme in operation today.

Organisation and success of cervical screening

The aim of the UK programme is to reduce the incidence of cervical cancer by performing regular cervical smears on every woman between the age of 25 and 65 years. Current national policy[8] is that all women between the ages 25 and 49 should be screened every three years and those between the ages of 50 and 65 every five years. Screening after the age of 65 is reserved for those who have not been screened since the age of 50 and those who have had recent abnormal results. In Scotland and Wales the policy is to screen all women between the ages of 20 and 65 (60 in Scotland) every three years.

The responsibility for cervical screening falls largely on the primary health care team. A computerised call and recall system organised by primary care workers (GPs, practice nurses and practice managers) ensures that every woman in the target population of each GP practice is offered a smear test. Full payment for smear testing is made to GPs if greater than 80% of their target population are screened.

Before 1987 around 40% of women in the then target age range 20–65 years were being screened. With the introduction of a national screening programme in 1988, coverage increased quickly. By 1994, 85% of the target population was being screened; this level of coverage has been maintained ever since. There is now much evidence that this increased level of cervical smear testing has had the desired effect on the incidence of cervical cancer.[9] In England between 1971 and 1987 the annual incidence stayed fairly steady, fluctuating between 14 and 16 per 100 000 women (i.e. on average 3900 cases a year). Since 1990, however, annual incidence has fallen steadily year on year; by 1995 the incidence was 10 per 100 000 women or 2900 new cases, and in 2003 just 2312 new cases were registered.[10] The screening programme since 1987 has also had an effect on the number of deaths attributed to cervical cancer. From 1950 to 1987, mortality due to cervical cancer fell steadily at the rate of 1.5% every year. Since 1987 this rate of fall has trebled. In 1987, 1800 deaths in England were attributed to cervical cancer; in 2003 this number had fallen to 888. A recent analysis[11] of trends in mortality before screening was introduced suggests that cervical screening prevents the death of 5000 women in the UK every year.

The cervical smear or 'pap' test

Around 80% of cervical smears are sampled in a primary care setting, most often by practice nurses.

Patient preparation

The best time to take a cervical smear is mid cycle to avoid contamination of the smear with menstrual blood. It is preferable to delay taking a smear for a few months following childbirth. The patient should be advised to avoid the use of vaginal creams and refrain from sexual intercourse for 24 hours before the test.

Table 23.1 Topics for discussion with patient prior to cervical smear test.

Why have the test?

- Cervical screening is recommended for all women between the ages of 25 and 65 years.
- Cervical screening is not a test for diagnosing cervical cancer but to confirm that the cervix (the lower part of the womb) is healthy.
- In 90% of cases the test confirms a healthy cervix.
- 10% of women have changes to the cervix, which in the vast majority of cases revert to normal with time. A small fraction of these 10% have changes that might lead to cancer in the long term.
- Simple out-patient treatment of these pre-cancerous changes prevents cancer developing.

About the test

- You will be asked to undress from the waist down, but if you wear a full skirt you will not have to remove it.
- The test is performed with you lying on a couch. A small instrument called a speculum is gently placed into your vagina to hold it open so that the cervix can be viewed.
- A small spatula is used to gently wipe some cells from the surface of the cervix.
- The cells are placed on a glass slide or into a small container of liquid and sent to the laboratory for examination under the microscope.
- The test takes just a few minutes; you might feel some discomfort. Take deep breathes to relax as it may hurt more if you are tense but tell the nurse or doctor if you experience pain.

After the test

- The doctor or nurse will tell you when and how you will receive the result of the test.
- There is no reason to be alarmed if you are asked to attend for a repeat test; about 1 in 10 tests have to be repeated usually for some technical reason such as insufficient number of cells or cells obscured by contaminating blood or mucus.

Many women will be anxious, especially on the first occasion they attend for a smear, so a calm reassuring manner is important. A brief explanation of the test, emphasising the points in Table 23.1, will help to allay fears. Any effort made to reduce the tension or anxiety a woman might experience at the time of smear sampling will increase the chance of obtaining a suitable sample. Furthermore, there is evidence to suggest that women who are dealt with in a sympathetic manner are more likely to re-attend for future testing or further investigation, if an abnormality is discovered.

Cervical sampling technique

The practical detail of collecting an adequate cervical smear is beyond the scope of this chapter but good technique is essential. A significant number of smears (up to 20% in some studies) are reported as inadequate in some way and have to be repeated. Expert technique, acquired through training and experience, can help to reduce the number of inadequate or unsuitable smears.

The cervix must first be visualised by passing a vaginal speculum. The cervix must be well illuminated. The object is to sample cells from the transformation zone and squamo-columnar junction, so a smear would normally contain squamous epithelial cells as well as some endocervical cells. Since the position of the squamo-columnar junction varies with age and parity, sampling technique must take account of these factors. Several sampling devices are routinely used. The endocervical brush and cotton-tipped swab is used to sample cells from the endocervical canal, while the Aylesbury spatula with its extended tip for insertion into the external os is used to sample cells from the transformation zone on the ectocervix. The full circumference of the transformation zone is sampled by rotating the spatula through 360 degrees. The sample is transferred to a glass slide (pre-labelled with patient details), by spreading the material from both sides of the sampling device or devices, evenly on to the glass slide. If more than one sampling device is used, sample material from both devices should be spread on to a single glass slide. It is vital that the cells in the sample are 'fixed' or preserved immediately. This is usually achieved by immersing the glass slide in 90% ethanol 'fixative' for 10–15 minutes. Spray fixative may be used. The slide is air dried and placed in a plastic slide box for transport to the laboratory. Alternatively, slides can be transported in the fixative solution. If the smear is found to be inadequate or unsuitable in some way, the laboratory will request that the test be repeated. The most common reasons for having to repeat the test are:

- inadequate number of epithelial cells due to:
  cervix not being scraped firmly enough
  sample not completely transferred to glass slide
- sample spread too thinly or too thickly on the glass slide
- cells poorly preserved due to:
  sample being allowed to air-dry before being 'fixed'
  inadequate time in the fixative solution
- sample contaminated with (for example) blood, lubricant, spermicide, inflammatory exudates.

Results of smear test

Around 90% of adequately collected smears are found on microscopical examination to be entirely normal and no further investigation, save recall in three or five years, is necessary. The remaining 10% have some degree of abnormality ranging from the benign (the vast majority), through entirely curable pre-malignant disease (CIN) to invasive cancer.

In the laboratory, cervical smears are stained with Papanicolaou stain and examined under the microscope. Having established that the smear is adequate, the main object of the examination is to search for the abnormal changes to epithelial cells associated with the pre-cancerous condition, CIN. These abnormal changes, which are known collectively as dyskaryosis (literally, abnormal nucleus), include an increase in the size of the nucleus compared with surrounding cytoplasm, along with irregularity in the shape and staining characteristics of the nucleus. There are three recognised grades of severity of dyskaryosis: mild, moderate and severe. In some cases, only slight changes to the nucleus are present which may not be sufficient to warrant a report of even mild dyskaryosis; these are reported as 'borderline nuclear abnormalities'. The severity of dyskaryosis correlates to some degree with the level of CIN that might be expected if a tissue biopsy were examined, so a report of a smear result from a patient with dyskaryosis implies a prediction of the level of CIN. In broad terms, CIN 1 would be expected if mild dyskaryosis were present; CIN 2 or CIN 3 would be expected if moderate dyskaryosis were present and CIN 3 would be expected if severe dyskaryosis were present. It is not possible to make a definitive diagnosis of CIN or invasive cervical cancer from examination of a cervical smear.

Follow up of abnormal smears

The cervical smear test is only a *screening* test; its value lies in its ability to exclude the 90% or so of women whose smear is negative. The severity of dyskaryosis found in an abnormal smear merely determines the next step in the diagnostic process. The majority of abnormal smears are either 'borderline nuclear abnormalities' or 'mild dyskaryosis'. There is a strong likelihood that these changes will regress to normal. However, there remains a risk that over time a pre-malignant lesion might develop. Such patients may require no treatment initially but more intensive monitoring. They might, for example, be advised to have a repeat smear test at three- or six-monthly intervals until the abnormality has resolved. For those whose smear shows signs of moderate or severe dyskaryosis, or mild dyskaryosis on two consecutive occasions, referral for colposcopy is indicated.

Colposcopy

Colposcopy is a usually pain-free, outpatient diagnostic procedure in which the cervix is viewed directly through a specially modified microscope, called a colposcope. A vaginal speculum is passed as for a cervical smear, and the cervix is 'painted' with acetic acid. Application of acetic acid turns CIN affected tissue white. With a colposcope, this area can be visualised and biopsied to determine the level of CIN or confirm the presence of micro-invasive cancer. The results of colposcopy and cervical tissue biopsy determine the treatment that may be offered. In the absence of invasive cancer, CIN can be treated in an outpatient setting by a variety of techniques which all involve the destruction (ablation) of abnormal tissue by extremes of heat (e.g. laser vaporisation, cryotherapy, loop diathermy). Surgical excision (cone biopsy) may be necessary, and rarely, in the absence of invasive disease, hysterectomy might be recommended. All patients who have been treated for CIN must be monitored for recurrence of disease. Instead of the normal three- or five-year interval between smears, such patients may be recalled every year for up to 10 years.

Other abnormalities in a cervical smear

Microscopic examination of a cervical smear may reveal incidental genital tract infections. In such cases an inflammatory exudate (accumulation of dead and dying white cells recruited to fight the infection and other cellular debris) may be present in the cervical smear, obscuring normal epithelial cells. The epithelial cells themselves may show signs of very mild dyskaryosis during an inflammatory process. All these effects of infection may make it difficult to identify those changes in epithelial cells that are due to CIN, and a repeat sample may be requested.

Specific infections that can be identified from microscopical examination of a cervical smear include:

Candida vaginitis. Infection caused by the fungus (yeast) *candida albicans*, which results in a thick purulent vaginal discharge and severe itching. The organism itself can be seen during microscopical examination of a cervical smear.

Trichomoniasis. Infection caused by the protozoon *trichomonas vaginalis*, which results in a thin watery discharge with offensive smell. Symptoms include itchiness. The organism can be seen during microscopical examination of cervical smears.

Genital herpes. Infection caused by the herpes simplex virus, gives rise to painful lesions (ulcers) on the genitalia. Recurrent infection (often asymptomatic) can result in chronic inflammatory disease of the cervix (cervicitis). The virus cannot be seen when examining a cervical smear, but virally infected cervical epithelial cells show characteristic changes, which are evident on microscopical examination.

Actinomycosis. Infection caused by the bacterium *Actinomyces israelii*. This organism is sometimes seen in cervical smears and is almost always associated with the use of an intrauterine contraceptive device (the coil). Infection can lead to pelvic inflammatory disease.

Human papilloma virus (HPV). Mention has already been made of HPV as a causative agent of cervical cancer. It is possible to see evidence of infection with this virus when examining a cervical smear. Epithelial cells infected with the virus have a particular appearance; such HPV-infected cells are called koilocytes.

A new technique: liquid-based cytology

The way smears are taken in the GP surgery as outlined above, as well as the way they are processed in the laboratory, has remained essentially unchanged for 40 years. A new, more reliable technique called liquid-based cytology (LBC) has been available for some years. In 2003, following extensive trials in several pilot studies across the UK, the National Institute for Clinical Excellence (NICE) recommended that LBC should replace the conventional smear test. That change is now well under way and is expected to be complete by 2008.

For LBC, cervical samples are collected as before, but rather than spreading the sample on a glass slide, the collecting device (spatula or brush) with the sample of cervical cells on it is placed directly into a vial containing a liquid preservative and fixative. The vial is then sent to the laboratory for processing. In the laboratory the liquid sample is first treated to remove extraneous obscuring cells (e.g. erythrocytes, leucocytes) and debris, before a thin and uniform film of cervical cells is applied to a glass slide for staining and microscopical examination.

The trials have demonstrated superiority of LBC over the conventional smear test in several areas. The process of taking a smear is simpler and quicker. Since all the cervical cells recovered from the patient are placed in the sample vial, the number of inadequate smears is greatly reduced. Consequently far fewer patients will have to re-attend surgery for repeat smear. No laboratory test is full proof, but LBC is associated with fewer false negative and false positive results than the conventional test.[1] Laboratory staff are impressed with the increased productivity associated with the new technique.

Case history 22

Sally Turnbull is a 23-year-old mother of three, who had her first cervical smear test five weeks ago. The report of the test arrived three weeks later and read 'borderline nuclear abnormalities'; it included the suggestion to repeat the test in six months' time. As soon as she received the appointment for the repeat test, Sally began to worry. She now telephones the surgery for a much earlier smear test booking insisting, 'If I have cancer I want to know now, not wait for five months.'

Questions

(1) What do you understand the laboratory report to mean?
(2) What can you say to Sally to allay her fears?

Discussion of case history

(1) The principal object of examining a cervical smear is to discover if the epithelial cells it contains shows any signs of dyskaryosis (literally 'abnormal nucleus'). The nucleus of a dyskaryotic cell is typically larger than normal, occupying an increased volume of the cytoplasm. It is irregular in shape and staining characteristics. Dyskaryosis is a signal that the cervical epithelial tissue from which the cells have been sampled has CIN, a condition that may progress to cervical cancer. There are three grades of severity of dyskaryosis: mild, moderate and severe, which broadly correspond to the severity of CIN. If there are only very slight abnormal changes to the nucleus of epithelial cells, insufficient in magnitude to warrant them being labelled even mildly dyskaryotic, a report of 'borderline nuclear changes' is made.

(2) You can assure Sally that she does not have cancer. While not normal, the changes seen in her smear are common; around 1 in 20 smears have such slight changes. You can say that in the majority of such cases the changes revert to normal over a period of months and that by the time of her next appointment, it is quite likely that her smear will be entirely normal. However, she must know that there is a chance that the abnormality will persist and could, if ignored, progress slowly over

many years to cancer. She should know that if the abnormality does persist, cancer can be prevented and a 'cure' achieved by a simple outpatient procedure. It is important that women presenting for routine cervical smear realise that the test is not to detect cancer, but to detect a curable condition (CIN), which if left untreated, might progress to cancer over many years.

References

1. NHS Health & Social Care Information Centre (2005) Cervical Screening Programme, England: 2004–05 *Bulletin: 2005/09/HSCIC.* ISBN: 1-84636-027-7. *www.ic.nhs.uk/pubs/cervicscrneng2005/*
2. Cervical Screening Wales Information Team (2005) *Cervical Screening Wales* Statistical Report. *www.screeningservices.org.uk/csw/results/KC53-61-65_04-05.pdf*
3. Scottish Health Statistics. *www.isdscotland.org*
4. Cancer Research UK (2005) Cancerstats Incidence: UK. *www.cancerresearchuk.org/statistics/*
5. Saseni P, Adams J & Cuzick J (2003) Benefit of cervical screening at different ages: evidence from the UK audit of screening histories. *Br J Cancer* 89: 88–93.
6. Cancer Research UK (2005) Cancerstats Mortality: UK. *www.cancerresearchuk.org/statistics/*
7. Bosch F & Iftner T (2005) The aetiology of cervical cancer. *NHSCSP publication No 22 NHS* Cancer Screening programme, Sheffield. ISBN: 1-84463 023 04. *www.cancerscreening.nhs.uk/cervical/publications/nhscsp22.pdf*
8. Koutsky L (1997) Epidemiology of genital human papilloma virus infection. *Am J Med* 102: 3–8.
9. Quinn M, Babb P *et al.* (1999) Effect of screening on incidence and mortality from cancer of cervix in England: evaluation based on routinely collected statistics. *Br Med J* 318: 904–907.
10. National Statistics (2005) Cancer Statistics. Registrations of cancer diagnosed *in 2003, England.* London: Office for National Statistics ISBN: 1-85774 617 1.
11. Peto J, Gilham C, Fletcher O & Matthews F (2004) The cervical cancer epidemic that screening has prevented in the UK. *Lancet* 364: 249–56.

Further reading

Bankhead C, Austoker J & Davey C (2003) *Cervical Screening Results Explained – a guide for primary care* London: Cancer Research UK. ISBN: 0-9508422 3 0. *www.cancerscreening.nhs.uk/cervical/publication/2003-csre.pdf*

Jolley S (2004) Quality in colposcopy. *Nurs Stand* 18(23): 39–44.

Mckie L (1993) Women's views of the cervical smear test: implications for nursing practice: women who have had a smear. *J Adv Nurs* 18: 1228–34.

Mckie L (1993) Women's views of the cervical smear test: implications for nursing practice: women who have not had a smear. *J Adv Nurs* 18: 972–79.

National Health Service Cancer Screening Programme (2004) Colposcopy and Programme Management: Guidelines for NHS Cervical Screening Programme. NHSCSP Publication

No 20 Sheffield: NHSCP. ISBN 1 84463 014 5. *www.cancerscreening.org.uk/cervical/publications/nhscsp20.pdf*

Patnick J (2000) Cervical cancer screening in England. *Eur J Cancer* **36**: 2205–2208.

Todd R, Wilson S *et al.* (2002) Effect of nurse colposcopists on a hospital-based service. *Hosp Med* **63**: 218–23.

Useful website

www.cancerscreening.nhs.uk A full list of NHSCSP publications relating to cervical cancer screening.

PART 7

Point of care testing

Chapter 24
DIPSTICK TESTING OF URINE

Urinalysis is a generic term for all those clinical tests that involve physical, microscopical, chemical or microbiological examination of urine. Microbiological examination of urine was the subject of Chapter 21. Another aspect of urinalysis, dipstick testing of urine, is the focus of this final chapter. In contrast to all other tests considered in this book, dipstick testing of urine is usually performed outside the laboratory, in clinics, on hospital wards and primary care surgeries by non-laboratory staff, usually nurses; it is a point of care test.

The value of the urine dipstick test lies in its ability to screen for serious renal, urological and liver disease as well as metabolic disorders such as diabetes. A positive result on dipstick testing is never sufficient to make a clinical diagnosis, although it may provide supportive evidence of one. More often, a positive result is used to inform what the next step in the diagnostic process should be.

After a general consideration of sample collection and what can be learned from physical examination of urine, attention will turn to the test itself. Each of the urine constituents tested for will be considered in turn, highlighting the most common pathological and non-pathological causes of abnormal results.

Urine sample collection

The ideal urine sample for urinalysis, including dipstick testing is a sample of uncontaminated bladder urine. The 'clean catch' midstream urine collection technique (Table 21.1) was designed for collection of such an ideal specimen. In practice, initial screening can be performed on a midstream urine sample collected without the exacting requirements of a 'clean catch' technique, although a chemically clean and sterile container is essential. The manner of sample collection is less important than its freshness. Urine should be tested within a few hours of voiding, because many urine constituents are unstable. The major changes in urine composition that occur after voiding are summarised in Table 24.1. If a delay in testing is unavoidable, the sample should be kept in a refrigerator, as reduced temperature slows the rate of these changes.

Table 24.1 Changes that occur in urine after voiding.

Physical

- Colour darkens
- Odour strengthens
- Turbidity increases

Chemical

- pH changes (may increase or decrease)
- Glucose decreases
- Bilirubin decreases
- Urobilinogen decreases
- Protein changes (may increase or decrease)
- Nitrite increases
- Ascorbic acid decreases

Microscopic

- Red blood cells haemolyse
- White blood cells lyse

Physical inspection of urine

Physical inspection of urine should focus on colour, clarity and odour. In health, freshly voided urine is usually a clear, pale yellow or straw-coloured fluid, with only slight, if any, odour. Urine appearance and odour can change if left to stand for more than a few hours, so it is important that freshly voided urine is used for physical inspection.

Colour

The pale yellow colour of urine is due to the presence of the pigments urochrome and urobilin. In health, the variability in intensity of the yellow colour of urine usually reflects varying urine concentration; the more concentrated the urine, the darker is the shade of yellow. The main physiological determinant of urine concentration is fluid intake. Overnight urine reflects a prolonged period without any fluid intake, so the urine passed first thing in the morning is usually the most concentrated and therefore the strongest coloured. Dehydration, whatever its cause, is associated with production of a concentrated urine that is consequently relatively dark in colour. After heavy fluid intake, a dilute urine is passed, which may be almost colourless.

Quite apart from these normal physiological changes in colour, urine may be abnormally coloured due to the presence of abnormal urine constituents.[1,2] These may be endogenous, in which case the abnormal colour reflects a pathological condition (e.g. bilirubin turns urine dark yellow, blood and haemoglobin turn urine pink/red). Alternatively, they may be exogenous in origin, simply reflecting ingestion of certain foods (e.g. acidic urine may be red after eating beetroot) or more frequently, prescribed drugs.

Clarity/turbidity

Freshly voided urine is usually clear, but urine from healthy subjects may become cloudy if left for more than a few hours due to precipitation of phosphates as urine becomes alkaline, or precipitation of uric acid if urine is acidic. The most common pathological cause of increased urine turbidity is urine tract infection. In such cases, turbidity is due principally to the presence in urine of the causative bacteria and white cells (leucocytes), recruited to fight the infection.

Odour

Ingestion of certain foods (e.g. asparagus, aromatic spices) can affect the odour of urine. Bacterially infected urine often smells characteristically fishy particularly if left to stand for more than a few hours. Certain species of bacteria (proteus, klebsiella and pseudomonas), elaborate an enzyme, urease, which acts on urea present in urine to produce ammonia. Urine infected with such organisms has a strong ammoniacal odour. A few metabolic disorders are associated with urinary excretion of odorous chemicals. The most significant of these is acetone excreted in the urine of diabetics during diabetic ketoacidosis.

Dipstick testing

Technical considerations

Commercially available reagent strips for urine dipstick testing consist of an inert plastic strip on which is mounted paper pads impregnated with chemical reagents. Each pad contains the chemicals needed for detection of a particular constituent of urine. A full list of the urine constituents that can be tested for using commercial dipsticks is listed in Table 24.2, but they vary according to the particular product being used. When the dipstick is dipped in urine, the reagents in each pad dissolve, initiating a chemical reaction that results in a colour change. After a set period of time (usually in the range 20–60 seconds) the colour change of each pad is compared with a colour chart provided by the manufacturer, and the result read. In the case of some urine constituents, the test is semi-quantitative, in that the more intense the colour change, the higher is the concentration of the particular urine constituent. If a semi-quantitative result is possible, results are typically reported as either trace (lowest detectable concentration), or 1+, 2+, 3+ or 4+ (very high concentration). If a semi-quantitative result is not possible then the report is either positive (the substance is present in urine) or negative (the substance is not present in urine).

Table 24.2 Urine constituents detectable by commercial dipstick testing.

- Glucose
- Bilirubin
- Urobilionogen
- Ketones
- Blood
- Leucocyte esterase
- Nitrite
- Protein
- Albumin
- Creatinine
- Trypsinogen
- pH
- Specific gravity

Each manufacturer of test strips provides detail of the test procedure that must be followed for accurate results, but some general points are made here.

- The chemical reagents contained on the strip pads have a limited shelf life governed by the expiry date on the container. Always check expiry date before use. Dipsticks should not be used if the expiry date has passed.
- The stability of the chemical reagents depend on the desiccant (which absorbs any moisture) provided either in a sachet or in the lid of the container. To maintain chemical stability, it is vital that dipsticks are stored in the container provided and that the lid is replaced immediately after use. Only remove enough dipsticks for immediate use.
- The chemicals on dipstick pads dissolve if left in urine long enough. The dipstick must be dipped in urine so that all reagent pads are immersed, and then immediately removed.
- It is important that the chemicals from one pad do not contaminate the next. To avoid this, excess urine must be removed as the strip is withdrawn from the urine sample, by dragging the edge of the strip against the urine container and then immediately blotting the side of the strip on an absorbent paper towel.
- Good lighting is essential for accurate reading of colour change.
- Ability to accurately differentiate sometimes subtle colour change is essential. It may be inappropriate for staff with colour blindness to perform dipstick testing.
- The timing of the reaction is vital for accurate results; always observe manufacturers' timing instructions.
- Urine is a biological fluid that must be treated as a potential source of pathogens, with risk to patient and staff of cross-infection. All staff performing dipstick testing must be familiar with local health and safety policy regarding work with body fluids (e.g. the need for protective gloves and apron, what to do in the event of a urine spillage, etc.).
- Results must be recorded on a worksheet and in the patient's notes.
- The quality of results using dipsticks should be regularly assessed by a local laboratory quality control scheme.[3]

Interpretation of results

Glucose

Although in health urine may contain very slight amounts of glucose, concentration is too low to give a positive result using urine dipsticks, and a negative result is normal. Glycosuria, the presence of abnormal amounts of glucose in urine, only occurs when blood glucose concentration rises above the renal threshold. For most people the renal threshold for glucose, i.e. the blood concentration above which glucose appears in urine, is around 10.0–11.0 mmol/l. A positive urine glucose result indicates that at some time since the bladder was last emptied, blood glucose concentration was in excess of 10.0 mmol/l. The test is semi-quantitative, allowing an indication of the degree of abnormality in blood glucose concentration.

The most common and significant cause of an abnormal rise in blood glucose, sufficient for glucose to be detected in urine, is diabetes mellitus. Other rarer endocrine disorders which result in raised blood glucose and resulting glycosuria include Cushing's syndrome (excess cortisol), acromegaly (excess growth hormone), phaeochromocytoma (excess adrenalin) and hyperthyroidism (excess thyroid hormones). Occasionally, a positive glucose urine dipstick may be found in an individual whose blood glucose concentration is within the normal range. This is due to lowering of the renal threshold for glucose. This most often occurs during pregnancy. It is also the defining feature of a rare and entirely benign defect of kidney function, known as renal glycosuria.

A positive urine glucose result raises the suspicion of diabetes, but this can only be confirmed or excluded by measurement of blood glucose concentration.

Once diabetes has been confirmed, the principal aim of treatment is to maintain near normal blood glucose concentration. Dipstick urine testing for the presence of glucose is sometimes used by diabetic patients to monitor blood glucose control. A positive result indicates raised blood glucose (at least above the patient's renal threshold) and therefore increasingly poor control. A negative result indicates either normal or reduced blood glucose concentration (hypoglycaemia). Only by measuring blood glucose concentration can hypoglycaemia be distinguished from normoglycaemia. Since the urine test is unable to distinguish hypoglycaemia from normoglycaemia, it is a less satisfactory way of monitoring diabetes than measuring blood glucose concentration directly.

Ingestion of large amounts of Vitamin C (ascorbic acid) can cause a falsely negative glucose result.

Bilirubin and urobilinogen

Bilirubin and urobilinogen are waste products of haemoglobin breakdown. Haemoglobin is the oxygen-carrying protein contained in red blood cells (erythrocytes). At the end of their 120-day life, red cells are removed from blood and degraded in the reticuloendothelial system, principally the spleen. Here the haemoglobin contained within them is broken to its constituent parts: haem and globin. Haem is converted to bilirubin. As a waste product of metabolism, bilirubin must be removed from the body. It is first transported in blood to the liver, where it is conjugated (joined) with glucuronic acid to form so called 'conjugated' bilirubin. The purpose of conjugation is to make bilirubin soluble in water. From the cells of the liver, conjugated bilirubin is excreted into the bile canniculi of the liver and out from the liver via the common bile duct, in bile, to the small intestine. During passage through the intestine, bilirubin is converted by bacteria to urobilinogen. Most of the urobilinogen is excreted in faeces but some is absorbed into blood. The urobilinogen that is reabsorbed to blood has two possible fates; some of it is taken up by liver cells and excreted in bile, thereby reappearing in the gastrointestinal tract, and some is excreted in urine.

In health, all bilirubin is excreted via the liver in bile and none is excreted in urine. A negative dipstick result for bilirubin is normal. The presence of bilirubin in urine is always pathological. By contrast, normal urine contains a small amount of urobilinogen and a negative urobilinogen dipstick result is pathological.

A positive urine bilirubin result indicates abnormal accumulation of conjugated bilirubin in blood. This can only occur if the normal excretory route (liver and biliary tract) is impaired. The causes of a positive result can be divided into those that result from liver disease (e.g. hepatitis, cirrhosis, primary biliary cirrhosis, liver cancer) and those that result from obstruction to bile flow in the biliary tract (e.g. gallstones, cancer of the head of pancreas). A positive urine bilirubin result indicates significant liver or biliary tract disease and requires further investigation; initially blood should be sampled for liver function tests. A falsely negative result can occur if urine contains large amounts of ascorbic acid (Vitamin C).

Normal urine contains some urobilinogen. A negative result indicates that conjugated bilirubin is not being excreted in bile to the intestine. Such a negative finding can be expected if the biliary tract is obstructed (e.g. gallstones, cancer of the head of pancreas). An abnormally high concentration of urobilinogen in urine occurs if urobilinogen cannot be excreted in bile due to liver disease (hepatitis, cirrhosis etc.). Additionally, increased excretion of urobilinogen in urine occurs if increased bilirubin is excreted in bile due to increased bilirubin production. Since bilirubin is derived from the haemoglobin in red cells, increased bilirubin production/excretion and therefore increased excretion of urobilinogen in urine are features of increased red cell destruction (haemolysis). A dipstick result indicating abnormally raised urobilinogen thus provides supportive evidence of the haemolytic process that causes haemolytic anaemia.

Ketones

Ketones (sometimes called ketone bodies) is the collective name for three chemical substances present in the body. Two are keto-acids (β-hydroxybutyric acid and acetoacetic acid) and the third is acetone. All three are produced during the oxidation of fatty acids, the metabolic process by which the energy contained in fat is released. Normally, ketones are quickly further metabolised. However, if fat metabolism is abnormally increased, the rate at which they are produced exceeds the rate at which they are metabolised. The result is accumulation of ketones in blood (ketonaemia) and excretion of ketones in urine (ketonuria). This abnormal metabolic state is known as ketosis. If the accumulation of keto-acids in blood is sufficient to overwhelm the homeostatic mechanisms that maintain normal blood pH, blood becomes abnormally acid; this pathological, potentially fatal, state is called ketoacidosis.

The principal causes of increased fat metabolism and resulting positive test for urine ketones are diabetes and starvation. In both of these conditions, there is a deficiency of glucose within cells to provide energy. In the case of the diabetic patient, the problem is a deficiency of insulin, the hormone required for entry of glucose into cells. In the case of the patient who is suffering from starvation, the deficiency of glucose is simply due to lack of dietary carbohydrate. In both instances, stored fat is metabolised to fill the 'energy gap' caused by glucose deficiency within cells.

The ketosis associated with starvation is usually mild and therefore very rarely associated with acidosis. By contrast, ketosis in diabetes can be severe, giving rise to the acute life-threatening complication of diabetes, known as diabetic ketoacidosis. If an insulin-dependent diabetic patient is unwell, the finding of a positive urine ketone test suggests possible diabetic ketoacidosis. Such a diagnosis can only be made by further blood testing.

A positive urine ketone test may also occur incidentally in normal pregnancy around the time of delivery, severe dehydration and alcoholism. The clinical significance in these cases is small compared with that associated with the same finding in a diabetic patient.

Nitrite

This is a screening test for urine tract infection (UTI). Normal urine contains no nitrite. However many species of bacteria can convert dietary nitrate, which *is* present in normal urine, to nitrite. A positive result for nitrite indicates that the urine contains bacteria. The test is highly specific, i.e. there are very few false positive results. In a typical study[4] only 4% of urines with a positive nitrite test did not contain significant numbers of bacteria. However, falsely negative results are a limitation of the test. In around 50% (range 45–60%) of urines containing significant numbers of bacteria, the urine nitrite test is negative.[5] The reasons for the false negative results are twofold. Firstly, some species of bacteria (mostly Gram-positive) can cause urine tract infection, but do not have the enzyme necessary for conversion of nitrate to nitrite. Secondly, urine must be present in the bladder for around four hours for complete bacterial conversion of nitrate to nitrite. Samples taken during the day may not have been in the bladder for a sufficient time. An early morning specimen, which has been in the bladder overnight, is more likely to result in a positive nitrite test than one taken during the day.

The presence of abnormally high amounts of Vitamin C (ascorbic acid) and urobilinogen in urine can affect nitrite detection resulting in falsely negative results.

Leucocyte esterase (white blood cells)

Like the nitrite dipstick test, this is a screening test for UTI. The test detects the presence of the enzyme leucocyte esterase, which is an enzyme present only in phagocytic white blood cells (leucocytes) called neutrophils. The test is thus a test for the presence of neutrophils in urine. Normally the test is negative; urine from a healthy individual does not contain sufficient neutrophils to produce a positive result. The presence of significant numbers of leucocytes (including neutrophils) in urine is called pyuria. The body's normal response to any bacterial infection is recruitment of neutrophils to the site of infection, where they engulf (phagocytose) and destroy bacteria. Pyuria and the resulting positive leucocyte esterase urine dipstick test is thus an indication of bacterial infection of the urine tract. In around 75% of UTI infections, the test is positive.

Pyuria and therefore a positive result can occur in the absence of bacterial infection of the urine tract; this is termed 'sterile pyuria'. Conditions associated with sterile pyuria include tuberculosis and inflammatory disease of the kidneys and urinary tract (e.g. chronic pyelonephritis, urethral syndrome). Although the most likely explanation, a positive result clearly does not necessarily indicate urine tract infection. If nitrite and leucocyte esterase tests are both negative, urinary tract infection can be reliably excluded.[5] However, a positive result in either or both is not sufficiently reliable to make a diagnosis of urine tract infection without laboratory confirmation.[5]

Blood

The presence of blood in urine is called haematuria. A distinction is made between macroscopic haematuria, the visible presence of blood in urine (this turns urine a reddish brown colour) and microscopic haematuria, the presence of blood in urine that is not obvious to the naked eye, and can only be detected by dipstick testing or examination of urine under the microscope. The number of red blood cells provides an index of the quantity of blood. Normal urine contains small numbers of red blood cells (fewer than 5000 per ml).[6] The sensitivity of the dipstick test is such that only those urines whose red blood cell concentration is greater than normal will give a positive result.

For women of reproductive age, a positive blood dipstick result may simply indicate that the specimen is contaminated with menstrual blood. If urine is very concentrated, the dipstick test may be positive despite the fact that a normal number of red cells are being excreted. Other causes of a false positive result include raised levels of ascorbic acid (vitamin C) in urine. Finally, since the dipstick test is detecting the haem part of haemoglobin, not red cells directly, rare conditions in which there is excessive urine excretion of free haemoglobin and myoglobin (which also contains the haem group) result in a positive result despite no increased excretion of red blood cells (i.e. no haematuria).

Although the dipstick test may be used to confirm the presence of visible blood in urine (macroscopic haematuria), its principal value is detection of microscopic haematuria.

Depending on the age of the population studied, between 0.2% and 22% of apparently well individuals test positive for microscopic haematuria.[7] A positive result is most likely to have a benign cause, for example exercise can result in transient microscopic haematuria. More rarely, it can be the first objective sign of serious urological or renal disease. The most common pathological cause of positive blood dipstick for blood is urine tract infection. Less common causes include inflammatory disease of the kidney (e.g. glomerular nephritis) and early bladder or renal cancer. A representative recent study[8] demonstrates just how rare it is for a positive dipstick to be associated with serious pathology. Of 368 patients with positive dipstick result, 40% did not even have significant haematuria when urine was examined in the laboratory. Of the remaining 225 in whom microscopic haematuria was confirmed, just 48 (13% of those with a positive dipstick result) were suffering any sort of pathology; just six were found to be suffering early malignant disease (all bladder tumours). A positive result should not be ignored, but confirmed by microscopical examination of urine before intensive urological (or renal) investigation.

Protein

The first step in urine production is filtration of blood at the glomerulus. The pores in the glomerular membrane are too small to allow proteins to pass, so that normally urine contains no protein. In health, urine dipstick protein result is negative. The presence of protein in urine is called proteinuria. Proteinuria, particularly mild proteinuria (trace/1+) is most often transient, benign and of no particular clinical significance. However it can be the first sign of serious renal disease and among pregnant women, the first sign of pre-eclampsia, a serious disease of pregnancy that can threaten both the life of the mother and health of her unborn child.

Fever, urine tract infection and strenuous exercise may all be associated with transient mild proteinuria, which resolves with time (days or weeks) and has no long-term consequences. Orthostatic proteinuria is a relatively common, entirely benign condition with particular prevalence among older children and adolescents. It is characterised by proteinuria in the standing position only and may be associated with positive dipstick result if urine is collected during the day. A morning specimen collected on rising is always negative. The condition usually disappears during adulthood.

Persistent proteinuria, i.e. positive dipstick results on three occasions separated by intervals of at least a week in an otherwise well patient without orthostatic proteinuria, is indication of possible renal disease and/or hypertension that warrants further investigation, including measurement of blood pressure, 24 hour urine protein estimation to quantify the protein loss, and serum creatinine.

All pregnant women have urine tested at first booking for the presence of protein to identify those at risk of pre-eclampsia, a condition characterised by the triad of hypertension, oedema and significant proteinuria (> 300 mg/24 hrs).

pH

In contrast to the tight control of blood pH, which is maintained between 7.35–7.45, urine pH may range from 4.0–8.0, although it is usually within the range 5.5–6.5. Extremes of urine pH can be due to diet. A vegetarian diet, for example, is generally speaking associated with an alkaline pH > 6.5. Pathological conditions associated with disturbance of acid-base balance and abnormal blood pH are reflected in urine, so that, for example, patients in diabetic ketoacidosis would tend to have an acidic urine pH < 5.0, whereas those with systemic alkalosis have an alkalotic urine (pH > 6.0).

Urine infections due to some bacterial species (proteus, klebsiella, pseudomonas) are associated with alkaline urine because they elaborate an enzyme, urease, that splits the urea present in urine to carbon dioxide and ammonia.

The pH of urine has little clinical significance except in two conditions – renal tubular acidosis and renal stone disease. Renal tubular acidosis is a defect of renal tubule cells characterised by failure of the kidneys to excrete hydrogen ions effectively. The consequent accumulation of hydrogen ions in blood results in reduced blood pH (acidosis) and inappropriately alkaline urine. Kidney stones are formed by the precipitation of urine constituents such as calcium phosphate and uric acid, a process that is dependent in part on the pH of urine. Drugs that modulate urine pH and thereby reduce mineral precipitation are used in the treatment of renal stone disease.

Specific gravity

Specific gravity (SG) is a measure of the concentration of solutes in a solution. The SG of water is 1.000. Urine SG can range from 1.001 (a very dilute urine) to 1.035 (a very concentrated urine). The actual level indicates state of hydration. A dehydrated patient should appropriately excrete urine of high SG, whereas a patient receiving too much fluid should excrete urine with low SG. Failure to concentrate urine appropriately when fluid is restricted can be an early signal of renal disease and diabetes insipidus.

References

1. Raymond J & Yarger W (1988) Abnormal urine colour: differential diagnosis. *South Med J* 81: 837–41.
2. Cone T (1968) Diagnosis and Treatment: Some syndromes, diseases and conditions associated with abnormal coloration of the urine or diaper. *Pediatrics* 41: 654–58.

3. Tighe P (1999) Laboratory-based quality assurance programme for near patient urine dipstick testing, 1990–1997: development, management and results. *Br J Biomed Sci* **56**: 6–15.
4. Ditchburn R & Ditchburn J (1990) A study of microscopical and chemical tests for the rapid diagnosis of urinary tract infections in general practice. *Br J Gen Pract* **40**: 406–408.
5. Deville W, Yzermans J *et al.* (2004) The urine dipstick test useful to rule out infection. A meta-analysis of the accuracy. *BMC Urol* **4**: 4–18.
6. Corwin H & Silverstein M (1988) Microscopic haematuria. *Clin Lab Med* **8**: 601–10.
7. Grossfield G & Carrol P (1998) Evaluation of asymptomatic microscopic hematuria. *Urol Clin North Am* **25**: 661–76.
8. Khan M, Shaw G & Paris A (2002) Is microscopic haematuria a urological emergency? *BJU Int* **90**: 355–57.

Further reading

Topham P, Jethwa A *et al.* (2004) The value of urine screening in a young adult population. *Fam Pract* **21**: 18–21.
Wingo C & Clapp W (2000) Proteinuria: Potential causes and approach to evaluation. *Amer J Med Sci* **320**: 188–94.

GLOSSARY OF SOME TERMS USED IN LABORATORY MEDICINE

Acidaemia	abnormal increase in acidity of blood, reduced blood pH
Acidosis	abnormal increase in the acidity of body fluids associated with reduced blood pH
Acetaminophen	alternative name for the drug paracetamol
Agranuloctyosis	complete or near absence of granulocytes in blood
Alkalaemia	abnormal increase in alkalinity of blood, increased blood pH
Alkalosis	abnormal increase in the alkalinity of body fluids associated with increased blood pH
Anaemia	the condition of reduced oxygen delivery to tissues that results from reduced haemoglobin concentration – many possible causes
Anisocytosis	red cells vary in size
Antibody	a protein (immunoglobulin) that circulates in blood plasma, binds specifically to the antigen that provoked its production
Antigen	a substance (protein or carbohydrate) present on the surface of cells that provokes specific antibody production
Anuria	failure to produce urine
Atheroma	disease of artery walls that leads to atherosclerosis
Atherosclerosis	thickening and hardening or arterial walls reducing blood flow, a common chronic condition that is the cause of coronary heart disease, strokes and peripheral artery disease
B-Cells	one kind of lymphocyte – matures to antibody producing plasma cell – one of many blood cells involved in the immune process
Bacteraemia	presence of bacteria in blood
Bacteriuria	presence of bacteria in urine
Basophil	one of five kinds of white blood cells
Benign tumour	abnormal growth of tissue whose margins are well defined – it may grow large but does not spread beyond its local site

Biopsy	a sample of tissue removed for microscopic examination to diagnose disease
Blast cell	immature white cell not normally present in blood
Cancer	general term for all malignant tumours
Carcinoma	a specific term for malignant tumours that originate in epithelial cells anywhere in the body
Commensal bacteria	bacteria that colonise the human body without causing disease
Dysplasia	tissue in which there is evidence of increased cell division
Ecchymosis	abnormal brown-red discoloration of skin caused by bleeding into tissues, a signal of coagulation defect or reduced platelet numbers
Endocervical cells	epithelial cells that line the internal surface of the endocervical canal, one of the cell types normally seen in cervical smear
Endothelial cells	the cells that line the internal surface of blood vessels
Eosinophils	one of five types of white cell normally present in blood
Erythrocyte	red blood cell
Erythropoiesis	process by which erythrocytes develop from bone marrow stem cell
Erythropoietin	hormone produced by the kidney that regulates red cell production
Euthyroidism	normal production of thyroid hormones by the thyroid gland
Exudate	fluid produced during inflammatory tissue damage
Factor V Leiden	common inherited defect in blood coagulation
Frozen section	rapid technique for preparation of biopsied tissue prior to microscopical examination, enables histopathological diagnosis within an hour or so
Glycolysis	the metabolic process by which glucose is oxidised to produce energy
Glycosuria	abnormal presence of glucose in urine
Gram Stain	staining technique that allows classification of all bacteria to one of two groups: Gram-positive and Gram-negative, the first step in identifying bacterial species
Granulocytes	white blood cells (neutrophils, eosinophils and basophils) that have granules in cytoplasm
Haematopoiesis	process of blood formation in bone marrow
Haematuria	the abnormal presence of blood in urine
Haemoglobin	oxygen carrying protein present in red blood cells
Haemoglobinopathies	a large group of inherited defects in haemoglobin structure
Haemolysis	rupture of red cell membrane, destruction of red cell – increased *in vivo* haemolysis is the cause of one kind of anaemia, haemolytic anaemia. Can occur during blood collection (*in vitro*) rendering samples unsuitable for analysis

Haemolytic anaemia	see haemolysis
Hepatitis	inflammation of the liver
Hypercalcaemia	raised plasma calcium concentration
Hypercapnia	increased amount of carbon dioxide in blood, raised PCO_2
Hyperglycaemia	raised blood glucose concentration
Hyperkalaemia	raised plasma potassium concentration
Hyperlipidaemia	raised blood lipid (cholesterol and/or triglycerides) concentration
Hypernatraemia	raised plasma sodium concentration
Hyperthyroidism	increased activity of thyroid gland
Hypocalcaemia	reduced plasma calcium concentration
Hypocapnia	reduced amount of carbon dioxide in blood, reduced PCO_2
Hypoglycaemia	reduced blood glucose concentration
Hypokalaemia	reduced plasma potassium concentration
Hyponatraemia	reduced plasma sodium concentration
Hypothyroidism	reduced activity of thyroid gland
Hypoxaemia	reduced amount of oxygen in blood, reduced PO_2
Hypoxia	reduced amount of oxygen in tissues
Infarction	necrosis of tissue due to ischaemia
Ischaemia	reduced blood flow to tissues usually the result of vessel blocked by thrombus and/or atherosclerotic plaque
Jaundice	yellow discoloration of skin and sclerae due to abnormal accumulation of the pigment bilirubin
Kernicterus	accumulation of bilirubin (unconjugated) in the brain which can cause permanent brain damage
Ketoacidosis	an abnormal metabolic state due to accumulation of ketoacids (ketones) in blood
Ketones	the collective name for three chemicals which accumulate in blood during increased fat metabolism
Ketonuria	the abnormal presence of ketones in urine
Lactic acidosis	an abnormal metabolic state that results from accumulation of lactic acid in blood
Leucopaenia	reduction in white blood cell numbers
Leucocytes	alternative name for white blood cells
Leucocytosis	increase in white cell numbers
Lymphocyte	one of five main types of white blood cells – two main types, B- and T-lymphocytes; both required for acquired immunity, they are cells of the immune system
Macrophage	a phagocytic cell present in tissues that is derived from a monocyte
Malignant tumour	a solid tumour that can spread (metastasise) to distant sites and grow
Megalobastic anaemia	anaemia caused by deficiency of B_{12} or folate

Metabolic acidosis	acidosis caused by the accumulation of metabolic acids (e.g. lactic acid) in blood
Microcytic anaemia	all those anaemias associated with reduced MCV
Microcytosis	red cells, on average, smaller than normal, reduced MCV
Monocyte	one of five types of white blood cell, matures to tissue macrophage
Necrosis	death of cells or tissue due to disease or injury
Neuroglycopaenia	reduced glucose in cells of the central nervous system (including the brain)
Neutrophil	the most abundant of five types of white blood cell, it is a phagocytic cell
Neutropaenia	reduced number of neutrophils in blood
Neutrophilia	increased number of neutrophils in blood
Nocturia	the need to urinate during the night
Nosocomial infection	hospital-acquired infection
Oedema	abnormal accumulation of fluid in the interstitial space
Pathogen	a microbial species (bacterium, virus or fungus) that causes disease
Platelets	formed particles present in blood, required for blood clotting
Pleural fluid	the fluid present in the pleural cavity
Pleural effusion	abnormal accumulation of pleural fluid
Poikilocytosis	red cells vary in shape
Polydipsia	increased thirst
Polyuria	increased urine production
Proteinuria	the abnormal presence of protein in urine
Respiratory acidosis	acidosis caused by failure to eliminate carbon dioxide from blood
Sepsis	systemic inflammation caused by bacterial or fungal infection
Thrombocyte	alternative name for platelets
Thrombocytopaenia	reduction in platelet number
Thrombocytosis	increase in the number of platelets
Thrombus	blood clot formed inappropriately within blood vessels

ABBREVIATIONS

A, B, AB, O	blood groups
AAFB	acid alcohol fast bacilli
ACD	anaemia of chronic disease
ACE	angiotensin-converting enzyme
ACS	acute coronary syndrome
ADH	antidiuretic hormone
ADP	adenosine diphosphate
AIDS	acquired immune deficiency syndrome
ALL	acute lymphoblastic leukaemia
ALT	alanine transferase
AML	acute myeloid leukaemia
ANF	anti-nuclear factor
ANP	atrial natriuretic peptide
AP	alkaline phosphatase
APC	activated protein C resistance
APTT	activated partial thromboplastin time
APR	acute phase reaction
AST	aspartate aminotransferase
ATP	adenosine triphosphate
ATPase	adenosine triphosphatase
AV	atrioventricular
BCSH	British Committee for Standards in Haematology
BMS	biomedical scientist
c, C, e and E	blood group systems
C3a and C5a C3b C6, C7, C8 and C9	complement proteins
Ca	calcium
CBC	complete blood count
CHD	coronary heart disease
CHF	chronic heart failure
CIN	cervical intra-epithelial neoplasia
CK, CKMM, CKBB and CKMB	creatine kinase and its isoenzymes
cl	centilitre (one hundredth of a litre)
CLL	chronic lymphatic leukaemia

CML	chronic myeloid leukaemia
CNS	coagulase negative staphylococci
CNS	central nervous system
CoA	coenzyme A
COPD	chronic obstructive pulmonary disease
CPK	creatine phosphokinase
CRP	C-reactive protein
CSF	cerebrospinal fluid
CSU	catheter specimen of urine
CT	computed tomography
cTnT, cTnI	cardiac troponin T and I
DIC	disseminated intravascular coagulation
DIT	di-iodotyrosine
dl	decilitre (one tenth of a litre)
DNA	deoxyribonucleic acid
DVT	deep vein thrombosis
ECF	extracellular fluid
ECG	electrocardiographic
EDTA	ethylenediaminetetraacetic acid
EMU	early morning urine
ERCP	endoscopic retrograde cholangiopancreatography
ESR	erythrocyte sedimentation rate
FBC	full blood count
fl	femtolitre (10^{-15} of a litre)
FT3	free triiodothyronine (T3)
FT4	free thyroxine (T4)
Fy	Duffy blood group system
GFR	glomerular filtration rate
GGT	gamma glutamyl transpeptidase
GH	growth hormone
GTT	glucose tolerance test
HAV, HBV, HCV	hepatitis A, B and C viruses
Hb	haemoglobin
HbA1	glycosylated haemoglobin
HCG	human chorionic gonadotrophin
HCl	hydrochloric acid
HCO_3^-	bicarbonate
HDN	haemolytic disease of the newborn
Hg	mercury
HIV	human immunodeficiency virus
HPV	human papilloma virus
hs	high sensitivity
Ht	haematocrit
ICF	intracellular fluid
IDA	iron-deficiency anaemia

IF	intrinsic factor
IgA	immunoglobulin A
IL-6	interleukin 6
INR	international normalised ratio
IPT	immunological pregnancy test
ISI	international sensitivity index
ITP	immune thrombocytopaenic purpura
IV	intravenous
Jk	Kidd blood group system
K	potassium
K	Kell K blood group system
kPa	kilo-Pascal
l	litre
LBC	liquid based cytology
Le	Lewis blood group system
LFT	liver function test
μl	microlitre (one millionth of a litre)
μmol	micromole (one millionth of a mole, 10^{-6})
M, C & S	microscopy, culture and sensitivity
MCHC	mean (red) cell haemoglobin concentration
MCV	mean (red) cell volume
mEq/l	milliequivalents per litre
Mg	magnesium
MI	myocardial infarction
MIT	monoiodotyrosine
ml	millilitre (one thousandth of a litre)
MLA	medical laboratory assistant
mmol	millimole (one thousandth of a mole, 10^{-3})
MRI	magnetic resonance imaging
MRSA	methicillin-resistant *Staphylococcus aureus*
MSU	midstream specimen of urine
N	Newton
Na	sodium
NAC	N-acetylcysteine
NAFLD	non-alcoholic fatty liver disease
NAPQI	N-acetyl-p-benzoquinone imine
NBS	National Blood Service
NH_3	ammonia
NHS	National Health Service
NICE	National Institute for Health and Clinical Excellence
NK	natural killer (lymphocytes)
nmol	nanomole (one billionth of a mole)
NSAID	non-steroidal anti-inflammatory drug
NSTEMI	non-ST elevation myocardial infarction
nvCJD	new variant Creutzfeldt–Jacob disease

P	partial pressure
P	phosphorus
PA	pernicious anaemia
PCO$_2$	partial pressure of carbon dioxide
PCV	packed cell volume
pH	*puissance hydrogen*
pmol	picomole (one trillionth of a mole, 10^{-12})
PO$_2$	partial pressure of oxygen
PT	prothrombin time
PTH	parathormone
PTHrP	parathormone-related polypeptide
PUO	pyrexia of unknown origin
QRS	Q, R, and S waves that represent the ventricular activity of the heart
RBC	red blood cell
RCN	Royal College of Nursing
RDW	red cell distribution width
RE	reticuloendothelial
Rh	rhesus
RNA	ribonucleic acid
SA	sino-atrial
SCID	severe combined immunodeficiency syndrome
SG	specific gravity
SHOT	serious hazards of transfusion
SI	Système International
SIADH	syndrome of inappropriate antidiuretic hormone
SIRS	systemic inflammatory response syndrome
SLE	systemic lupus erythematosus
STEMI	ST elevation myocardial infarction
T3	triiodothyronine
T4	thyroxine
TATT	tired all the time
TB	tuberculosis
TBG	thyroid binding globulin
TFT	thyroid function tests
TIBC	total iron binding capacity
Tn, TnC, TnI, TnT	troponin (C, I and T)
TRALI	transfusion-related acute lung injury
TRH	thyrotropin-releasing hormone
TSH	thyroid-stimulating hormone
TT	thrombin time
U&E	urea and electrolytes
UA	uric acid
U/l	units per litre
ULRR	upper limit of reference range

UTI	urine tract infection
UV	ultraviolet
VRSA	vancomycin-resistant *Staphylococcus aureus*
WBC	white blood count
WCC	white cell count
WHO	World Health Organization

Appendix 1
ADULT REFERENCE RANGES

The column headed 'Local laboratory reference range' is left blank for you to fill in the precise reference range that is used in your hospital.

Test	Approximate reference range	Local laboratory reference range
Sodium	135–145 mmol/l	
Potassium	3.5–5.2 mmol/l	
Bicarbonate	25–30 mmol/l	
Urea	2.5–6.5 mmol/l	
Creatinine	55–105 µmol/l	
Fasting blood glucose	3.0–6.0 mmol/l	
pH	7.35–7.45	
Hydrogen ion	35–45 nmol/l	
PCO_2	4.7–6.7 kPa	
Bicarbonate	22–28 mmol/l	
PO_2	10.6–13.3 kPa	
Base Excess	−3.0–+3.0	
Lactate	0.5–2.0 mmol/l	
Bilirubin	< 20 µmol/l	
Alanine aminotransferase (ALT)	10–40 U/l	
Aspartate aminotransferase (AST)	10–40 U/l	
Gamma glutamyl transferase (GGT)	< 50 U/l	
Alkaline phosphatase (AP)	30–150 U/l	
Albumin	35–50 g/l	
Amylase	< 200 U/L	
Magnesium	0.7–1.0 mmol/l	
Calcium (total)	2.20–2.60 mmol/l	
Calcium (ionised)	1.15–1.30 mmol/l	
Phosphate	0.80–1.40 mmol/l	
Parathyroid hormone (PTH)	10–70 ng/l	
Total cholesterol	NSF Target* < 5.0 mmol/l JBS Target* < 4.0 mmol/l	

Test	Approximate reference range	Local laboratory reference range
LDL-cholesterol	NSF Target* < 3.0 mmol/l JBS Target* < 2.0 mmol/l	
HDL-cholesterol	> 1.2 mmol/l	
Thyroxine – free (FT4)	9–26 pmol/l	
Triiodothyronine – free (FT3)	3.0–9.0 pmol/l	
Thyroid Stimulating Hormone (TSH)	0.3–4.5 mU/l	
Uric acid	150–400 µmol/l	
Cortisol (9.00 am)	150–680 nmol/l	
(midnight)	< 100 nmol/l	
Adrenocorticotrophic hormone (ACTH) (9.00 am)	< 50 ng/l	
Cardiac troponin T (cTnT)		
Cardiac troponin I (cTnI)		
CK(MB)		
Myoglobin		
Haemoglobin (Hb)	Male 13–17 g/dl Female 11–15 g/dl	
Red cell count	Male 4.5–6.5 × 10^9/l Female 3.9–6.5 × 10^9/l	
Packed cell volume (PCV)/Haematocrit	Male 40–52% Female 36–48%	
Mean cell volume MCV	80–95 fl	
Mean cell haemoglobin conc. (MCHC)	20–35 g/dl	
Red cell distribution width (RDW)	10–15%	
White cell count	Male 3.7–9.5 × 10^9/l Female 3.9–11.1 × 10^9/l	
Erythrocyte Sedimentation Rate (ESR)	Male 1–10 mm/hr Female 5–20 mm/hr	
C-Reactive Protein (CRP)	< 10 mg/l	
Platelet count	150–400 × 10^9/l	
Prothrombin time (PT)	10–14 secs	
Activated partial thromboplastin time (APTT)	30–40 secs	
Thrombin time (TT)	14–16 secs	
Iron	10–30 µmol/l	
Total iron binding capacity (TIBC)	40–75 µmol/l	
Ferritin	10–300 µg/l	
Vitamin B_{12}	150–1000 ng/l	
Folate	150–700 µg/l	

* See text p. 128

INDEX OF TESTS

INDEX